Dangerous Drugs

Dangerous Drugs

The Self-Presentation of the Merchant-Poet Joannes Six van Chandelier (1620–1695)

Ronny Spaans

Translated by Ciarán Ó Faoláin

Routledge
Taylor & Francis Group
LONDON AND NEW YORK

The publication of this book has been made possible by: Programredaktør Andor Birkeland og hustru Halinas legat, Dr. C. Louise Thijssen-Schoute Stichting, and Nord University.

The translation of the book has been possible by a grant from the Norwegian Research Council.

First published in 2020 by Amsterdam University Press Ltd.

Published 2025 by Routledge
4 Park Square, Milton Park, Abingdon, Oxon OX14 4RN
605 Third Avenue, New York, NY 10158

Routledge is an imprint of the Taylor & Francis Group, an informa business

ISBN: 9789462982543 (hbk)
ISBN: 9781041177906 (pbk)
ISBN: 9781003693642 (ebk)
NUR 694

Cover illustration: Egbert van Heemskerk, *An Alchemist in His Study*, 17th century. Oil on canvas. (© Science History Institute, Philadelphia).

Cover design: Kok Korpershoek

DOI 10.5117/9789462983543

Knowing oneself is a reason,
That fell down from Heaven.
Blessed is the one, that in his mind
Knows what he is, and what he does.
– Joannes Six van Chandelier[1]

The terrifying sight of sword hanging
from the gilt panelled ceiling over purpled necks beneath.
– Persius[2]

1 'Sich self te kennen is een reên, / Die, van den Heemel viel beneên. / Wel saaligh, wie in syn gemoed Kent, wat hy is, en wat hy doet', 'Myn antwoord, aan den selven' (J258), l. 1–4.

2 'Et magis auratis pendens laquearibus ensis / purpureas subter cervices terruit', Persius, Satire 3, l. 40. In *Juvenal and Persius*, trans. by Susanna Morton Braund, 2004, pp. 76–77.

Table of Contents

Part III Divine Blood for Sale

List of Illustrations

Colour plates

Figures

Acknowledgements

Joannes Six van Chandelier is considered one of the most difficult poets in Dutch literature. Compared to Constantijn Huygens, who is usually considered to be 'the puzzle' of seventeenth-century Dutch poetry, 'Six is difficult squared; many passages in his poems can only be called sequences of riddles', writes the critic C. Kruyskamp.[1] The poet himself even thematises the high degree of difficulty in his poems. In 'Raad aan den Geenen, die myn rymen mishaagen' ('Advice to the ones who dislike my rhymes') (J393), Six describes his verses as hard nuts on which the reader will break their teeth, only to find them empty when they are cracked open. With this study, however, I want to show that the tough 'nuts' of Six's poetry are not empty, but contain substantial experiences of a human being in a time rife with changes and contradictions.

My interest in Six began with a fascination for the metaphorical and playful language he used as a Dutch *metaphysical poet*, but I soon found out that there were also exciting aspects to his work that had not been explored. The key to any new understanding would be to read him not only as a poet, but also as a druggist. His so-called hard poetic nuts, then, were not so empty after all. They contained insights that could cast new light not only on early modern Dutch art and literature, but also on medicine, trade, and science. These insights also have a further relevance beyond Six's own time. The reader will easily be able to transfer the discussions in Six's texts to our own time – not just moral and medical arguments against drug abuse, but also discussions of ecology, and on the local food movement, as an alternative to the global food model, which often sees food travelling long distances before it reaches the consumer. We can also recognise discussions on materialism, on the artificial versus the authentic, and on the cult of personality within politics and culture. In addition, a debate in Six's poetry about the chemical use of drugs, in which concepts such as the artist/artisan as 'a creator', and the human body as God's 'work of art' are important, has parallels with today's ethical discussions on genetic engineering.

But cracking open these nuts has not been easy. This study started as a PhD project at the University of Oslo in 2006. Over the years, I have been working continually, with breaks both long and short. I have consulted with a number of people along the way. Without their help, I would not have been able to crack open these nuts. First, I would like to thank Kirsti Sellevold, Knut Stene-Johansen, and Terence Cave for their excellent advice on the approach to Renaissance poetry

1 C. Kruyskamp, 'Poësy van J. Six van Chandelier. Bloemlezing uit zijn dichtwerk met inleiding en aantekeningen door Dr. G.A. van Es', *Tijdschrift voor Nederlandse Taal- en Letterkunde*, 1954, p. 79.

as I was starting my research. I would also like to thank the late Jan Karlsen at the Department of Pharmacy at the University of Oslo for the keen insights he offered on pharmacy in the early modern period. Henrik Keyser Pedersen of the University Library of Oslo deserves my special thanks for purchasing books of a wide variety relevant to my research. I would also like to thank a number of Dutch scholars who were of considerable assistance during my six-month residence at the University of Utrecht in 2007. Lia van Gemert provided important materials for my research and offered many keen insights into Dutch Renaissance culture, particularly medicine and the life and work of the doctor Johan van Beverwijck. Lia also put me in touch with other Dutch researchers, including Nina Geerdink and Helmer Helmers, who were also kind enough to offer their own insights and share their considerable expertise. The e-mail correspondence I had with Saskia Klerk, Marlise Rijks, and Gary Schwartz on the history of drugs, medicine, and art in the Netherlands was of considerable help to me. I thank Anne Goldgar for sharing information with me on Abraham Six and Maria de Haen. I would also like to thank Riet Schenkeveld-van der Dussen for the valuable expertise and insights she shared in our e-mail correspondence, and Vincent Buyens and Monique A.F. Peters for allowing me to read their unpublished theses. Monique also gave generously of her time to discuss her extensive knowledge of Six van Chandelier and his contact network, in sometimes lengthy conversations at the Amsterdam Stadsarchief. I would also like to mention here – and thank – another expert on the historical archives of Amsterdam, Wim Heijnen, whom I got to know accidentally, having ordered a book at his antiquarian bookshop, Antiquariaat Academia. I was pleasantly surprised to discover that Wim was a virtual mine of information on Six van Chandelier and his family and network, and I am most grateful to him both for our extensive conversations, and his for the access he gave me to his rich archive.

I would also like to thank Carmen Verhoeven and Phil Dehing for their indispensable help with my research on the Ledger of the Wisselbank. The latter has my special thanks for the clear introductions he offered to trade and financial transactions in the Netherlands in the seventeenth century – territory that is not readily understandable to a scholar of literature. Through my good friends Guido van Rijkom and Ron Wiebolt, I came into contact with Inge Fraters, whose language corrections in the original Dutch manuscript of this book were of immense help. I am also grateful to Inge for sharing with me her own study of tea in the early modern Netherlands. Jessica Allen Hansen deserves my thanks for the language corrections she made on an earlier version of Chapter 7. It gives me great pleasure to think back to my visit to the Six Collection in Amsterdam, where Jonkheer Six van Hillegom showed me treasures from his collection of books and art, and also shared a wealth of helpful and interesting information on Six van Chandelier. I would like to thank Håkan Sandell and Eirik Lodén for their stimulating comments on the analysis of Six's poems; Giuliano D'Amico and Rune Spaans for helping me with the illustrations included in the book; Roar Kjærnstad and Hans de Boeck for their inspiring conversations on Renaissance art; and Hilde Norrgrén, Mikael Males, and Tor Ivar Østmoe for their help with the Latin texts I have consulted for this book. In 2015, I defended my thesis at the University of Oslo. I would like to thank my opponents, Freya Sierhuis and Harold J. Cook, and the chair of the defence, Jon Haarberg, for all the further input they gave at that point, and which has only enriched this book further.

Just as the writing process has taken a long time, the path from my first contact with Amsterdam University Press to the publication of the book has also been long and sometimes tortuous. And throughout this process, several people have given generously of their time, and their assistance has been indispensable. I would like to thank Benjamin Roberts for the pleasant and informative discussions we had in Amsterdam on early modern drugs and academic publications. I am grateful, too, to Inge van der Bijl, Erika Gaffney and Chantal Nicolaes just as much for their patience as for the guidance they offered in shepherding the manuscript through to final publication. My thanks also go to Thijs Weststeijn and Nelleke Moser, members of the Editorial Board for the series Studies in the Dutch Golden Age, for their enlightening comments on the manuscript. And I am most grateful to the translator of this book, Ciarán Ó Faoláin, not only for producing a fine translation, but also for the many helpful comments and suggestions for improvement he offered along the way.

In closing, I would like to say a special thank you to my dear friends Gudmund Harildstad, Per Thorvald Larsen, Raf De Saeger, Klaus Johan Myrvoll, and Lars Pharo for their invaluable support, their constructive critiques and, yes, their occasional gentle nagging: 'How's that manuscript coming along?' Well, here it is! And last but by no means least, I would like to express my deepest gratitude to my wife, Maria, and our son, Stefan. Without their nearly infinite patience, this book would not have been possible.

I dedicate this book to my father, Leen Spaans (1948–2010), in loving memory.

Part I

Introduction

1. Theory and reception

Abstract
In the seventeenth century, the Dutch Republic dominated global trade. Historical research has stressed the positive effects of exchanges of goods and knowledge. In literary criticism, the merchant-poet Joannes Six van Chandelier (1620–1695) is similarly presented as a poet with an interest in the material world. But Six's work includes a number of poems on exotic materials that not yet have been examined. These texts show that global trade, to a greater extent than previously understood, gave rise to a certain moral anxiety. I argue that Six's approach to exotics drugs is therefore determined by a process of self-criticism, but that it also contributed to an important shift in early modern science, from drug lore based on mythical concepts, to botany based on experience and observation.

Keywords: Global trade, early modern, poetry, exotic drugs, history of science, botany

> [I]t gives me [...] pleasure to watch the ships arriving,
> laden with all the produce of the Indies and all the rarities of Europe.
> Where else on earth could you find, as easily as you do here,
> all the conveniences of life and all the curiosities you could hope to see?
> – Descartes in Amsterdam[1]

'Rarities for Sale'

'Rariteiten te koop' ('Rarities for Sale') (J158) is one of the most remarkable poems of Dutch literature. I will therefore use this poem as a point of entry to the study of Six's poetry. The text was printed in the collected poems of the merchant-poet Joannes Six van Chandelier, *Poësy* (1657).[2] The poem was printed in red ink, and thus

1 Descartes, letter to Balzac, 5 May 1631. René Descartes, *The Philosophical Writings of Descartes*, 1991, vol. 3, pp. 31–32.

2 The number preceded by a 'J' refers to the order of Six's poems in A.E. Jacobs's annotated edition of the poetry of Six van Chandelier: Joannes Six van Chandelier, *Gedichten*, 1991. I include Jacobs's numbering

Spaans, R., *Dangerous Drugs: The Self-Presentation of the Merchant-Poet Joannes Six van Chandelier (1620–1695)*. Taylor & Francis Group, 2020
DOI 10.5117/9789462983543_CH01

attracts the reader's attention at once (Plate 1). 'Rariteiten te koop' probably refers to more exotica than any other literary text in the early modern Dutch Republic. And that's not all: the poem introduces a new item that surpasses all these exotica: an eccentric substance that has an irresistible appeal to Dutch consumers. The text, which comprises 162 lines, is a panegyric to a new, and until then unknown, commodity that has appeared on the market. The text begins, 'Maar nu is, op Hollands stroomen, / In myn handen, stof gekomen,/Ongehoort, en ongesien' ('But now, there has come a commodity onto Dutch streams, and in my hands, /which no one has heard of or seen before') (l. 7–9).

The new article distinguishes itself from other foreign goods by its really unusual origin. This time it is not aromatic resins, beautiful precious stones, or plants from desolate regions in the East or West Indies (l. 10–19 and 25–30):

Niet als quam se, uit verre landen,
Van de west, of oosterstranden,
  Uit een landschap sonder liên.
Als een gomboom afgedroopen,
Als een beekjen fyn ontloopen,
  Als een duuren bergh ontschaakt,
Als van boomen, of van planten,
Neevens soete waaterkanten,
  Of van seldsaam kruid gemaakt.
Neen, se komt, van 't ryk der Britten,
[...]
S'is van 't bloed van Kooningh Karel
Schynende een robyne paarel,
  Gloênden ink, en purpre verf,
Steen, en hout, en roode roosen,
Rooder dan het wroegend bloosen,
  Om het kooninghlyk verderf.

It did not come from distant lands,
From the shores of the West or the East [Indies],
From a landscape without people.
As from a tapped rubber tree,
As from a nicely panned brook,
Or extracted from a hard mountain,

of the poems throughout the book. The poet spelled his name Joannes Six van Chandelier, but in the research on his poetry, the name 'Jan' has also been used. I will use the former spelling.

Or from trees, or of plants,
By freshwater shores,
Or made of a rare herb.
No, it comes from the British kingdom.
[...]
It is the blood of King Charles,
Shining [as] a ruby pearl,
Glowing ink, and purple dye,
Stone, wood, and red roses,
Redder than the blushing outrage
Of the ruin of the king.

Paradoxically enough, this is an exotic product that originates from within Europe itself, produced by political disturbances in a country right next door to the Netherlands. The red ink used in this poem thus suggests the blood shed by Charles I. 'The sun never saw something so precious', 'the blood is a shining ruby pearl', according to the poem.

'Rariteiten te koop' is a paean to the attractiveness of this blood. The merchant, who speaks in the poem, turns to all sorts of participants on the market, retailers and consumers alike, and boasts about the exceptionally beautiful red colour of his product. The blood is a luxurious dyestuff that, in its lustre and radiance, surpassed various rare and exotic red commercial products that were on the market, whether dyes, gemstones, red flowers or varieties of fragrant wood. Altogether, about 25 different precious exotic goods are mentioned in the text. In Appendix I to this book, I give a more detailed overview of all the exotic drugs that it mentions. One of these substances will be listed here: Tyrian purple, the legendary dye of the Roman Empire (l. 41). Purple was the most expensive and most exclusive colour in antiquity. The *toga picta*, which was worn by Roman generals in their triumphs, and by Roman consuls, was dyed purple. But the substance was therefore also associated with opulence and decadence. The embodiment of the city of the antichrist, the whore of Babylon, was, according to the Book of Revelation (Chapter 17), 'dressed in purple and scarlet'. The blood is presented as a wondrous substance that can be put to all kinds of uses. Among other things, the blood delivers social mobility. By wearing clothes dyed with this blood – 'kingly costumes', as splendid as those of the biblical Solomon – one grows in stature (l. 37–51). At the same time, the text shows the sensory and physical reactions that consumption of the new commercial product arouses. Drinking wine that is mixed with this blood tastes like the 'blood of saints' (l. 61–66). The seductive praises speak to the most secret dreams of consumers. The blood produces an ecstasy, a collective daze, among consumers in the Dutch marketplace for exotica.

An interesting moment in the text comes when the merchant-poet Six includes himself among the avid consumers. Six presents himself in the poem as a merchant, as a poet and as someone in love: he says he feels 'his heart opens / At the sight of the bouquet / Of early flowers from that precious martyr's blood' (l. 121–123). The blood would be a lovely rosary for a certain Roselle – the recipient of Six's love poems – and in the form of ink, the blood could do wonders for his career as a poet – it would give life force to his verses – and also for other poets who write only 'rhymes'. In the lines that immediately follow, he advises his fellow rhymesters to follow his example. By using wonderful human blood as ink, Dutch rhymesters could bring the ideal of a Golden Age to fulfilment (l. 141–146).

All these ambivalent statements give us a clear picture of the poem. It is not, of course, a straight-up praise poem, but an ironic one – a satirical text. The blood is not a wondrous substance, but a diabolical product. When we read the following lines of poetry, this becomes quite obvious: Six tells us what must be done with their wondrous poems if no one recognises their brilliance: royally gilded poetry is worth no more than 'gilded' toilet paper (l. 147–150). The last lines of the text compare the seller of the king's blood with the one who sold Jesus: Judas. The merchant asks 'thirty stivers' for the 'wondrous blood', 'a good deal less than the amount for which Judas hanged himself' (l. 159–162). This first discussion of the poem in this chapter will be decisive for the approach I take in my research. The problems and questions that 'Rariteiten te koop' raises will determine the approach to and method of this study. 'Rariteiten te koop' is about the representation of material objects in the Netherlands of the early modern period, especially exotic drugs. At the same time, it is about the self-presentation of an early modern merchant. As we have seen, the text does not give a positive image of the trade in exotica. But as I see it, the text has not only a satirical, but also a self-critical function, given the place that the poet assigns himself within it.

The self-presentation of a druggist-poet

Within the research that has been done on early modern Dutch culture, a lot of attention has been paid to the trade in, and the exchange of, exotic materials. However, this attention is not consistent with the depiction of such materials in 'Rariteiten te koop'. Historical research has stressed the positive effects of global trade, and how these effects are expressed through objects of art. This tells us how Amsterdam became a centre for global exchanges of tastes, techniques and knowledge, demonstrating the curiosity and the engineering of the Dutch.[3] The representation of materials in Six's poetry has been presented in similar terms. In

3 For example, recent scholarship on the introduction of Asian lacquerware, porcelain and banyan (morning gowns) into the Dutch Republic shows how these novelties were praised and even copied by

Dutch literary criticism, Six is regarded as a poet with a conspicuous interest in the material world. He represents a so-called realistic poetics. This attention includes a love for food and a curiosity about foreign things. 'Rariteiten te koop' has been treated separately from these questions; it has been interpreted as a satire on Oliver Cromwell's beheading of the English king.[4]

In this study, by contrast, I argue that Six himself is an example of the very phenomena he ridicules in his satires. The function of the poem is, in my view, self-criticism and self-examination. This applies not just to 'Rariteiten te koop', but to a large group of poems in *Poësy* (1657). The prominence Six accords himself in 'Rariteiten' can, as we shall see, also be found throughout his entire poetic *oeuvre*.

In this book, I make two arguments: first, I oppose the view that this and other poems of Six only have a satirical function, and argue that they are motivated by self-confrontation. Second, I show that this self-confrontation is followed by a process of purging, which is expressed both in religious and in medical terms. Six suffered from a spleen disease, and I argue that his perception and treatment of his illness must be understood in the light of his ambivalent perception of his merchandise. These two hypotheses share the premise that exotics in the Dutch Republic were regarded with greater ambivalence than we see in the latest historiography. This points to a secondary hypothesis: I hope to show that exotic materials – both as rhetorical figures and tropes and as physical objects – are perceived as a source of moral and medical unease. Here it is important to emphasise that this applies to the exotics in which the early modern *koopman-drogist* traded – *drogerijen*. By means of an investigation of the historical definition of 'drogerij', I argue that this moral unease is related to problems which a modern reader would associate with drug abuse: intoxication, lust and illness. In this discussion, I will take as starting point a debate on foreign versus local medicines that engaged physicians and intellectuals in the early modern Dutch Republic.

The notions 'drogist', *druggist*, 'drogerij', *drug*, and also 'droog', *dry* – the term underlying both *drogist* and *drogerij* – are therefore central to this research. As for Six's self-presentation, I argue that he uses a variety of names for his profession in order to portray himself as a reliable and honest merchant, but also as a patient under treatment and as a penitent sinner. In line with these literary self-portrayals, I will show that Six gives *dry* different meanings, from 'sober' and 'rational', through 'insipid' and 'weak' in accordance with the theory of humours, to *thirsty* ('dorst' is derived from 'dor', a synonym for 'droog'), in the religious sense, thus 'thirsty

Dutch artisans. See Karina Corrigan, Femke Diercks & Martine Gosselink, *Asia in Amsterdam: The Culture of Luxury in the Golden Age*, 2015.

4 G.A. van Es & Edward Rombauts, *De letterkunde van renaissance en barok*, 2, 1952, pp. 172–173; Riet Schenkeveld-van der Dussen & Willemien B. de Vries, *Zelfbeeld in gedichten. Brieven over de poëzie van Jan Six van Chandelier (1620–1695)*, 2007, p. 159. For other interpretations of the poem, see Chapter 9.

for God'. As I have noted, my study includes drugs both as rhetorical figures and ornaments and as physical objects. I have therefore adapted a method for my inquiry into the authorial self-presentation of Six – a method that takes into account early modern theories of emotions, the body, and the physical properties of materials on the one hand and of rhetorical and literary notions and concepts, on the other. The sections on material and literary drugs in this chapter offer an overview of the theories and concepts that are relevant here. And this book has a fourth goal: as an importer of foreign drugs, Six relates his self-presentation not only to his own body but also to that of his country. This notion of a link between Six's own body and the so-called body politic is built on the early modern concept of a micro- versus a macrocosmos. I argue that Six's process of self-criticism, following a process of medical purging and moral penance, also has to do with the bodily and spiritual 'health' of the Dutch Republic.

It is thus a matter of the literary self-portrayal of a merchant-poet, where self-criticism and self-examination are important ingredients. I will be emphasising in this connection that these terms are problematic, given that they are concepts that emanate from our own time. Even though Six van Chandelier offers no *autobiographical* texts in the modern sense of the word, the texts in *Poësy* are a unique source of information on his life: the number of literary self-portraits is high in Six's case, and he presents himself as a merchant-druggist in a surprisingly high number of them, even in occasional poems dedicated to others, such as wedding poems to close family and friends, and panegyrics to official events. Although these texts are not autobiographical in the strict sense of the word, they do allow us to reconstruct Six's self-image.[5] This research is based on many of the insights of New Historicism: the emphasis on the historically situated social and cultural context, on history as cultural production, and on the idea that literary and non-literary texts influence each other. Even according to the father of New Historicism, *self-fashioning* is a problematic concept: Stephen Greenblatt is sceptical about the possibility of an early modern poet's creating their own identity, but he demonstrates all the same that their works offered them various opportunities to construct a public persona, among other things by identifying with classical poets.[6] Nina Geerdink shows in her research into the authorial self-portrayal of Six's colleague, the glassmaker-poet Jan Vos (1612–1667), that he used his professional identity in his literary and social self-promotion. On the basis of theories such as 'career criticism' and of the institutional research inspired by Pierre Bourdieu, she analyses how Vos

5 See Margaret C. Jacob & Catharine Secretan (eds.), *The Self-Perception of Early Modern Capitalists*, 2008, pp. 75–97; Willem Frijhoff & Marijke Spies, *1650. Hard-Won Unity*, 2004, p. 4.

6 Stephen Greenblatt, *Renaissance Self-Fashioning: From More to Shakespeare*, 1980. For a recent discussion on subjectivity in Renaissance literature, see Brian Cummings & Freya Sierhuis, 'Introduction', in: Brian Cummings & Freya Sierhuis (eds.), *Passions and Subjectivity in Early Modern Culture*, 2013, pp. 1–13.

shapes his own authorship based on authors' strategies. If we go by this mode of interpretation, it is a matter, not of the identity of the author's 'self', but of the way a distinct public profile was created, both by himself and others. What is interesting in this context is the way in which Vos uses materials from his profession as design elements in his image. For instance, he has the transparency of his windows serve as a symbol for the purity and openness of everything he does as a glassmaker-poet.[7] As noted above, I will also be looking at how Six actively uses the names of the commodities he trades in, and his profession, in his authorial self-representation. But as this book will show, creating a distinct profile of oneself in terms of one's profession is more problematic for a druggist than it is for a glassmaker, in view of the negative connotations that 'drug' and 'druggist' have. Another distinction lies in the audience for Six's poems. Whereas Vos offers his poems to the Regents of Amsterdam in order to promote his social career as a poet, theatre manager, and glassmaker, Six addresses many of his texts to doctors and pastors of the Reformed Church who are concerned for Six himself – a young, travelling trader suffering from an ailment of the spleen. Taking account of self-knowledge as an inner somatic process, these doctors and pastors were interested in how Six created a public profile of himself as a religiously and medically healthy person. This approach implies a break with New Historicism. I am basing myself here on Michael C. Schoenfeldt, who has done research on the body and the self in early modern English literature:

> Where New Historicism has tended to emphasize the individual as a victim of the power that circulates through culture, I stress the empowerment that Galenic physiology and ethics bestowed upon the individual. This is a book, then, about control, but not the authoritarian state that so frequently characterizes New-Historicist descriptions of Renaissance England; I emphasize rather the self-control that authorizes individuality. It is about how to fortify a self, not police a state. Its focus is a regime of self-discipline which an earlier culture imagined as a necessary step towards any prospect of liberation.[8]

Six's process of self-analysis is characterised as much by a certain humoral self-control as by coming into contact with, and taking, exotic drugs. As mentioned above, I also suggest that this process of self-control included not only the borders of the individual body, but also those of the country it found itself in. That does not

7 Nina Geerdink, *Dichters en verdiensten. De sociale verankering van het dichterschap van Jan Vos (1610–1667)*, 2012, p. 140. *Cf.* also the self-portrayal of the ferryman-poet, who also uses his materials in the process of creating a public profile for himself, in: Laurie Ellinghausen, *Labor and Writing in Early Modern England, 1567–1667*, 2008, p. 109.

8 Michael Schoenfeldt, *Bodies and Selves in Early Modern England*, 1999, p. 11.

mean, however, that Six was invoking the power of an 'authoritarian state': that would presuppose a unanimous and homogeneous state, and there was no such thing in the Netherlands of the early modern period.

Material drugs

Before I turn to Six's poems, I would like to discuss the state of affairs regarding other concepts that this study is building on and responding to, such as 'drugs', 'drug use', 'druggist', and 'spice merchant'/'grocer' (*kruidenier* in Dutch). I will go into the development of the theory of drugs as material goods, and then of drugs as literary ornaments. This is followed by a brief discussion of Joannes Six van Chandelier and his collection of poems, *Poësy.* I conclude this section with a discussion of the reception of Six's *oeuvre*. Finally, I offer an overview of the main part of this book, specifying which literary self-profiling strategies of Six's we find in which chapters.

We usually associate drug abuse with the post-industrial age. However, in this study, I would argue that there were also discussions about the individual and social dangers of drugs in the Netherlands of the early modern period. According to Marxist and poststructuralist theory, drugs are symbols of capitalist consumption and the fragmented modern individual.[9] This brings us to more recent research on drugs. Andrew Sherratt underlines the importance of psychoactive drugs in older cultures: he says the modern definitions of drugs and drug culture are not specific to modernity and the Industrial Revolution. He has it, however, that these definitions are 'misleading as a framework for approaching the great variety of ways in which organic substances have been used by human beings to alter their mental states'.[10] Sherratt points to a 'genealogy' of substances that included an extensive knowledge of other cultures. He regards 'peculiar substances' as part of an 'anthropology of consumption', where psychoactive substances 'thus take their place alongside a variety of other meaningful consumables'. He stresses that these substances 'can therefore be considered not so much a category in themselves but as one aspect of a potentially wide range of social activities.' Sherratt argues that one also has to take into account the meaning of drugs not only under capitalism, but also in indigenous, traditional, and prehistoric economies. On the basis of an analysis of pre-modern and indigenous practices, he protests against current medical and legal definitions of drugs, which reduce them to their psychoactive

9 *Cf.* the concepts 'magical commodity' and 'commodity fetish' in the writings of Marx, and *la drogue* as a representation of the Western conception of 'the other' in Derrida: 'Plato's Pharmacy', in: Jacques Derrida, *Dissemination*, 1981, pp. 61–171.

10 Andrew Sherratt, 'Introduction: Peculiar Substances' in: Jordan Goodman, Paul E. Lovejoy & Andrew Sherratt (eds.), *Consuming Habits: Drugs in History and Anthropology*, 1995, pp. 1–10; quote on p. 1.

effect and declare their legal status legitimate or illegitimate. Sherratt defines drug use as a form of consumption whose meanings are as numerous as those who engage in it, from soft drugs to narcotics. He sees it as an act that can take place just as easily in very different settings, from taking a coffee in the morning to the abuse of opiates.

Sherratt's insights have influenced newer research into the role of drugs in early modern culture, but the work has also received some critical comments.[11] First, *Consuming Habits* focuses primarily on pre-modern, non-Western drug consumption. Second, it goes along with the idea of drug use as part of a 'civilising process'. In the discussion of colonial drugs in *Consuming Habits* – referred to as *excitantia* – Jordan Goodman argues that the introduction of these commodities was accompanied by the rise of bourgeois culture with its tobacco, coffee, tea, chocolate and sugar, which were 'commercial capitalistic substitutes for indigenous European drugs and alcohol', and also for European plants associated with demonological purposes. These commodities were thus regarded as embodiments of moderation and frugality, by contrast with excess, drunkenness and witchcraft. This interpretation of colonial commodities fits well with the portrayal of the Netherlands of the early modern period as a level-headed bourgeois society.[12] One would then expect foreign drugs to be welcomed by early modern medical authorities as sober alternatives to indigenous European intoxicants such as beer. Goodman admits that the process is not so simple as that. He stresses that a foreign drug as tobacco had to be adapted to pre-existing European medical concepts, and in this way be made understandable and desirable to European consumers. But instead of dwelling on early modern medical concepts and ideas, he places greater emphasis on economic mechanisms, such as supply and demand, and chemical properties of plants, revealed through empirical modern chemistry, such as the side effects of various drugs. But beer and other European products were actually highlighted as healthy substitutes to dangerous, exotic food by many physicians in the seventeenth century. The process of introducing foreign drugs into the European market was intertwined with early modern physiological, social and political concepts and ideas. That is clear from the intriguing study of the history of coffee by Brian Cowan, who asks why coffee succeeded in entering the European consumer market while other exotic drugs that were popular within the rarefied circles of early modern scientists, the so-called *virtuosi*, did not. While coffee does not have the same sort of intoxicating effect as, say, opium, the physiological discourses surrounding drugs

11 Phil Withington, Introduction: *Cultures of Intoxication*, in: Past & Present, 2014, pp. 9–33.

12 See Jordan Goodman, 'Excitantia: Or, How Enlightenment Europe Took to Soft Drugs', pp. 121–141, and see also Woodruff D. Smith, 'From Coffee-House to Parlour: the Consumption of Coffee, Tea, and Sugar in North-Western Europe in the Seventeenth and Eighteenth Centuries', pp. 142–157, in: Jordan Goodman, Paul E. Lovejoy & Andrew Sherratt (eds.), *Consuming Habits*, 1995.

in the early modern period 'extended into areas far beyond the "natural" – that is to say, the ahistorical and the noncultural – mechanics of brain and body chemistry. Exotic drugs were often attributed mind-altering or body-affecting qualities that had no basis in biological fact', Cowan writes. One important reason why coffee, and not betel nut or *datura*, for example, became successful, is that stories were told about them by early modern physicians and moralists: these narratives associated other drugs with 'licentious sexuality' and 'drunken disorder'. In this study, I am interested in similar stories that were told by doctors and moralists in the early modern Dutch Republic.[13]

Another important critical comment on *Consuming Habits* comes from Phil Withington, and it concerns the use of concepts. To get away from the ideological connotations that 'drugs' can have, Withington argues instead for the use of the term 'intoxication', which includes the effects not only of alcohol, but of all kinds of other intoxicating substances, and at the same time also covers concepts such as 'bewitchment'. Withington then refers to Samuel Johnson's dictionary and says about this 'broad meaning of intoxication' that it:

> was in almost direct contradistinction to the Old French term 'drug', which until the end of the nineteenth century was used primarily to describe 'An ingredient used in physic; a medicinal simple' and less commonly to denote 'anything without a value'. Different medicines had different qualities – including stupefaction and stimulation – but these qualities varied according to the drug and were not inherent to the word. It is only relatively recently that 'drug' has acquired its presiding connotations of illegality, addiction, danger, and harm on the one hand and subversion, counter-culture, and hedonism on the other.[14]

However, by contrast with Withington, I suggest in this book that the concept of 'drug' is just as productive as 'intoxication' when it comes to research into drug culture in the seventeenth century. In his interesting study on drugs in the early modern Portuguese and British empires, Benjamin Breen emphasises that Samuel Johnson's definition of 'drugs' was coloured by a 'decidedly moralistic slant' that the term had acquired in the eighteenth century. According to Breen, it is striking, given the widespread assumption that drugs played a role in modernity, to observe the relative silence on the subject from early modern historians.[15]

13 Brian Cowan, *The Social Life of Coffee: The Emergence of the British Coffeehouse*, 2005; quote on p. 54.

14 Withington, 2014, p. 13.

15 Benjamin Breen, *The Age of Intoxication: Origins of the Global Drug Trade*, 2019, p. 48. For a survey of recent works on the history of drugs in the early modern period, see also Benjamin Breen, *Drugs and Early Modernity*, in: *History Compass*, 2017, pp. 1–9.

I hope this book can go some way towards filling this gap in the history of drugs. The cultural and moral complexity of drugs becomes clear to us if we include the Dutch origin and use of the term in its 'genealogy'. This shows that the original meaning of 'drugs' – 'dried goods' (in Dutch, *drogerijen*) – that is, products that were preserved so they could be shipped over longer distances – evokes associations with a number of concepts and phenomena such as strangeness, craving, and disease. The fact that drugs were transnational commodities means that we must also take into account concepts such as 'spices' (*kruiden, specerijen*) and 'exotica' in our research into the early modern trade in drugs. I will return to the semantic relationship between 'drugs' and these latter terms in Chapter 2.

The plethora of meanings that 'drugs' has also applies to terms derived from it, such as 'druggist'. And in Dutch, 'grocer'/'spice merchant' (*kruidenier*) and 'druggist' (*drogist*) also have pejorative meanings, even if these are not as common. *Kruidenier* also means 'a narrow-minded or bigoted person', while *drogist*, with its etymology in *droog* – 'dry' – also means 'a bore'.[16] Eduard Douwes Dekker plays on the latter meaning in his caricature of the straitlaced Dutch businessman in *Max Havelaar*, Batavus Droogstoppel. These negative traits also have concepts in common with 'merchant', a word that Six also uses in naming his profession.[17] The figure of the merchant has been viewed with ambivalence since the days of antiquity: Aristotle argues in his *Politics* that trade for the sake of accumulating wealth is 'unnatural', and this view finds echoes in Cicero's condemnation of the 'vulgarity' of trade. The biblical condemnation of usury and worldly riches contributes to this anti-commercial ethics. Thinkers of the Renaissance repeat these arguments: Erasmus pointed to the meanness of the methods that merchants used: 'their lying, bearing false witness, thievery, and treachery'. But just as old is the view of the merchant as a positive figure, as long as they – as Cicero put it – emulate positive qualities, especially *honestum* and *utile*. If they do that, they will be honest in their trade and work towards the common weal. In the early modern Dutch Republic, this position was defended from a Christian standpoint by Dirck Volckertszoon Coornhert in *De Coopman* (*The Merchant*) (1580), and from a humanistic viewpoint by Caspar Barlaeus in *Mercator sapiens* (*The Wise Merchant*) (1632).[18] This ambivalent perception of a merchant's traits – a selfish miserliness versus a thriftiness that was positive for society – colours research into the social conception of the early modern merchant. On the other hand, we know Max Weber's views on the Protestant work ethic as an

16 See these terms in *Woordenboek der Nederlandsche Taal* (WNT).

17 Judit Gera, 'The grocer as a stereotype in Dutch culture', *Praagse perspectieven*, 2005, pp. 33–43.

18 Caspar Barlaeus, *The Wise Merchant*, ed. by Anna-Luna Post & Corinna Vermeulen, 2019; D.V. Coornhert, *De Coopman*, [1580] 1969. See also Arthur Weststeijn, *Commercial Republicanism in the Dutch Golden Age: The Political Thought of Johan & Pieter de la Court*, pp. 141–204; Steven Shapin, *A Social History of Truth: Civility and Science in Seventeenth-Century England*, 1994, p. 94.

ideal type on the one hand and, and on the other, the image of the Dutch, Protestant merchant as a phlegmatic, petty trader.[19] An intellectual-historical examination of these words will help us avoid falling into old social prejudices. In this study I will, therefore, draw attention to how Six uses the concepts not only of 'druggist', but also of *koopman* ('merchant') and *kruidenier* ('grocer', 'spice merchant').

Even though little research has been done on drugs in early modern Dutch culture, studies have been done on assertions of the moral dangers of amassing material goods. The iconological method has been central to research on luxury and opulence in Dutch society. One well-known study is Simon Schama's *Embarrassment of Riches* (1987).[20] I will build on the findings of these works. But my methodological approach will also include medical and scientific, as well as iconological, discussions.

This book is about the merchant as a trader in exotic drugs, and in this connection I would mention three books in particular: in *Matters of Exchange,* Harold J. Cook shows how the interests of merchants and of university-educated physicians overlapped in the early modern period, and how natural history contributed to the scientific revolution as much as natural philosophy did: merchants were particularly interested in collecting, transporting and exchanging both things and ideas. They were thus interested, not primarily in the economic value of the materials, but just as much in how material goods were interpreted by the senses. This insistence on objectivity is understood as an ambition to acquire 'the knowledge of objects

19 *Cf.* Immanuel Kant's view: 'Der Holländer ist von einer ordentlichen und emsigen Gemüthsart [...] so hat er wenig Gefühl für dasjenige, was im feineren Verstande schön oder erhaben ist' ('The Dutchman is of an orderly and diligent disposition [...] He has little feeling for what, to a more refined mind, is beautiful or sublime'). Roland Barthes argues that intellectual life in the Netherlands in the early modern period was limited to material and commercial matters, to the 'patient weighing of property or of merchandise'. The quotes come from Dorothee Sturkenboom, 'Staging the Merchant: Commercial Vices and the Politics of Stereotyping in Early Modern Dutch Theatre', *Dutch Crossing,* 2006, p. 212; Anne Goldgar, *Tulipmania: Money, Honor, and Knowledge in the Dutch Golden Age,* 2007, pp. 11 and 12. As these scholars emphasise, such characteristics should be seen in light of the Anglo-Dutch wars. The negative view of the Dutch merchant was coloured by English war propaganda. An extreme case is John Milton's comparison of a Dutch fleet of Indies vessels with Satan: 'close sailing from Bengala, or the isles / of Ternate and Tidor, whence merchants bring/their spicy drugs', John Milton, *Paradise Lost,* 2007, p. 141.

20 In his research Simon Schama emphasises the symbolism and iconology of painting, but the sometimes liberal iconographic analyses in his research have met with criticism. One of Schama's main hypotheses is that trade was a source of moral unease with Dutch, merchants included. This claim is contested by other historians. For instance, C.M. Lesger writes: 'Their self-assurance in the economics, political, and social realm seems not to have been undermined by doubts about the salvation or by embarrassment over their riches', C.M. Lesger, 'Merchants in charge: The self-perception of Amsterdam merchants, c. 1550–1700', in: Margaret C. Jacob & Catharine Secretan (eds.), *The Self-Perception of Early Modern Capitalists,* 2008, pp. 75–99, quote on p. 91. *Cf.* also Mariët Westerman, *A Worldly Art: The Dutch Republic, 1585–1718,* 1996. A more recent study on luxury goods in the Netherlands: Rengenier C. Rittersma (ed.), *Luxury in the Low Countries: Miscellaneous Reflections on Netherlandish Material Culture, 1500 to present,* 2010.

without reference to intuition or innate knowledge, the corporeal knowledge of things that can be experienced by the bodily senses, information which can be exchanged'. This new objectivity was indispensable when it came to gathering knowledge from abroad, especially as regards exotica and marvels. I also include Cook's methodological approach in this book. The main weakness of his approach is that the role of religion and the knowledge of antiquity in the rise of empirical research are not treated in any depth. Reflections on epistemology, on the conditions for, and the scope of, knowledge, by the ancient philosophers Plato and the Stoics, and by the Church fathers, especially Augustine, are treated superficially.[21]

One researcher who does take the moral implications of global trade into account is Julie Berger Hochstrasser. Taking Marxist and post-colonial theory as a starting point, she defines still-life paintings featuring exotica as 'pictorial capitalism', and breathes new life into the myth of the unscrupulous Dutch merchant. Admittedly, she includes in her discussion the polemic *Inleydinge tot de Hollandtsche Genees-middelen* (*Introduction to Dutch Medicines*) (1642) by Johan van Beverwijck – a book that criticises the use of exotic medicines. Her argument also stresses, on the other hand, that Van Beverwijck's other books praise exotica as medicines: 'Judging from this conflicting evidence, questions of morality could not have weighed all that heavily on the matter of foreign luxuries being imported and consumed in Dutch households.'[22] In Chapter 4, I delve further into Johan van Beverwijck's polemic. Here I argue that, on the contrary, the *Inleydinge tot de Hollandtsche Genees-middelen* had considerable influence on Dutch society.

In this connection it should be emphasised that Dutch merchants brought back to Europe from 'exotic lands' not only novelties such as porcelain or Maldivian coconuts, popular in recent research on exotica in the Dutch Republic, but also spices, incense and gems – products with a long history of reception in Europe. A product like incense was so closely interwoven with Asia that it had become an epithet of the continent (Fig. 1.1). Since ancient times, these categories of exotica have had a variety of meanings. The large distance between the producing countries meant that exotica were subject to illusory and mystifying processes. It was not so much the spices themselves that were appealing, but the mythical knowledge they were connected with. Even in the age of discovery, herbals were still full of marvellous classical fables, religious myths and Bible stories.[23] The process of mystification introduces us to concepts related to *exotica* such as *curiosity,*

21 Harold J. Cook, *Matters of Exchange: Commerce, Medicine, and Science in the Dutch Golden Age*, 2007, quote on p. 19. Also, compare Pamela H. Smith & Paula Findlen (eds.), *Merchants and Marvels: Commerce, Science, and Art in Early Modern Europe*, 2002.

22 Julie Berger Hochstrasser, *Still Life and Trade in the Dutch Golden Age*, 2007 – quote taken from p. 241.

23 See Paul Freedman, *Out of the East: Spices and the Medieval Imagination*, 2008, and Stefan Halikowski Smith, 'The Mystification of Spices in the Western Tradition', *European Review of History*, 2001, pp. 119–136.

mirabilia and *wonder.*[24] Lorraine Daston and Katherine Park emphasise that these last two terms blur the boundary between the marvellous on the one hand and the miraculous on the other – between the earthly and sacred connotations of 'wondrous substance'. They also emphasise that 'wonder' was also a cognitive passion. It had as much to do with 'knowing' as with 'feeling'. Thus 'being amazed' can be seen as a process of acquiring knowledge. It is thus important to investigate how theologians and scientists maintained the distinction between these spheres – that of the Wunderkammer, or cabinet of curiosities, and that of the Church. Similarly, the concept of 'curiosity', especially with regard to occult and magical philosophy, was intertwined with 'enthusiasm'. In Greek, *enthousiasmos* originally meant 'possession by a god'. In the early modern period, it was connected to a radical form of Protestantism and also with the concept of the inspired poet.[25]

Drugs as exotica and wondrous substances served as markers of social status and aspirations. They were exchanged among kings and statesmen as 'political gifts'.[26] And they served as offerings in the religions of antiquity. In addition to discussions that certain authorities held on therapeutic properties, we find warnings against exotica as substances that lead to temptation, lust and decadence. The satirical poets Persius, Juvenal and Horace, whom Six imitates, were critical of the influence of the 'decadent East' on 'the simple and honest character' of the Romans. Here, the extensive *Naturalis Historia* by the Roman naturalist Pliny the Elder, who is one of the most important sources in Six's poetry, serves as a paradox. The work exhibits a strong fascination with *mirabilia*, exotic animals and plants, and natural phenomena. But he also warns against importing luxury goods into the Roman Empire. These thoughts were later taken up by the Church Fathers Jerome, Augustine and Tertullian. Moralists in the seventeenth century drew from both

24 In addition, the mystification of drugs is linked to the concept 'orientalism'. Since the publication of Edward Said's *Orientalism* (1978), orientalism has become a commonplace to discuss western attitudes toward Asian culture and people. For a discussion of early modern drug culture versus Said's interpretation of orientalism, see Brian Cowan, *The Social Life of Coffee*, 2005. Cowan uses the term 'consumer orientalism', and argues that this 'orientalism' of the seventeenth century 'was not the hegemonic imperialist discourse that is the subject of [Said's] *Orientalism*' (p. 116).

25 The meaning of exotica comes originally from the Latin *exōticus*, from Greek *exōtikos*, 'foreign', from *exō* 'outside' (Oxford English Dictionary), while concepts such as marvels, *mirabilia* and *miracula* are etymologically related and can be traced back to the Latin *miror* (be amazed, wonder) and *mirus* (marvellous, extraordinary); see Eric Jorink, *Reading the book of Nature in the Dutch Golden Age, 1575–1715*, 2010, p. 7. For further analyses of these the semantic development of these concepts, Lorraine Daston & Katharine Park, *Wonders and the Order of Nature, 1150–1750*, 1998; R.J.W. Evans & Alexander Marr (eds.), *Curiosity and Wonder from the Renaissance to the Enlightenment*, especially the Introduction by Alexander Marr, pp. 1–20; and Michael Heyd, *'Be Sober and Reasonable': The Critique of Enthusiasm in the Seventeenth and Early Eighteenth Centuries*, 1995.

26 *Cf.* Claudia Swan, 'Birds of Paradise for the Sultan: Early Seventeenth-Century Dutch-Turkish Encounters and the Uses of Wonder', *The Seventeenth Century*, 2013, pp. 49–63.

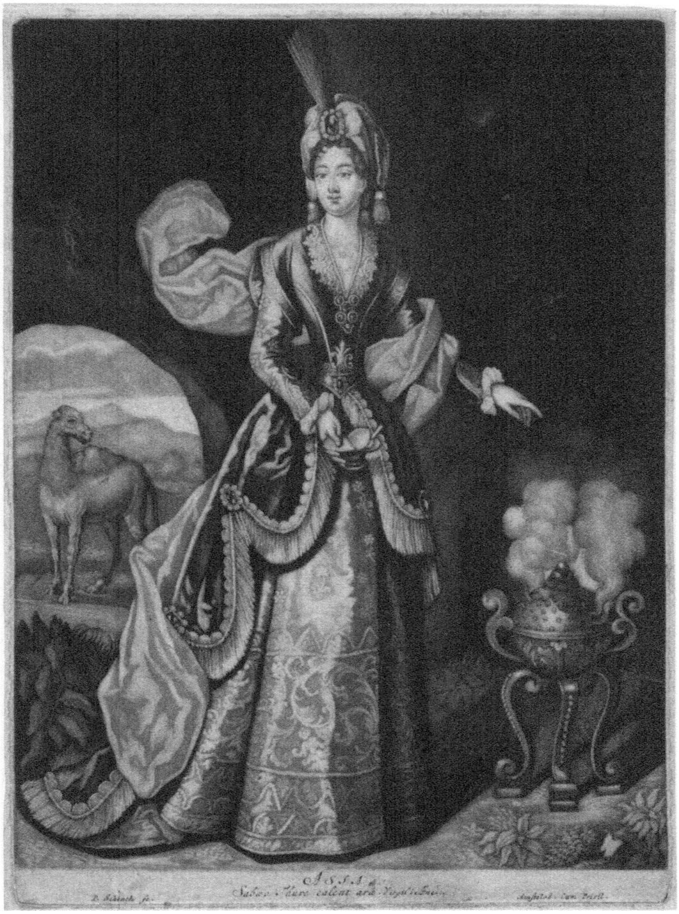

Fig. 1.1: Pieter Schenk, *Asia*, c. 1670–c. 1713. Engraving. (© Rijksmuseum, Amsterdam).

the classical and Christian knowledge traditions. And when Six uses Pliny both as a moral and a scientific counsellor, he follows the advice that Caspar Barlaeus gives to merchants in his aforementioned *Mercator sapiens* (Fig. 1.2).[27] The classical resonance of the concept of exotica clashes with the formation of the idea that the discovery of strange parts of the world entailed a total re-evaluation of the European culture of knowledge, as well as with the idea that a new, modern world image was accepted only when Europeans took a dislike to an unproductive passion for the past – the humanistic dependence of the ancient world – and adopted an open, objective approach to the perception of the cultural 'other'. Revisionist analyses of the Renaissance, especially the work of Anthony Grafton, however,

27 Freedman, 2008; Barlaeus, 2019, p. 105.

have undermined this image of humanistic culture as an intellectual limitation. The discoveries produced no shock of the new and no displacement of old methods, but led to the beginning of a slow process of adaptation; the humanistic culture of knowledge was vital well into the seventeenth century.[28] Thus, the physical effects of both tobacco and heavier drugs such as opium were understood in light of long-established concepts such as drunkenness.[29] This is the message from Christine R. Johnson's research. She studied the discussion on moral versus immoral trade in German-speaking countries in the sixteenth century, and showed that German authorities based themselves on classical moralists in making their case for economic independence and against the consumption of tropical spices, and that an aversion to foreign plants was based on domestic manifestations of greed and wealth.[30] Moralists regarded the trader in exotic drugs and spices as a carrier of disease. They believed that the trade in drugs created a direct physical connection between the strange substance that was ingested and the body itself. But Johnson also showed that some New World plants were interpreted as having an enriching effect rather than constituting an invasion, once they had become acclimated to German soil and included in the humoral system of the classical authorities, such as Dioscorides and Galen. That is because these novelties were not found on the lists of ancient moralists on foreign commodities.

The 'indigenous body' is a central notion in the writings of early modern moralists. It refers both to the individual body and to the 'body politic', one of the oldest metaphors in the history of ideas: philosophers from antiquity to the early modern period, from Plato to Thomas Hobbes, conceived of the state as a body and thus fitted out political and social discourse with anatomical and medical concepts.[31] Historians make reference to various medical concepts to explain how spices could cause disease: Jonathan Gil Harris has it that early modern debates on the spice trade in England anticipated the modern concept of infectious, invasive diseases. Harris's interpretation of spices as *semina* is based on what was then Paracelsus's new medical doctrine, and implies a break with an important mindset within the classical tradition of knowledge: Galenic medicine. By contrast, Margaret Healy relates the sick body, both of the individual and of the state,

28 Anthony Grafton, *New Worlds, Ancient Texts: The Power of Tradition and the Shock of Discovery*, 1992. See especially the section on medicine that he wrote with Nancy Siraisi: pp. 260–291.

29 Benjamin Roberts, *Sex and Drugs Before Rock 'n' Roll: Youth Culture and Masculinity during Holland's Golden Age*, 2012, pp. 171–184.

30 Christine R. Johnson, *The German Discovery of the World: Renaissance Encounters with the Strange and Marvelous*, 2008, pp. 123–164.

31 David Hale, *The Body Politic: A Political Metaphor in Renaissance English Literature*, 1971. Not much research has been done on this concept in early modern Dutch culture. For an introduction, see Helmer Helmers, 'Illness as Metaphor: The Sick Body Politic and Its Cures', in: J. Grave & B. Noak (eds.), *Illness and Literature in the Early Modern Low Countries*, 2015, pp. 97–120.

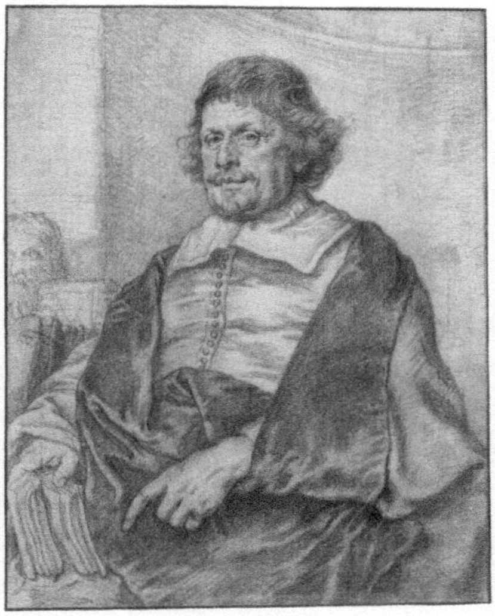

Fig. 1.2: Joachim von Sandrart, *Portrait of Caspar Barlaeus*, c. 1637–1643. Brush on paper. (© Rijksmuseum, Amsterdam).

to Galenic theories about excessive appetites. She speaks of an interaction between two medical concepts; an 'exopathic' one (disease as an external, invasive force) and an 'endogenous' one (disease as an inner disorder). She also introduces the idea of a 'glutted, unvented body', and uses it to show how the consumption of luxury goods was associated with the court and was conceived of as a threat to physical well-being.[32] In this book, I want to keep in mind the notion of exotic drugs as potentially pathogenic infectious agents, and of the merchant-druggist as a potential 'source of infection'.

No systematic study of this kind has yet been done on the critique of exotic materials in the early modern Netherlands. In this sense, then, this book can claim to be innovative. While the criticism of exotic drugs had little impact on the economic development of the Dutch Republic, it did influence the country's cultural, social and scientific life. Benjamin Schmidt and Benjamin Roberts have shown how tobacco imported from America was a source of moral concern in the Netherlands, while Alix Cooper has looked at how Johan van Beverwijck's polemic influenced discussions among Dutch physicians such as Lambert Bidloo and Jan Commelin, as well as those from other European countries.[33] Her main thesis is that, given the reaction against exotic imports, scholars urged their readers to

32 Jonathan Gil Harris, *Sick Economies: Drama, Mercantilism and Disease in Shakespeare's England*, 2004; Margaret Healy, *Fictions of Disease in Early Modern England: Bodies, Plagues and Politics*, 2001.

33 Benjamin Schmidt, *Innocence Abroad: The Dutch Imagination and the New World, 1570–1670*, 2006; Roberts, 2012. Van Beverwijck's Latin translation, for instance, was a model for the polemic *De medicina danorum domestica*, 1666, by the Danish physician Thomas Bartholin. *Cf.* also the moral unease that

discover the flora in their own country. We should also not forget the cultural shock of tulip mania: this plant, imported from Turkey, gave rise to a moral crisis in the Netherlands, even though fewer people than has previously been supposed actually lost money on tulip mania, as Anne Goldgar has shown in her study.[34] In this study of the literary self-presentation of the merchant-druggist Joannes Six van Chandelier, I must thus take into account the moral discourse around native versus non-native plants. Merchants were constantly looking for a moral identity in the quest to win social recognition, according to Margaret C. Jacob and Catherine Secretan.[35] My hypothesis is, then, that Six – in addition to the traditional critique of the merchant as a representative of avarice and the pursuit of profit – is conceived of as a representative of products that moralists considered to be morally, socially and medically dangerous. I would like to show through my research that the perception of the merchant-druggist Joannes Six van Chandelier was integrated into complex medical, social and religious discussions that had their roots in the classical culture of knowledge. That does not mean, however, that ethical concerns precluded progressive scientific insights into material culture: Anthony Grafton and Nancy Siraisi show how morally intoned warnings against the use of tobacco in the early modern period anticipate medical condemnations of nicotine in our day, while Alix Cooper shows how the emergence of the first Dutch reference book on indigenous wild plants, *Catalogus plantarum indigenarum Hollandiae* by Jan Commelin (1683), was a direct result of the debate on native versus exotic plants.[36]

To make the picture even more complicated: it is important to emphasise that the alarm to which contact with the foreign gave rise did not manifest itself in only one direction – far from it. It also gave rise to a critique that was focused on European society. And that criticism came from a quarter one would least expect – from moralists connected with the pietistic movement within the Dutch Reformed Church, the Further Reformation. In the Calvinistic literature, we find works that show not only a surprising openness to foreign peoples and ethnographic

tobacco and chocolate aroused in Spain: Marcy Norton, *Sacred Gifts, Profane Pleasures: A History of Tobacco and Chocolate in the Atlantic World*, 2008.

34 Alix Cooper, *Inventing the Indigenous: Local Knowledge and Natural History in Early modern Europe*, 2007; Anne Goldgar, *Tulipmania: Money, Honor, and Knowledge in the Dutch Golden Age*, 2007. *Cf.* Benedict Robinson's research on 'cultural anxieties' linked to the introduction of the tulip to the English market: Benedict S. Robinson, 'Green Seraglios: Tulips, Turbans, and the Global Market.' *The Journal for Early Modern Cultural Studies*, 2009, pp. 93–122.

35 Margaret C. Jacob & Catherine Secretan (eds.), *The Self-Perception of Early Modern Capitalists*, 2008. On the importance of honour and reputation to early modern merchants, see also L. Kooijmans, 'De koopman', in: H.M. Beliën, A.Th. van Deursen & G.J. van Setten (eds.), *Gestalten van de Gouden Eeuw. Een Hollands groepsportret*, 1995, pp. 78–83.

36 Grafton (with Nancy Siraisi) 1992; Cooper, 2007.

information, but also a globally oriented curiosity that warrants a critical re-evaluation of their European, Christian culture. This revisionist view of orthodox Protestantism is expressed in the analysis by Jos Gommans and Ineke Loots of *De conversione Indorum et Gentilium* (1669) by the pastor and theologian Johannes Hoornbeeck (1617–1666), on the conversion of pagans to Christianity. Gommans and Loots also stress 'the long-term intellectual roots of a much wider movement of Enlightenment' rather than radical ruptures.[37] Hoornbeeck is an important name in this context, because he was one of the recipients of Six's poems. According to 'Rariteiten te koop', it is not an exotic luxury article that constituted a considerable danger, but 'exotica' from a European country. I want to take into account in this book the insights offered by Gommans and Loots.

Literary drugs

In the research on exotic materials in the early modern Netherlands, literature has received less attention than the visual arts. But a look at 'Ontrouwe vrienden: Op de wyse van den 88 psalm' ('Unfaithful Friends: in the manner of Psalm 88') (J461) by Joannes Six van Chandelier presents another view of the matter. The title gives us a hint of what the poem contains: Six wants to take his revenge on friends who have left him in the lurch. The poem is thus a satire. This form apparently requires a particular kind of ink, l. 1–4:

> Myn heil, myn trooster, wat voor ink
> Myn klaaghsche pen nu zal ontvallen,
> Dat die van kooperrood, en gallen,
> Wel swarter, dan de steenkool blink [...]
>
> My salvation, my consolation, what other sort of ink
> Would fall from my complaining pen
> Than vitriol and gall [or: bile]
> Blacker than the shine of coal [...]

Six's 'complaining pen' contains vitriol and bile, a mix that is apparently of quite a spiteful nature. The negative connotations of these concepts are well known to us. 'Copper red', better known as vitriol, indicates 'violently caustic sharp words or expressions', while Dutch 'gal', which means both 'bile' and 'gall' in English, connotes

37 J. Gommans and I. Loots, 'Arguing with the Heathens: The Further Reformation and the Ethnohistory of Johannes Hoornbeeck (1617–1666)', *Itinerario*, 2015, pp. 45–68, quote on p. 46.

'seething rage, malice' – *cf.* expressions such as 'baptise his words in bile'.[38] These figurative meanings determine our understanding of the passage cited. But what a modern reader would fail to notice is the extent to which Six also bases himself on the literal reality behind these concepts. *Kooperrood*, a kind of 'mineral salt', is an older name for a sulphate (sulphuric acid) of heavy metals – and a gall nut is a nut-shaped growth on oak leaves that have been infected by the sting of a gall wasp. For the early modern poet, rather than being exclusively frivolous images, both were directly observable materials, because they formed the ingredients of so-called gall-nut ink, the most common writing ink in Six's day, which was sold at druggists such as Six's. The bitterness of these substances should thus be understood literally. Just like other early modern goods found at a druggist's, they were suitable for many purposes, especially as medicines. That makes it likely that people living in the seventeenth century also had a sensory perception of the 'caustic' and 'corrosive' effects of ink, and thus of writing. The Dutch botanist Dodonaeus describes the gall nut as 'pungent and sour when taken' and therefore effective against a slew of complaints.[39] This materiality apparently concerns not only the target of the mockery, but also the one doing the mocking. Before Six writes out his lethal satire, he reflects, according to the sequel to the text: he realises the danger his revenge entails, and prays to the Holy Spirit – the one to whom the poem is dedicated ('My salvation, my consolation') – for help in resisting the temptation, because Six 'salf, en troost / Des heilgen geest verhoop t'ontfangen, / Op prikkels, die myn boesem prangen, / Met meenigh sucht, om lucht, geloost [...]' ('hopes to receive salve and consolation from the Holy Spirit, against thorns that press into my bosom, which heaves many a sigh for air [...]') (l. 7–10). Six hopes that the salve from the Holy Spirit will calm the desire for revenge in his heart. He ascribes to the redemptive salve of the Holy Spirit, just as to the ingredients of the ink, not just a spiritual but also a somatic function.

According to some literary historians, the large number of medical references is one of the features of early modern literature, especially in satire.[40] This is the subject of the study done by Tanya Pollard on the chemical vocabulary used in the early modern English theatre.[41] She discusses the physiological powers that

38 Six borrowed the figurative meaning of bile from the yellow or black bile in the human body: *cholē* in Greek. The literal meaning of the word is based, however, on the nut-shaped growth on the leaves of an oak tree, the oak tree. *Cf.* also the metaphorical meaning of vitriol in English.

39 Rembertus Dodonaeus, *Cruydt-boeck* (*The Book of Herbs and Spices*), 1644, pp. 1292–1294, quote on p. 1293; Nicolas Lemery, *Woordenboek of algemeene verhandeling der enkele droogeryen*, 1743, pp. 76, 299, 751–753, 'Writing ink is made from gallnuts and vitriol, to which a little arabic gum is added' (p. 76).

40 See for example Mary Claire Randolph, 'The Medical Concept in English Renaissance Satiric Theory: Its Possible Relationships and Implications', *Studies in Philology*, 1941, pp. 125–157.

41 Tanya Pollard, *Drugs and Theater in Early Modern England*, 2005, especially pp. 1–22.

early modern writers attributed to language. Central to her study is the dominant medical paradigm of the early modern period: the Galenic theory of humours. Literary works were thought to exert as much influence on the body as on the mind of the reader, Pollard argues, because humoral physiology made no clear distinction between mental and physical processes: thoughts, emotions and the imagination were perceived as parts of the human body. A change to one's state of mind, she tells us, was thought to cause a corresponding change in one's body. Psychological processes were understood in corporeal terms, as a 'physiology of inner emotion', in the words of Michael Schoenfeldt.[42] The emotional impact of literature on the human mind, then, also had consequences for the human body. Whether it was material or literary drugs were involved, Pollard shows how pigments and aromatics were perceived as powerful transformative substances. Etymologically, the concept of the pharmacy was intrinsically ambiguous, she tells us: the Greek word *pharmakon* itself means poison, remedy *and* love potion.[43] Pollard's emphasis on the senses, the body and emotions is of a piece with a wider interest in emotions in the study of early modern culture, the so-called emotional turn.[44] I follow this research tradition in this book. But, as Brian Cummings and Freya Sierhuis have shown in their studies, the passions were understood not only in the light of the Galenic ideas of restraint and physical balance, but were also defined by social, literary and religious concepts. As we will see, in his poems Six speaks positively about 'Christian excesses', namely a Christian enthusiasm and even a Christian cannibalism.[45]

Not only the vitriol in ink, but drugs that were more closely linked with foreignness and luxury, such as ambergris, ivory, incense and gems, were popular as metaphors in poetry in the early modern period. These materials bring us closer to the exotic materials portrayed in 'Rariteiten te koop' and to the aforementioned discourse of local as opposed to foreign drugs. This is the subject of Farah Karim-Cooper's study of cosmetics in English Renaissance drama. She writes that 'the fear of a diminishing Englishness in an ingredient culture that thrived upon foreign commerce is quite central to the anti-cosmetic case.'[46] The transformative power ascribed to foreign drugs gave rise not only to a medical anxiety, but also to an

42 In this theory of a 'humoral self', Pollard builds on Gail Kern Paster, *The Body Embarrassed: Drama and the Disciplines of Shame in Early Modern England*, 1993, and Schoenfeldt, 1999.

43 Pollard, 2005, p. 4.

44 See for example Susan Broomhall, *Early Modern Emotions: An Introduction*, 2017; H.W. Roodenburg, *A Cultural History of the Senses in the Renaissance, 1450–1650*, 2014; and Gary Schwartz (ed.), *Emotions: Pain and Pleasure in the Dutch Golden Age*, 2015.

45 For a critical review on body, passion and emotion in the early modern period, see Cummings & Sierhuis, 2013, pp. 1–13.

46 Farah Karim-Cooper, *Cosmetics in Shakespearean and Renaissance Drama*, 2006, p. 41.

ethnocentric fear and to religious unease. Here, the concept of *ethnicity* needs to be understood in the light of the early modern discourse surrounding the term. The physicality of emotions indicates that ethnicity was defined more by emotional differences than by external characteristics such as skin colour. Mary Floyd-Wilson has coined the term *geohumoralism* to talk about how ethnicity was defined through humoral-climatic theories, in accordance with what she calls a 'regionally framed humoralism'. In the early modern period, 'race' was a flexible concept: a change in diet and lifestyle could lead to a radical change in identity.[47] Just like human bodies, materials had humoral qualities ascribed to them. For example, tropical dyes and fragrances were generally considered to be hot and dry. For a person with the opposite humoral constitution, however, consuming these drugs could cause an unhealthy change in the balance of the humours, thus causing the arousal of immoral appetites and desires, and even a change in their identity. 'Hot' foreign products were thus held to exert a negative impact on the 'cold' bodies of Northern Europeans. In the same way, then, I will show how the exotic substances in Six's pharmacy were perceived as a threat to his Dutchness.

The theological opposition to ornaments was based on a central concept in the anti-cosmetic argument: of the human body as God's 'work of art'. Moralists argued that substances such as face paint, pigments and perfumes, which altered the body, jeopardised God's handiwork. And since there were no clear distinctions between the mental and the physical, this fear also entailed an anxiety about the effects on that handiwork at a spiritual level. Cosmetics, it was held, thus undermined God's work and distracted from spiritual meditation and reflection. In this context, it is useful to look at Karim-Cooper's definition of 'cosmetic'. She offers a broad reading of the term: 'it is material and symbolic; it is that which beautifies. It refers not only to make-up, but also to perfumes, herbs, and even aesthetic commodities such as tapestries, which "beautify" a room'.[48] I will use the same definition here: as we shall soon see, this broad field of application was also typical for exotic drugs in the early modern period. And as I will show, even explosives were perceived as 'cosmetics' in early modern Europe.

The juxtaposition of exotic smells and colours with literary composition is not new: it has been used in rhetoric since antiquity. Classical writers define *ornatus* (adornment) as the culmination of the skills of the speaker: Cicero writes that speakers should adorn their texts with *colores rhetorici* (rhetorical colours – that is,

47 According to Floyd-Wilson, 'Ethnicity in the early modern period is defined more by emotional differences than by appearance: distinctions rest on how easily one is stirred or calmed – on one's degree of emotional vulnerability or resistance – or one's capacity two move others', see 'English Mettle', in: Gail Kern Paster, Katherine Rowe & Mary Floyd-Wilson (eds.), *Reading the Early Modern Passions in the Cultural History of Emotion*, 2003, pp. 130–146, quote on p. 133.

48 Karim-Cooper, 2006, pp. 41 and 42.

tropes and figures) to win their listeners' attention. These linguistic 'pigments' can help bring the text to life for the audience. In poetry, this ability has been linked to terms such as *ut pictura poesis*, 'as is painting so is poetry' – a statement from Horace's *Ars Poetica* – and *energeia*, the liveliness or force necessary to engage and involve the reader. The view of rhetorical metaphors and tropes as pigments reappears in Renaissance literary theory. In his influential book on poetics, *The Art of English Poetry* (1589), George Puttenham echoes Cicero in defining rhetorical devices as 'coulours in our arte of Poesie'. He compares writing poems to applying paint: 'a Poet setteth [...] upon his language by arts [...] as th'excellent painter bestoweth the rich Orient coulours upon his table of pourtraire'. The prominent position Puttenham accords to 'rhetorical colours' gives a sense of the power he felt they had to bring lines of verse to life. According to Elizabeth D. Harvey, implicit in these arguments is the idea that colours are not simply ornamental trappings in, but constitutive elements of, poetry.[49] Thijs Weststeijn shows that the same ideas were promoted by art theorists in the Dutch Republic – scholars who also took the rhetoric of the antiquity as a starting point for their discussions. In his *De Schilder-konst der Oude* (*On the Painting of the Ancients*) – in his Dutch translation of the Latin original from 1641 – Franciscus Junius links the Greek term *kosmos* with the Latin *ornamentum* – 'cosmos' literally means *ornament* – and points to the important role colours are given in the act of creation: the creator 'embellished' his creation with colour, light and other ornaments. When Junius refers to 'veruw-cieraeten' ('coloristic ornaments'), he thus means not only outer ornamentation but colours with a life-giving, 'bewitching' force. In this context, other terms that occur in Renaissance art treaties have to be understood, such as *incarnazione* – incarnadine or flesh colour – a term that was accorded a special position within Italian art theory. According to Weststeijn, this concept of an incarnating, or even transubstantiating, power of colour forms a basis for the thoughts of other Dutch art theorists as well: he tells us that Samuel van Hoogstraten's comparison of colour to the 'divine fire' that gave life to the first man is in line with this idea.[50]

49 George Puttenham, *Arte of English Poesie*, 1589, p. 115; Elizabeth D. Harvey, 'Flesh Color and Shakespeare's Sonnets', in: Michael Schoenfeldt (ed.), *A Companion to Shakespeare's Sonnets*, 2007, pp. 314–329, quote on p. 322. Other have also written, of course, of the meaning of ornaments in Renaissance literature – for instance, Mary E. Hazard, 'An Essay to Amplify "Ornament": Some Renaissance Theory and Practice', *SEL*, 1976, pp. 15-32; Frances E. Dolan, 'Taking the Pencil out of God's Hand: Art, Nature, and the Face-painting Debate in Early Modern England', *PMLA*, 1993, pp. 224–239.

50 See Thijs Weststeijn, *The Visible World: Samuel van Hoogstraten's Art Theory and the Legitimation of Painting in the Dutch Golden Age*, 2008, pp. 219–265, especially pp. 220–226. For further discussion of rhetorical colours in Dutch literature, see also Nelleke Moser, *De strijd voor rhetorica: poëtica en positie van rederijkers in Vlaanderen, Brabant, Zeeland en Holland tussen 1450 en 1620*, 2001, pp. 38–43.

However, as Pollard and Karim-Cooper have shown, just as old as the link between language and cosmetic materials are the linguistic, medical and religious warnings against the 'narcotic power' of literature. Cicero warns against an extensive use of *flores*, saying that this is typical of a sophistic style. Quintilian likewise warns against an abuse of artistic ornament, saying that it will have the effect of deception. Dionysius of Halicarnassus, a classical teacher of rhetoric, depicts a style abundant in ornaments as a prostitute who is installed in the house of language after having ousted the legitimate bride, a simple and virtuous Attic muse. In a passage in his famous *An Apology for Poetry* (1595), where Philip Sidney talks about an excessive use of *energeia*, he compares a 'honey-flowing' eloquence with dishes covered with 'sugar and spice', and with Indians wearing too many jewels.[51] These warnings are based on an older critical attitude to literary composition. One commonplace is the rejection of rhetoric in Plato's *Gorgias*, where rhetoric is included in the same category as cosmetics, cooking, and sophistry. Plato's criticism also concerns poetry, given that the poetic forms mentioned in *Gorgias*, the dithyramb and the tragedy, are considered subcategories of rhetoric – and the opposite of philosophy, the means of knowledge chosen by Socrates. The purpose of rhetoric is merely to please and satisfy the listener – it is nothing but flattery. The dithyramb is important here. It was a hymn to Bacchus, the god of wine, whose praises were sung during the Bacchanalian festivals. The hymn was thus associated with categories that are important for this research: intoxication and ecstasy. In his notorious attack on poetry in *The Republic*, Plato refers to the falsehood of literature as a *pharmakon:* a dangerous blend of poison and remedy, which only the rulers of the city are able to control. Michael A. Rinella tells us that Plato was in fact one of the first to address the problem of drug-induced ecstasy as dangerous to the society. An important assumption in his study is that the Greeks included mind-altering substances in their wine. This has been confirmed by recent archaeological research.[52]

In order to understand Six's ambivalent writing strategy, we need to study the Dutch parallels to this discourse. Like the English moralists whom Pollard discusses in her inquiry, Dutch moralists attached great importance to the senses and bodily organs in warning of the dangers of theatre. For example, the Calvinist preacher Petrus Wittewrongel labelled the theatre as a 'schadelijk vergift' ('harmful poison'). The pernicious words of plays, he wrote, corrupted the senses and bodies of 'beyde de Speelers ende de aenschouwers ('actors and audience alike'):

51 See Jacqueline Lichtenstein, 'Making up Representation: The Risks of Femininity', *Representations*, 1987, pp. 77–87; quote on p. 79; Philip Sidney, *An Apology for Poetry*, [1595] 1965, p. 138.

52 *Gorgias*, 502a-c12. Michael A. Rinella, *Pharmakon: Plato, Drug Culture, and Identity in Ancient Athens*, 2011. See also Pollard, 2005, pp. 13–14.

> What could such a bitter root produce, but gall and the wormwood of sins. Such a tree, such a fruit. People are infected inside and out: their eyes and their ears are polluted by it, their hearts and their deeds are drawn to unchaste lusts, when they behold all these new spectacles of sin, and are amused by them.[53]

The discourse of the deceptive power of poetry can also be found in the poetic works of humanist poets in early modern Dutch literature, especially in discussions of mythological decoration in poetry. Marijke Spies tells us that Dirck Volckertszoon Coornhert (1522–1590) and later Joachim Oudaen (1628–1692) were fiercely opposed to the use of religious ornaments in Renaissance poetry, and that they labelled this adornment a vicious attempt at persuasion (Fig.1.3). Coornhert, she argues, promoted an 'argumentative-rhetorical' poetics in opposition to the 'musical-fictional' poetics of contemporary writers, which, she says, was affiliated with a mythological repertoire. In the opening poem of *Comedie van lief en leedt* (*Comedy of Love and Suffering*) (1582), 'Coornherts rymerien aenden rymlievenden leser' ('Coornhert's Rhymes to the Rhyme-Loving Reader'), Coornhert distances himself from the 'hoge Parnasser spraken' ('the language of the high Parnassus'), full of 'gonst-zuchtige pluymstruykeryen' ('flattering toadyism'), and references to 'onreine' ('unclean') Roman gods such as Bacchus and Venus – a 'pronckelyc' ('flaunting') style that serves 'yemandt te behagen met logens soet' ('to please people with lies so sweet'). He made a distinction between 'Poeetsche fabrijcken' ('poetic products'), which contain no truth, and artistic writing that is shorn of mythological fiction, written in good Dutch and about things that are true.[54] This criticism includes references not only to gods and religious myths, but also to material aspects of pagan religion, as is apparent from 'Godsdienst- en het Godendom ontdekt: aan de Hedendaagsche Dichters' ('Religion and the Idolatry of Gods Disclosed: to the Poets of the Present Day') by

53 'Wat soude sulcken bitteren wortel, anders als een galle ende alsem der sonde konnen voort-dringhen. Sulcken boom, sulck een vrucht. De mensche werdt uytwendigh ende inwendigh besmet, de ooghen, de ooren werden daer door verontreynight, het herte tot onkuysche lusten, en de daden afghetrocken, wanneer hy alle dese nieuwe vertooninghen der sonde aenschouwt, / ende sich daer in vermaeckt', Petrus Wittewrongel, *Oeconomia christiana ofte Christelicke huys-houdinge*, 1661, vol. II, p. 1168.

54 D.V. Coornhert, *Het roerspel en de comedies van Coornhert*, 1955, pp. 156–159. For a discussion of Coornhert's poetics and of 'argumentative/rhetorical' versus 'mythological-fictional' poetics, see Marijke Spies, 'Between Ornament and Argumentation: Developments in 16th-Century Dutch Poetics', in: Jelle Koopmans, Mark A. Meadow, Kees Meerhoff & Marijke Spies (eds.), *Rhetoric-Rhetoriqueurs-Rederijkers*, 1995; Marijke Spies, '"Helicon and Hills of Sand": Pagan Gods in Early Modern Dutch and European Poetry', in: Helen Wilcox, Richard Todd & Alasdair MacDonald (eds.), *Sacred and Profane: Secular and Devotional Interplay in Early modern British Literature,* Amsterdam, 1996, pp. 225–236; see also Johan Koppenol, 'Een tegendraadse poëtica. De literaire ideeën van Jan van Hout', in: K.J.S. Bostoen *et al.* (eds.), *Jan van Hout, Voorrede tot het gezelschap. Voorrede bij zijn vertaling van Buchanans Franciscanus*, 1993, pp. 3–25.

the poet Joachim Oudaen.[55] The poem attacks the representation of 'Wierook, Ooster-kruideryen, Oliën, en dierb're geuren' ('Incense, Eastern Spices, Oils and Expensive Fragrances') (l. 10–11) in early modern poetry. Oudaen held that, with 'het zoet vergift der woorden' ('the sweet poison of words') (l. 22), the Renaissance poet kept ancient paganism alive. It is here that Six's rhymester-poetics, so to speak, becomes relevant. M.A. Schenkeveld-van der Dussen has already pointed to Six's critical comments on Joost van den Vondel's notion of universal poetry – though we can also see Six's poetics as following on from Coornhert's 'rymerien' and the discourse of ornamental poetry. A comparison between Six's poetics and the literary programme of Coornhert and Oudaen has not yet been undertaken, but it could be fruitful. In fact, there are many parallels between 'Coornherts rymerien aenden rymlievenden leser' ('Coornhert's rhymes to the rhyme-loving reader') and one of Six's poetic texts, 'Het boek, aan den leeser' ('The Book, to the Reader') (J119).

An analysis of Six's rhymester-poetics in the light of the ornamental-cosmetic vocabulary of Dutch Renaissance poetry might help shed light on his relationship to Vondel's poetics and show that Six's own position is more ambivalent than has been assumed. Taking the definition of Marijke Spies as a starting point, I argue that the contrast between Six and Vondel perpetuates the opposition between the 'argumentative-rhetorical' and the 'musical-fictional' poetics of sixteenth-century Dutch literature. I have therefore opted to use the notion of 'the language of the high Parnassus' in reference to Vondel's poetics, in accordance with the terminology promulgated by Karel Porteman and Mieke B. Smits-Veldt. They define Parnassian language as a literary mode written in an epic register and suffused with references to the sacraments and the sacrifices found in classical mythology. This mode also characterises the writings of poets who were influenced by Vondel's aesthetics, such as Jan Vos and Reyer Anslo. The view of poetry as an elevated form can also be found in theoretical writings from the period. In his *Aenleidinge ter Nederduitsche dichtkunste* (1650) (*Introduction to Dutch Poetry*), Vondel makes a distinction between, on the one hand, the practice of rhymesters, who study classical writers in antiquity, and, on the other, 'heavenly poetry'. I will come back to this in Chapter 8.[56]

The implications for cosmetics of this Parnassian language become clear if we look at Vondel's poem 'Wieroock voor Cornelis en Elizabeth le Blon' ('Incense for Cornelis and Elizabeth le Blon').[57] The theme of this short poem is simple: Vondel showers Cornelis and Elizabeth le Blon with a poetic 'wieroockgeur van danckbaerheit' ('scent of the incense of gratitude') because they brought him a

55 Joachim Oudaen, *Poëzy*, I, 1712, p. 32.

56 Karel Porteman & Mieke B. Smits-Veldt, *Een nieuw vaderland voor de muzen: Geschiedenis van de Nederlandse Literatuur 1560–1700*, 2008, pp. 401–403.

57 J.F.M. Sterck *et al.* (eds.), *De werken van Vondel*, vol. 5, 1931, p. 472.

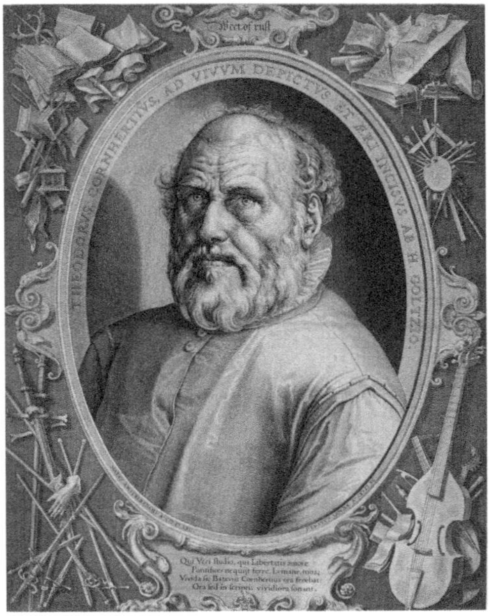

Fig. 1.3: Hendrick Goltzius, *Portrait of Dirck Volckertsz Coornhert*, c. 1591–1592. Engraving. (© Rijksmuseum, Amsterdam).

medal that he had been awarded by Queen Christine of Sweden. Naturally, Vondel means this showering with incense to be understood figuratively. In modern Dutch, this figurative meaning still lingers on in the verb 'bewieroken', from 'wierook', incense – meaning 'praise to the skies' or 'fawn over'. The spiritual connections that exotic aromatics awaken with religious rituals form the basis of the argument. 'Wierook' comes from 'gewijde rook' – 'holy smoke' – and refers to resins that release fragrant smoke when burned, especially frankincense (also known as olibanum) and myrrh, which is a resin found in trees native to the Arabian Peninsula.[58] These references give Vondel's text a certain feeling of solemnity and exoticism. At the same time, I would suggest that we must also take into account in this poem the physical perception of incense. A prominent feature of the literary representation of exotic ornaments is the emphasis on the senses and sense impressions, as is apparent from such phrases as 'wieroock*geur* van danckbaerheit' and 'het *zoet* vergift der woorden' ('the *sweet* poison of words'). This makes it clear that aromatic materials were used more widely in the early modern period. For example, incense was used not only in religious sacraments, but also as a perfume and for therapeutic

58 See the entry in the WNT. See Carolus Clusius's description of exotic plants in Dodonaeus, 1644, pp. 1366–1367.

purposes. Even a staunch Calvinist such as Gisbertus Voetius used this 'holy smoke' to fumigate his room in Utrecht when the city was swept by the plague.[59] More than people do today, early modern individuals thus had a strong sense of the physical characteristics of many of the items – whether dyes or fragrances – that featured as literary adornments in literature. Voetius knew the smell of incense just as well as his Catholic countrymen, such as Vondel. Given Six's work as a druggist, it makes even more sense to include early modern medical and physical theories of exotic drugs in discussions of his poems. We get a sense of the latter if we compare the literary representation of amber in his 'Dankdicht aan Jakob Breine te Dantsich, voor een paar barnsteene hechten' ('Poem of Thanks to Jacob Breyne of Dantzig for a Couple of Amber Handles') (J165) with that offered by a contemporary poet, Jan Vos, 'Barnsteene koffertje door Haare Keurvorstelyke Doorluchtigheidt van Brandenburg, aan Mejoffrouw Leonora Huidekoopers van Maarseveen, gemaalin van den E. Heer scheepen Joan Hinloopen, vereert' ('Amber Chest Offered by Her Princely Serenity of Brandenburg, to Mademoiselle Leonora Huidekoopers van Maarseveen, Consort of the Alderman Joan Hinloopen'). Six's treatment includes references to theories about the origin of amber (see l. 15–24). But the Calvinist also plays, more or less ironically, on the emotional and religious connotations of the exotic: 'Ik neem het aan, als soete lucht /Van wierook, uit geneegen sucht, / My opgeoffert, sonder schulden' ('I accept it as the sweet smell of incense, which you have offered out of affection though you owe me nothing') (l. 35–37). The gift smells so heavenly that the Protestant businessman imagines himself as a deity to whom a fragrance has been brought as a sacrifice! By contrast, Jan Vos contents himself with a play on words around 'barnsteen' ('amber') and 'brandsteen' ('burning stone').[60]

This emphasis on emotions and the physical perception of materials legitimates a broader approach in our analysis of how exotic materials are represented in Six's poetry. At the same time, it makes his position as a satirist more ambiguous. In taking account of the physical and religious theories connected to the early modern discourse on foreign drugs, I argue that Six's self-criticism derives from his involvement with exotic materials.[61]

59 M.J. van Lieburg, 'Voetius en de geneeskunde', in: J. van Oort *et al.* (eds.), *De onbekende Voetius: Voordrachten Wetenschappelijk Symposium*, 1989, pp. 168–180, quote on p. 178.

60 The olfactory impression amber made was based on both its wide use in early modern Europe and on its being fossilised resin, which releases fragrant smoke when heated. Among other things, Catholic rosary beads were often made of amber, and the scent that they gave off when touched was regarded as holy. See Rachel King, '"The beads with which we pray are made from it": Devotional Ambers in Early Modern Italy', in: Wietse de Boer & Christine Göttler, *Religion and the Senses in Early Modern Europe*, 2013, pp. 153–175. Rosaries were among the commodities Dutch merchants traded in – see Hermann Wätjen, *Die Niederländer Im Mittelmeergebiet Zur Zeit Ihrer Höchsten Machtstellung*, 1909, p. 254.

61 I will be looking in the early going here at the reference books on natural history that Six himself used. As I noted, *Naturalis Historia* by Pliny the Elder seems to have been a major source for Six, if one

A merchant-poet

Before I discuss the reception of Six's poetry, I would like to offer a brief overview of his life and of the contents of his book of poetry. Joannes Six van Chandelier was born on 19 February 1620 in Amsterdam, the eldest of 10 children. His father, Jacob Six van Chandelier, was a trader in spices and drugs who had a drugstore in Amsterdam, 'De Vergulde Eenhoorn' ('The Gilded Unicorn') on the Kalverstraat (Fig. 1.4). His mother's name was Sara Juliens. She was descended from a wealthy family: her mother, Catharina Jeheu, to whom Six addresses a number of poems, had a country house built in 1643 on the Middenweg, in the Diemermeerpolder, southeast of Amsterdam. Six inherited the country house and spent a lot of time there in his later years. Both sides of Six's family had moved from the Spanish Netherlands. His maternal grandparents, Joost Juliens and Catharina Jeheu, came from Ninove and Brussels, respectively, while Wesel is listed as the city in which Jacob Six's father lived before the family settled in Haarlem and Amsterdam. The quasi-aristocratic name 'Van Chandelier' dates from a later period. Jacob Six was able to add this name to 'Six' thanks to an aristocratic diploma that was granted to him and his brothers in 1617 in Prague by the Emperor Matthias.[62]

From what we know of Six's education, it seems possible that he and his brothers were originally destined for careers other than as merchants. Like his five brothers, Six attended the Latin school in the Oudezijds neighbourhood near the centre of Amsterdam. This career path was in any case interrupted by the early death of his

looks at all the references that Six made to it, as traced by A.E. Jacobs. Indeed, Six cites Pliny as a reliable informer in 'Ter eere van de fonteine Pouhon' ('In Honour of the Spring at Pouhon') (J104), l. 8–20. The medical works that I have consulted are as follows: Rembertus Dodonaeus (1517-1585) *Cruydt-boeck* (*The Book of Herbs and Spices*) (1644), which discusses only substances of vegetable origin; Johan van Beverwijck (1594–1647), *Alle de wercken, zo in de medicyne als chirurgie* (*Complete works, on Both Medicine and Surgery*), 1656, in particular the description of medicines in *Schat der ongesontheyt* (*Treasure of Ill-Health*); Pierre Pomet (1658–1699), *Histoire générale des drogues* (1694) (I use the English translations, *A Compleat History of Druggs*, 1737); and Nicolas Lémery (1645–1715), *Dictionnaire universel des drogues simples*, 1698 (I use the Dutch translation, *Woordenboek of algemeene verhandeling der enkele droogeryen*, 1743). It may be that these last two works were not available to Six, but the early modern approach they took to drugs does represent the state of pharmacological knowledge in *Poësy*. I also refer a number of times to Carolus Clusius (1526–1609) *Exoticorum libri decem*, 1605), and to the Dutch translation of the works of Ambroise Paré (1510–1590), *De chirurgie, ende alle de opera, ofte wercken* (*Surgery, and Complete Works*, 1636). Six discusses both Clusius and Paré.

62 Jacobs, 1991 II, p. 232; Joh. C. Breen, 'Geschiedenis van het huis keizersgracht 676', *Jaarboek van het genootschap Amstelodamum*, 1915, p. 88. See also Appendix II. Unfortunately there is no portrait of Joannes Six van Chandelier. There is a drawing of him made by Jan Stolker, but this image is not authentic, see Gerdien Wuestman, 'Een portret van Jan Six van Chandelier?', *Maandblad Amstelodamum*, 2011, pp. 147–154.

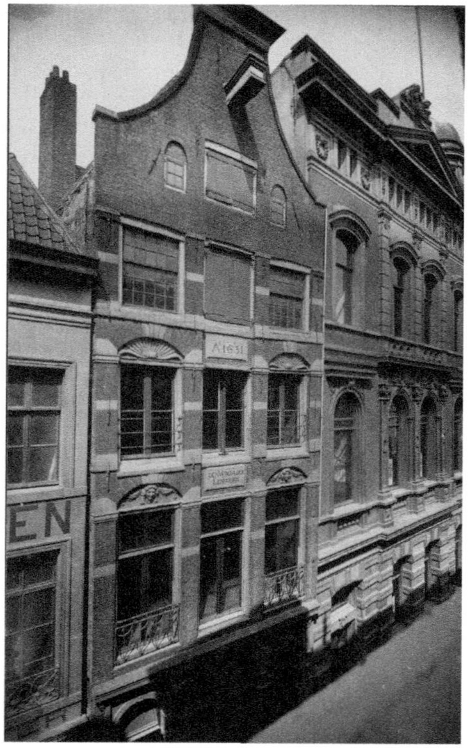

Fig. 1.4: *Kalverstraat 2–4, with 'De Vergulde Eenhoorn'.* 'De Vergulde Eenhoorn' was demolished at the beginning of the 20th century, 1900. Photograph. (© Amsterdam Stadsarchief).

father in 1639, when Six was 19. As the eldest son, he was given responsibility for the drugstore together with his mother. On the one hand, he took business trips in Europe and, on the other, he corresponded with trading partners such as the above-mentioned business contact, and the family of Jacob Breyne, who originally came from Brabant and was located in Danzig.[63] Many of Six's poems were thus addressed to merchants. The drugstore stayed under his mother's name, 'Widow of Jacob Six', in the registers at the Exchange Bank until her death in 1666. From 1668 on, the family business was listed under the name 'Joannes Six van Chandelier'. In addition to his activities as a merchant, Six was involved in investments outside the trade. Thus, in 1647 he sold a 'huys ende seeperie' ('a soap factory'), while in 1671 he was working as a moneylender. This is in line with the activities of many

63 Alette Fleischer, 'Breyne's Botany: (Re-)locating Nature and Knowledge in Danzig (circa 1660–1730)', in: Fokko Jan Dijksterhuis, Andreas Weber & Huib J. Zuidervaart, *Locations of Knowledge in Dutch Contexts*, 2019, pp. 107–135.

early modern merchants; they engaged in these kinds of activities to ensure their families' future.[64]

Six's family business traded in drugs – that is, exotic medicines, dyes, perfumes and so on – and had trading interests both in Europe and farther afield. The registers of the family firm at the Exchange Bank in Amsterdam list a wide range of trade contacts in both the Dutch East and West India Companies, family names such as De Smeth and Kemp, the names of wealthy Amsterdam businessmen such as Peter Trip and Jan de Neuville, of the Amsterdam ruling elite such as Jacob Bicker and Frans Banning Cocq, and of Sephardic Jews living in Amsterdam such as Bento Osorio and Antonio Lopes Suasso. Although the family firm was not one of the richest merchant families in Amsterdam, it did carry out trades involving considerable sums, sometimes amounting to more than 10,000 guilders. Unfortunately, the Exchange bank does not specify which spices Six traded in (Fig. 1.5). The same goes for other sources, which list items only generically – 'spices', 'drugs' and so on.[65] But one poem tells us the origin of the commodities he was trading in: here Six refers to 'Spices from the Ganges' ('Aan Raimond de Smeth') (J70, l. 10). And in a trade contract, a commodity of Six's firm is explicitly named, opium, which Six's father probably got from Bengal, and sold to Morocco.[66] Joannes's brother, Joost Six, who worked as an assistant with the Dutch East India Company, was stationed near the Ganges in Bengal.[67] In addition, Six had family members stationed in other Dutch trading outposts, such as the Dutch East Indies, and Isfahan, Iran. Moreover, Six's company was listed as one of the major Amsterdam trading firms in the Mediterranean region.[68]

64 Jacobs, 1991 II, p. 232; Joh. C. Breen, 'Geschiedenis van het huis keizersgracht 676', *Jaarboek van het genootschap Amstelodamum*, 1915, p. 88; L. Kooijmans, 'De koopman', in: H.M. Beliën, A.Th. van Deursen & G.J. van Setten (eds.), *Gestalten van de Gouden Eeuw. Een Hollands groepsportret*, 1995, pp. 86–92. For the Exchange Bank in Amsterdam, see Pit Dehing, *Geld in Amsterdam. Wisselbank en wisselkoersen, 1650–1725*, 2012. Six also wrote a poem to the Exchange bank: 'Wisselbank' (J216).

65 The registers of 'Jaquis Six wed.' and 'Joannes Six van Chandelier' in the Exchange bank in Amsterdam, Amsterdam City Archives, see Appendix II. Not all the bank's transactions were linked to trade. Some also involved loans and converting cash into bank funds and vice versa.

66 See Appendix II.

67 Abraham and Johannes Six van Chandelier – the first a brother of the poet, the latter a nephew and namesake, worked in the Dutch East Indies – see Appendix II. One of Joannes's nieces, Sara Jacoba Six van Chandelier, was married to the head of the Dutch East India Company in Isfahan, Iran – see Jacobs, 1991 II, p. XXXVI. Another relative, Cornelis van der Loeff, travelled in 1668 with the poet Willem Godschalck van Focquenbroch to Fort Elmina on the Dutch Gold Coast as an assistant ('ondercommis'). He died there in 1671 – see 'Zijn er nog vragen? Een speurtocht in de archieven van de Oude Westindische Compagnie', *Fumus*, 2017, pp. 23–32.

68 Wätjen, 1909. Wätjen also lists other Dutch traders who were active in the Mediterranean region and whom I discuss in this book, such as Hendrik Spiegel, Joost de Smeth, Jonas Abeels, and Isaak Fokquier. See also the list of products that Dutch merchants bought and sold in Southern Europe: Wätjen, pp. 242–329 and 333–346.

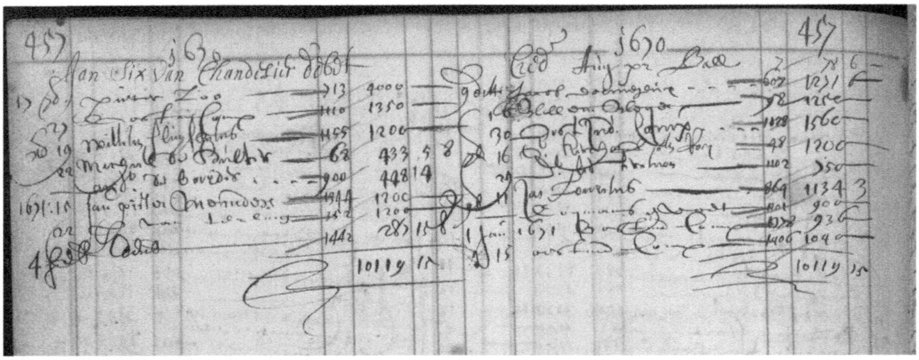

Fig. 1.5: *The ledger of the Exchange Bank in Amsterdam*, 1670, nr. 71, p. 457. Photograph. (© Amsterdam Stadsarchief).

Six himself travelled around Europe. From 1649 to 1651 he made a long journey through Southern Europe, travelling through France to Spain before crossing to Sardinia and visiting various cities in Italy. The peace with Spain had opened up new trading opportunities, both in Spain and in Italy, and that is probably why Six made this journey.[69] In 1651 he visited Italy again, this time travelling along the Rhine to Innsbruck and then on to Venice. Between 1652 and 1657, he made further trips – one to Germany and two to England (1654 and 1655). He also combined business trips with humanistic activities. For instance, he did a study of a Horace's codex, probably in a library in Paris, where he compared the variants he found there with his own copy of his favourite poet.[70] The company name also turns up in archives in Sweden.[71] In this context, it is worth mentioning that the poet's uncle, Abraham Six van Chandelier, was commissioned in 1630 by the Swedish King Gustav II Adolf to establish a Swedish colony in Ingria, an area along the southern shore of the Gulf of Finland. Abraham became a member of the Swedish nobility, named Abraham Six von Sandelier, and received the permission to build a manor, Sixenburg, in the area where St. Petersburg is today. However, the plans for a Swedish colony ruled by enterprising Dutchmen failed after a few years.[72]

Six's father died of an ailment. Six's anxiety that he would suffer the same fate is reflected in his poems. As we have seen, he himself was sick: he had an ailment

69 The peace with Spain opened up the possibilities for both the import of American drugs to the Netherlands and the export of Eastern specimens to Spain. See Jonathan Israel, *Dutch Primacy in World Trade 1585–1740*, 1989, pp. 202 and 232–33.

70 Jacobs, 1991 II, p. 49–50. On Six's travels to Italy, see also Maartje van Gelder, *Trading Places: Netherlandish Merchants in Early Modern Venice*, 2009, p. 106.

71 Jacobs, 1991 II, p. XXXVI.

72 Bertel von Bonsdorff, *Abraham Six van Chandelier & consortes: en kolonisationsplan i Ingermanland 1629/30*, 1997.

of the spleen – an 'obstructed spleen', as he himself put it. The ailment also posed a problem both for the social reputation of the poet and for the family business. This will become clear from many of the poems I will be discussing in this book.[73] Six wrote many amorous poems to a loved one he calls Roselle, but he never married, and he blames his ailment for this, saying it made it impossible for him to live with a woman. He went to see the doctor Simon Dilman (or Dilleman), a good friend and a relative of Six. The poet addressed a series of occasional poems to him and his family. One of the doctor's sons, Jacob Dilman, did his apprenticeship in Six's family business. But the friendship was not without its conflicts. In some of his writings, Six expresses disappointment at Dilman's medical methods. In 1656, Six started on another course of treatment, taking a nine-week-long cure in Spa, in what was then the Spanish Netherlands. In a series of poems that he wrote there, he praised the positive effects that the mineral water was having on him. But those effects were apparently not strong enough to return him to full health. Years later, in 1659 and 1669, he went through what he called a 'spa season' – a summer cure with bottles of spring water imported from Spa in the Ardennes.[74] He also kept in touch with others who had a medical background: botanists and surgeons. The Six van Chandelier family were Reformed Protestants. In addition to commercial and medical connections, it appears from Six's poems that Reformed pastors belonged to his circle of friends. In addition to names such as Petrus Wittewrongel and Jacobus Hollebeek, Johannes Hoornbeeck, a preacher and professor at the University of Utrecht, seems to have played an important role in Six's life. He was also a relative of Six's. Six sent poems to Hoornbeeck, and the theologian responded with religious writings.

Six van Chandelier's collection, *Poësy*, appeared in 1657. Biographical information on the druggist-poet for the years after its publication becomes harder to come by. Apart from individual pamphlets and poems, he produced no more literary texts of his own. Having retreated to Ceulen, his country house, he devoted himself to a literary work of a more serious character: a newly rhymed version of the Psalms of David, which he undertook in the hope that they would replace the older version by Petrus Datheen. Six was 'oover de twintig jaaren swanger, en ontrent de tien jaaren in swaaren arbeid' ('was pregnant for twenty years, and about ten years in heavy labour') with the translation, according to the foreword to this work, which

73 In addition, the relationship with the family of Jan Willemsz Bogaert caused problems for Six. This fierce contra-remonstrant was banned in 1629 from Amsterdam because of his agitation. Bogaert's son was married to an aunt of Six's, and the two families were in conflict because of inheritance issues – see Appendix II. But where Six's medical reputation is treated in several poems, he mentions the Bogaert in just two poems. One of these is 'Wensch des Eenhoorns' ('Wish of the Unicorn') (J182).

74 See 'Prinsselijk inhaal, t'Amsterdam' ('Princely Reception in Amsterdam') (J612), and a letter from Six to the theologian Johannes Coccejus, reproduced in Schenkeveld-van der Dussen & De Vries, 2007, p. 387.

appeared in 1674.[75] In 1690, a second, revised edition of the Psalms appeared. Six van Chandelier died in 1695, and was buried in the family grave in the Zuiderkerk in his hometown, Amsterdam.

Corpus

Poësy by Joannes Six van Chandelier appeared, according to the title page of the book, in 1657 'in Amsterdam. Published by Joost Pluimert, on the Dam, in Seneka'. Pluimert (or Pluymer) is the name of the publisher and seller of the book. He was just 23 years old at the time, and this was the first book he had published. Pluymer's bookshop was called 'Seneca' and would have specialised mainly in classical literature, which is interesting when we think of the many classical allusions in Six's poetry and, as we shall see, his self-presentation as a *poeta doctus* or learned poet. No indication is given of who the printer was.[76] As is clear from the full title, *Poësy verdeelt in ses boeken en eenige opschriften* (*Poetry Divided into Six Books and a Number of Inscriptions*), *Poësy* is in fact a collection.[77]

The subtitles indicate that the division of *Poësy* is somewhat formal. Genre and length are the determining factors for the first two sections, and for the last part, which is added on: 'Sonnets' and 'Inscriptions' contain sonnets and epigrams, respectively, while the section 'Five poems' includes the five longest poems in the collection. The title of the third book, 'Poems from Spa', shows that an organising principle is at work here, too: Six wrote the poems in it while he was staying in Spa. It seems that these are the last poems that Six wrote for this collection, because their contents show that it was in 1656 that he took the treatment in Spa. A certain chronological sequence can also be found in the first section – the collection of sonnets – and in the three largest books in the collection, those with 'Dichtbosch' ('Forest of Poems') in their titles. It seems from that term that the reader should see these sections as 'bundles of poems', a mix of texts that pay scant regard to chronology and genre.[78] And this is indeed the primary impression we get from

75 Joannes Six van Chandelier, *Davids Psalmen*, 1674, p. VI.

76 Monique A. F. Peters, *Van miskend tot geprezen: Het beeld van de koopman-dichter Jan Six van Chandelier (1620-1695) in de Nederlandse literatuurgeschiedschrijving*, 2012, pp. 23–24.

77 These books are: 'Klinkdichten', 'Het tweede boek / Vyf gedichten', 'Het derde boek / waar in Spadichten', 'Het vierde boek / genaamt Dichtbosch / Het eerste deel', 'Het vyfde boek / genaamt bos/ Het tweede deel' and 'Het seste boek / genaamt Dichtbosch / Het derde deel'. ('Sonnets', 'The Second Book/Five Poems ', 'The Third Book/including Poems from Spa', 'The Fourth Book/Entitled Forest of Poems /Part I', 'The Fifth Book/Entitled Forest of Poems/Part II', and 'The Sixth Book/Entitled Forest of Poems/Part III'.) The book concludes with an appendix, entitled 'Opschriften' ('Inscriptions'/'epigrams').

78 For 'bos' ('forest') as a genre determination, see the definition of 'de sylvis' in Vossius, *Poeticarum institutionum libri tres / Institutes of Poetics in Three Books* [1647] (2010), p. 1214.

reading *Poësy*. Thus in earlier literary research, scant attention was paid to the way in which *Poësy* was put together. And in interpreting *Poësy*, I will also be looking primarily at other principles according to which its parts have been arranged.[79]

The subtitles of the six parts of the collection give us no indication about the themes of Six's poems, except in the case of the Spa poems in the third part, which are as thematically varied as they are formally rich. Certain themes and motifs do come up more often than others. Thus, on the one hand, there are a large number of erotic poems in the collection, while on the other it also contains impressions of travel in other countries. The first category includes both love poems that Six wrote to Roselle, and wedding poems to family members and fellow merchants. There are also numerous texts in the second category. One of the longest poems in the collection is devoted to Venice, 'Schetse van Venecie' ('Sketch of Venice') (J97). This poem is also interesting in light of Six's business as a druggist. In it, he argues that Amsterdam has taken over Venice's role as the leading European centre for the trade in perfumes, drugs and spices. In Rome, Six found himself in the company of the Dutch painters the *Bentvogels* (*Birds of a Feather*) and also met with the Amsterdam poet Reyer Anslo, among others. He devotes a number of poems to these individuals. A series of poems is dedicated to the Joyous Entry into Madrid of Queen Mariana of Austria, second wife of Philip IV, on 15 November 1649. Six was there on a business trip, and was probably at the procession. A large number of texts were

79 For the transmission of Six's texts, see Jacobs, 1991 II, pp. XI–XX. Of the vast majority of poems, just one version has come down to us – that in *Poësy* (1657). Six involved himself personally in the printing of the collection, because he made author's corrections to the edition (Jacobs, 1991 II, p. XIV). A small number of texts had previously been published as a pamphlet. Changes were made to them before they were included in *Poësy*. We do not know whether Six edited them when he was preparing the book. Another interesting question is whether he had a particular goal in mind in organising *Poësy* in the somewhat chaotic way we have seen. Thus a number of long poems have been included in 'Het tweede boek/Vyf gedichten' ('The Second Book/Five Poems'), J96 and J97, while the introduction poems to these long texts appear in the collected-poems sections, J308 and J289. The inclusion of the poems Six wrote on the occasion of the Peace of Münster, and that had previously appeared in the pamphlet *Vreughde-Zangen* (*Songs of Joy*) (1648), is more radical. Not only are some of these heavily edited, but Six also had them included in really different spots in *Poësy*: J215, J327, J219, J220, J218, J227, J213, J270 and J223. This list follows the original order of the *Vreughde-Zangen* (*Songs of Joy*). Parts of the pamphlet that were not printed in *Pöesy* were included in the edition put out by A.E. Jacobs: J608, J609 and J610. I will return in Chapter 7 to Six's adaptation of the *Vreughde-Zangen* (*Songs of Joy*). In addition to *Poësy*, we know of 22 individual poems by Six, which he wrote after 1657 and that appeared as pamphlets or were published in seventeenth-century anthologies. Nineteen of these were included in the study published by Jacobs. Two texts were printed, with commentary, in: Schenkeveld-van der Dussen & De Vries, 2007, pp. 189–191 and P.E.L. Verkuyl, 'Een dichterlijk pamflet naar aanleiding van de komeet van 1664', *Tijdschrift voor Nederlandsche taal- en letterkunde*, 1996, pp. 30–43. The last text, an epigram entitled 'Schijnheiligheyt' ('Hypocrisy'), with calligraphy by L.W. Coppenol, was sold at a Dutch auction in November 2013. It is quite possible that more poems by Six will be found. Some of these poems are discussed in this book.

written to Abraham Grenier, a lawyer from Zeeland and a close friend of Six's, who accompanied him on two of his trips. There are also a large number of anti-English poems, written after the execution of Charles I and as the First Anglo-Dutch War was being fought. The longest poem in the collection, ''s Amsterdammers winter' ('Winter in Amsterdam') (J96), a literary winter scene that is set in the poet's hometown and that emphasises in particular the fun that skaters in Amsterdam are having, also stands out.[80] Finally, what stands out on the one hand are the number of poems devoted to the poet's illness and its treatment, and, on the other, the large number of texts about meals and culinary delicacies, including exotic medicines such as bezoar stone. The latter theme is seen as a hallmark of *Poësy*. Compared with the contents of other seventeenth-century Dutch poetry, the contents of Six's poems are remarkable for the absence of tributes to one or another luminary – possible patrons or benefactors. M.A. Schenkeveld-van der Dussen regards this as a particular feature of the collection: Six dissociates himself from any kind of patronage.[81]

As far as language and form are concerned, given Six's aforementioned affinity for a scholarly, mannered style of writing, *Poësy* differs from the poetry of many of his peers, especially those who called themselves adherents of Vondelian language – but even in this regard Six is not an exception in early modern Dutch literature. In this respect he was heavily influenced by Constantijn Huygens. In many texts, he expresses his admiration for Huygens's poetic language.[82]

Reception

We have now named the main features of *Poësy*, and have also, in fact, addressed in outline its literary-theoretical reception before the twentieth century. The only critical response to Six's poetry that we know of from his own time is found in correspondence from 1671 between two pastor-poets, Joannes Vollenhove and Geeraerdt Brandt. A letter from the former to the latter contains a list of the names of poets who recognised the greatness of P.C. Hooft; Vollenhove counts Joannes Six among these. Brandt misunderstands Vollenhove: he assumes that Vollenhove means the Amsterdam regent Jan Six, Rembrandt's patron and the author of *Medea*. Brandt's response is surprising, because not only did he himself exchange a series of sonnets with Six van Chandelier, but when Brandt was accused of plagiarism the druggist had even

80 This text is in an edition that comes with commentaries: M. Schenkeveld-van der Dussen & Hans Luijten (ed.), *'s Amsterdammers winter*, 1988.

81 M.A. Schenkeveld-van der Dussen, 'De anti-idealistische poëtica van een christen-burger, Joannes Six van Chandelier', *De nieuwe taalgids*, 1983, pp. 291–316.

82 For example, 'Op de leedige uuren, van C. Huigens, ridder & c.' ('In the Idle Hours, by C. Huygens, Ridder *et al*') (J408) and 'Op K. Huigens Oogenblikken' ('On C. Huygens's *Momenta desultoria*') (J439).

defended him. Vollenhove's aesthetic judgment is also odd, because, as we shall see, in his poems Six expresses his opposition to the poetics of P.C. Hooft. Evidently, Brandt let Vollenhove know this, but for Vollenhove those traits of P.C. Hooft's style that can be discerned in Six outweigh the signs of an individual, distinctive poetics: 'If he is not such a great lover of the Bailiff [P.C. Hooft], he ought to be at least, and could not, I think, have written so much great poetry, which I believe I have read in his book'.[83]

Vollenhove's and Brandt's assessments are indicative of Six's reception: over the centuries, Six van Chandelier has always been seen as one of the important names of seventeenth-century poetry, but without attracting the same level of interest as many of his contemporaries. For example, only one edition of *Poësy* has appeared. It is true that Six was rediscovered in the nineteenth century.[84] But it is only in the second half of the last century that he acquired the elevated status we accord him these days. The credit for this goes to G.A. van Es, and especially to M.A. Schenkeveld-van der Dussen. My observations about the study of material culture in the early modern Republic also apply to the perception of Six van Chandelier in the history of literature: Six's poetry takes a particular interest in everyday life and shows an openness to material objects. 'Realism' is the keyword in studies on Six.

G.A. van Es was the first literary researcher to write several articles on Six. In the literary-historical standard *Geschiedenis van de letterkunde der Nederlanden* (1952), Van Es describes the poet as 'simple in spirit, loyal, open, and sincere to the point of being naïve' and as representing a kind of harmonic and realistic poetry: 'He barely runs into or raises problems [...]. Six has a rarely poignant lyricism. The dominant feature of his poetry is a healthy realism.' Van Es later nuances his description of Six. His introduction to an anthology of Six's poetry in 1953 conveys a gloomy tone. He now discerns in Six's texts an inner development that contains a swing from joy to grief, and that results, in a sense, in religious reflection. They lead 'finally to the suspected turn in his life's path, which unfortunately made him stop writing poetry.' He reads the book that followed *Poësy*, Six's rhyming psalms, in the light of this religious turning point, which according to him resulted in the silence of Six van Chandelier as a poet. He proposes, therefore, that the publication of the psalms was a 'reckoning with the past'. This thesis is interesting when it comes to the hypothesis of this book: does 'Rariteiten te koop' have such a self-critical function?[85]

83 'Is hy [Six] zoo groot een liefhebber van den Drost niet, hy behoort ten minste te zijn, en kon, mijns dunkens, zonder dat zoo veel goets, als ik 'er meen van gelezen te hebben, niet schryven', J. de Haes, *Het Leven Van Geeraert Brandt, Beschreven Door Joan De Haes* [...] (*The life of Geeraert Brandt, as Recounted by Joan De Haes* ...) 1740, p. 150. I have the reference from Jacobs, 1991 II, pp. 17–18.

84 Thanks to favourable articles on his writings by Jeronimo de Vries and Dirk Groebe (1823) and by Johannes Godefridus Frederiks (1883), see Peters, 2012.

85 G.A. van Es & Edward Rombauts, *De letterkunde van renaissance en barok*, 2, 1952, pp. 161 and 175; G.A. van Es, 'Introduction', *Poësy van J. Six van Chandelier: bloemlezing uit zijn dichtwerk*, 1953, pp. 10–12.

The next generation of researchers will go by Van Es's first impression: that of Six as a realist. M.A. Schenkeveld-van der Dussen has made the main contribution to research on Six; her most important article on him, 'De anti-idealistische poëtica van een christen-burger, Joannes Six van Chandelier' (1983), provides a theoretical foundation for the many articles on Six she has since written.[86] We can see two different but mutually related approaches in Schenkeveld to Six's poetry. On the one hand, she speaks of Six as a distinctly realistic poet: he pays great attention to reality. The other approach has to do with what she calls Six's 'anti-idealistic' poetics. Schenkeveld-van der Dussen was the first to note, and study, the large number of metapoems Six wrote – that is, poems about writing poetry. She has also pointed to Six's particular use of irony, and notwithstanding the many intellectual references in his poems, to his role as a *poeta doctus*. Based on these two points, she shows us what an exceptional position Six occupies in the literary landscape of the Dutch Golden Age: his was a powerful dissenting voice against the pretentious poetic ideal his contemporaries strove for. As Schenkeveld-van der Dussen sees it, Six speaks the naked truth. And if he is not doing that, that is so he can poke fun at others' grandiose words and pretensions. He positions himself as a sceptic, an anti-idealist.[87]

In her article, Schenkeveld-van der Dussen makes an interesting argument that culminates in her vision of Six's writing. In her research into the rationale behind Six's particular poetics, she takes as her starting point three central poems in *Poësy*.[88] Here she discusses several poetic standpoints that Six presents, and two of which address poetry as a vocation. The first relativises the value and status of poetry from both a social and a religious perspective: poetry is no more important than 'neeringe in de droogen' ('trading in drugs') – 'Begin met God' ('Beginning

86 Here I follow Schenkeveld's most important works: M.A. Schenkeveld-van der Dussen, 'Joannes Six van Chandelier: Realist Jaarrede door de voorzitter, mevrouw Dr. M.A. Schenkeveld-van der Dussen', *Jaarboek van de Maatschappij der Nederlandse Letterkunde*, 1981, pp. 3–15; M.A. Schenkeveld-van der Dussen, 'De anti-idealistische poëtica van een christen-burger, Joannes Six van Chandelier'; M.A. Schenkeveld-van der Dussen, 'Ut pictura poesis: de paragone tussen dicht- en schilderkunst bij Jan Vos en Jan Six van Chandelier', *Nederlandse letterkunde*, 2001, pp. 101–112; Riet Schenkeveld-van der Dussen & Willemien de Vries, *Zelfbeeld in gedichten. Brieven over de poëzie van Jan Six van Chandelier*, 2007. For the image of Six in more recent literary-historical retrospectives and guides: M.A. Schenkeveld-van der Dussen, 'Najaar 1649, Jan Six van Chandelier overnacht in Toulouse – Drie anti-idealistische dichters', in: M.A. Schenkeveld-van der Dussen, *Nederlandse Literatuur, een geschiedenis*, 1993, pp. 255–260; Theo Hermans (ed.), *A Literary History of the Low Countries* 2009. The section on Six, pp. 277–279, was written by E.K. Grootes & M.A. Schenkeveld-van der Dussen.

87 M.A. Schenkeveld-van der Dussen, 'De anti-idealistische poëtica van een christen-burger, Joannes Six van Chandelier'.

88 'Het boek, aan den leeser' ('The book, to the Reader') (J119), 'Afscheid aan myn rymen' ('Farewell to My Rhymes') (J120), and 'Begin met God' ('Beginning with God') (J121). See the following chapter for my interpretation of the poems.

with God') (J121) (l. 33) – and, like any other occupation, the writing of poems needs God's blessing. The second point concerns 'an apparent incompatibility between being a druggist and being a poet'. The contrast between druggist and poet could lead to an interesting contextualisation of *Poësy*, but instead Schenkeveld-van der Dussen points to 'a deeper reason why Six did not expect a better reception for his poems', to be found in an opposition between rhyming and writing poetry.[89] Six's particular views on poetry can, according to her argument, be explained in the first instance by literariness itself and not so much by the socio-historical context in which the poetry was written. Six's social identity comes up again at other points in the article, but here Schenkeveld-van der Dussen interprets the profession of druggist not as something problematic, but as a mundane, everyday job through which Six learned what really mattered in life.[90] The rest of the article is about Six's poetics in relation to the literary-aesthetic hierarchies to be found in influential Renaissance poetics, especially that of Joost van den Vondel. Schenkeveld-van der Dussen finds it noteworthy that these hierarchies also contain extratextual references to a social ranking, and that they are even rooted in social divisions in the medical world – but she does not find this important enough to study in the context of Six's own social background. Both the famous distinction offered by Pierre de Ronsard between the 'venerable Prophete', the true poet, and 'un Charlatan vendeur de triacles', and Vondel's repetition of this in his influential statement, 'Rijmers die eerst hun AB opzeggen, vallen verwaendelijck aen 't zwetsen, gelijck de quackzalvers, om hun zalfpotten' ('Rhymesters who have just left finished learning their ABCs, grow presumptuously prolix, like quacks peddling their jars of ointment') – principles of 'universalist' poetics to which Six was opposed and which Schenkeveld-van der Dussen discusses in her article – can be seen against the backdrop of a medical-social reality.[91]

Schenkeveld-van der Dussen also discusses the receipt of materials in Six's poetry. An older article of hers contains an interpretation of 'Dank, voor een gerookten salm, aan Pieter Loones' ('Thanks for a Smoked Salmon – to Pieter Loones') (J357). She calls the piece of Russian smoked salmon in the text 'a trivial gift from a poetic perspective'.[92] The question, however, is whether the goods that come up for discussion in Six really were so trivial: smoked salmon – or other products such as olive oil and dates – are now ordinary items that we come across every day. But was that the case yet in the early modern period? Asking such questions offers new points

89 Ibid., p. 298.
90 Ibid. p. 299 and 311.
91 Ibid., p. 305; Pierre de Ronsard, *La Franciade*, ed. by Paul Laumonier, 1983, p. 335; Joost van den Vondel, *Aenleidinge ter Nederduitsche dichtkunste* (*Introduction to Dutch poetry*), 1977, p. 44. I will return to this point in Chapter 10.
92 Schenkeveld-van der Dussen, 1982, p. 311.

of entry into Six's poetry. I will argue that the large number of exotic products that Six describes transcends the paradigm of realism.[93]

The more serious sides of Six, his illness and his religious musings, have also come in for attention in scholarly research. An article from before Van Es discussed this theme is particularly enlightening: 'Johan Six van Chandelier' by J. Koopmans, from 1915.[94] All the elements of *Poësy* that I find important are discussed in this book: Six's 'culinary interests' and his 'knowledge [...] of all kinds of strange products from East and West'; his anti-Vondelian poetics and warnings of the temptations encountered on his journey through Southern Europe; the ailment he had in his spleen and the break with his regular doctor Simon Dilman in favour of a Spa cure; his Calvinist sympathies and his identification with biblical figures; and his correspondence with Calvinist preachers who are concerned about the state of his soul, especially the theologian Johannes Hoornbeeck. Even if the textual analyses done by subsequent researchers on Six who are familiar with new methods of literary analysis such as close reading are more thorough, the overall picture they give of Six as a writer is not as good as the picture we get from Koopman.

These factors are also raised in the first monograph on Six, *Zelfbeeld in gedichten. Brieven over de poëzie van Jan Six van Chandelier* (2007). The book consists of an exchange of letters between Schenkeveld-van der Dussen and her fellow literary historian, Willemien B. de Vries. In one chapter, the ailment Six had in his spleen is discussed in the light of early modern medical theories. With reference to his profession as 'druggist', Six calls himself a 'dry' person in several texts. This prompts Schenkeveld-van der Dussen to wonder whether 'dryness' is also a reference to the theory of the humours. According to Galen's teachings, melancholics possess the qualities 'dry' and 'cold'. Did Six, then, regard himself as a melancholic? Schenkeveld-van der Dussen's answer is no. She does not detect any great inner struggle in him.[95] I will argue for a different vision: I intend to show, on the one hand, that Six refers directly, and several times, to the doctrine of the humours, and on the other, that melancholy was a fairly elastic concept in the early modern period: thanks to the rediscovery of Aristotle's idea that all great intellectuals and artists were inspired by the qualities of black bile, melancholy lost many of its negative connotations. But at the same time, Protestant theologians and doctors associated a morbid form of melancholy with inappropriate religious behaviour, ranging from

93 Compare also Vincent Buyens, 'Joannes Six van Chandeliers "Schetse van Venecie". Meer dan een reisindruk'. In *Spiegel der Letteren*, 2005, pp. 21–51. Buyens argues that we should not take terms like 'sketch' and 'rhymes' too literally, he also shows that Six in his poetry connects with national-mythological traditions within the Dutch culture which undermines the view of Six as an anti-idealist.

94 *De nieuwe taalgids*, 1915, pp. 25–49.

95 Schenkeveld-van der Dussen, 2007, p. 117.

ecstatic 'frenzy' to introverted pondering.[96] For a good sense of the profile of Six's ailment, we would therefore do well to avoid the stereotypes in the doctrine of the humours. The paradigm of realism has thus made a deeper understanding of Six's poetry more difficult.

In connection with the discussion of *melancholia*, I would also like to discuss another example. In the comments on Six's 'Horatius Liersangen, in Hollands vertaalt door J. v. Vondel. Aan den selven' ('The Odes of Horace, Translated into Dutch by J.v. Vondel. To the same person') (J363), A.E. Jacobs asks, for example, whether Six's concept of 'sinloos' ('without the senses') (l. 11) with respect to Vondel's poetic style refers to the old doctrine of enthusiasm. In my methodological approach, in which I pay attention to humanistic concepts, I want to look more closely at this interesting suggestion. I will return to this point in Chapter 8, on drugs as a source of inspiration.[97] But *Zelfbeeld in Gedichten* also contains observations that shed new light on Six. As we have seen, in several texts Six presents himself as a sinner. He writes religious meditations on vices such as greed and hubris. Many of these poems are addressed to Calvinist preachers. Willemien B. de Vries places the strikingly self-critical attitude of Six in a broader context: 'In Reformed belief, self-examination falls under the question of sin and grace in one's own life. In the Republic in the course of the seventeenth century, this was manifest in the movement of the pietistic Further Reformation'.[98] According to De Vries, this self-examination can be found in Six's poetry. De Vries touches on an interesting point that I will go into more fully in this book. in addition to the issues of morality and illness, I will focus on morality and material in *Poësy*.

How this book is organised

The main part of this book is organised by theme. I follow the same structure as other historical studies on *materia medica* whose starting point is the multi-faceted use of

96 Dorothee Sturkenboom, 'Understanding Emotional Identities. The Dutch Phlegmatic Temperament as Historical Case Study', *BMGN*, 2014, pp. 163–191; see, in particular, p. 179; M.J. van Lieburg, *De ziekte der geleerden. Een hoofdstuk uit de geschiedenis van de melancholie en hypochondrie*, 1989; Michael Heyd, *'Be Sober and Reasonable': The Critique of Enthusiasm in the Seventeenth and Early Eighteenth Centuries*, 1995.
97 Jacobs, 1991 II, p. 642. More problematic is Jacobs's use of a concept such as popular belief – see, for instance, his commentary on 'Op de reedenstryd, oover de kooninghlyke siekte' ('On the disputation on the King's Evil') (J423). Jacobs has clearly been influenced here by natural-scientific and historical works that have appeared in the centuries since Six, such as that by Noel Chomel, *Algemeen Huishoudelijk-, Natuur-, Zedekundig- En Konstwoordenboek*, 1778, and M.A. van Andel, *Klassieke wondermiddelen*, 1928. The magical ideas that Jacobs links to popular belief were, however, scholarly concepts in Six's day.
98 Schenkeveld-van der Dussen & De Vries, 2007, pp. 131 and 132.

drugs in the early modern period.[99] This schema reflects the various roles that Six adopts in 'Rariteiten te koop': as a merchant, a poet of love, an inspired poet, a city poet, as the harbinger of a Golden Age, and indirectly as a patient. In Chapter 2, I discuss the meaning of 'druggist' and 'drugs' in Six's day, with a view to locating Six within a particular socio-medical landscape. Six's ambivalent relationship to his own trade in drugs constitutes a common thread in the remaining chapters, each of which covers a different way in which drugs, spices and perfumes were used. Chapter 3 is devoted to a non-medicinal use of drugs: drugs as collector's items and objects of research in the Wunderkammer, which was popular in the early modern period. Here I discuss *curiositas*, an eagerness for knowledge about exotic drugs as rarities in the cabinet of curiosities. In both of these chapters, I argue that Six's self-portrayal as a modest druggist cannot be traced back to the presentation of the druggist as engaging in a simple, run-of-the-mill activity, but that it involves a rewriting of the negative connotations associated with 'druggist'.

Chapter 4 discusses the use of exotic plants and spices as medicines and foods in Six's poetry. I will explain the close relationship between these two domains at the beginning of that chapter. The discourse on native versus exotic drugs plays a large role in this section. Chapter 5 covers how drugs were used outside the kitchen and the pharmacy: drugs as cosmetics, as both material and literary ornaments. This part deals with drugs as substances that have a transformative effect and thus as threats to the human body, in both the medical and the religious senses. Chapter 6 builds on the argument in Chapter 5 on drugs as cosmetics, but focuses on gunpowder and fireworks as material and as literary ornamentation. The last two chapters discuss religious and ceremonial uses of goods from the early modern drugstore. Thus in Chapter 7 I discuss incense and perfumes as holy offerings – both in the literal and figurative senses – in Joyous Entries by political leaders into cities. Here I show how Six associates the alleged apotheosising power of drugs with idolatry and pride. In Chapter 8 I discuss the use of drugs for artistic inspiration – uses that are alluded to in Renaissance poetry. These chapters present us once again with the self-image of the sober, self-critical druggist, but I also show that Six uses another literary strategy that yields yet other redefinitions of identity: he presents himself as a weak and fragile rhymester, but in a positive sense, to distance himself from associations that drugs give rise to with divinity and perfection. But at the same time, we get to know Six as a pragmatic poet. By using exaggeration, irony and the

99 Compare, for instance, how the chapters are arranged in Alfred Schmidt, *Drogen und Drogenhandel im Altertum*, 1924; A.M.G. Rutten, *Blue Ships: Dutch Ocean Crossing with Multifunctional Drugs and Spices in the Eighteenth Century*, 2008; and Holly Dugan, *The Ephemeral History of Perfume. Scent and Sense in Early Modern England*, 2011.

figure of speech *praeteritio,* Six still manages to make use of material and literary ornaments without actually being identified with them.

In the main part of the book, drugs from all 'three kingdoms of nature' are discussed: plant substances such as cachou ('*terra japonica*'), gum resin and olive oil; animal substances such as bezoar stone, musk, horn, civet and ambergris; and minerals such as saltpetre, gems and gold. I also discuss a number of *composita* – what Van Beverwijck would call 'mengelmiddelen' or 'mixed materials'. In addition to gunpowder, I will also discuss the classic cure-all theriac.

In the third and final part of this book, I will look at another category of drugs, classified not according to how they are used but by their origin: drugs with a fourth origin or, more precisely, a subcategory of *animalia*. These substances come from the 'animal endowed with reason': the human body. We will look at a number of poems by Six in which three types of human 'drugs' play a role: the so-called *mumia* (ground Egyptian mummies), Catholic relics, and human blood. This last substance takes us back to the 'miracle medicine' from 'Rariteiten te koop', the blood of King Charles I. I offer a new reading of this poem, based both on the knowledge we now have of early modern pharmaceutics and on discussions related to it from the main part of the book. Also in this section, I will shift my attention from the sick bodies of individuals to the sick body of the state, and I will look at a new interpretation of the name Six gives his profession: 'thirsting', in the sense of longing for God.

Part II

Medicinal and Sacred Drugs

2. The sober druggist

Abstract
In this chapter, I discuss the meanings of 'druggist', 'drug' and 'spice' in the early modern Dutch Republic, with a view, on the one hand, to locating the druggist-poet Joannes Six van Chandelier within a socio-medical landscape and, on the other, to determining what associations the druggist's 'dry spices' had for his contemporaries. In contrast to the view that literary historians have taken of Six's profession, as an everyday activity from which he derived his realistic view of life, I argue that the drug trade was a cause for concern among readers of his poems who were focused on whether it was morally acceptable. 'Spices' and 'drugs' were associated with strangeness and opulence, and even the miraculous. In order to avoid these negative associations, then, Six presented himself in many of his poems as a sober and rational druggist-poet.

Keywords: Drugs, spices, medical profession, panacea, hemp, self-presentation

Wat mannen sie ik in dit boek,
Wyl ik syn geestenhof doorsoek!
Hier schynt een heemelsch hof vol licht
Van sonne, maane, en stargesigt,
En alles geeft zo schoonen glans,
Slechts tot meer luisters eenes mans.
Hoe past myn naam in deese saal?
Syn kaars licht niet by zulk gestraal.
Neen, Heiblok, ik blyf hier van daan:
Een koopman mag by koopmans staan.

What men do I see in this book,
As I search through this court of spirits!
A heavenly court full of light is shining here
From faces of the sun, the moon and the stars,
And everything gives off a beautiful sheen,
Which only strengthens the illustriousness of these men.

Spaans, R., *Dangerous Drugs: The Self-Presentation of the Merchant-Poet Joannes Six van Chandelier (1620–1695)*. Taylor & Francis Group, 2020
DOI 10.5117/9789462983543_CH02

How does my name belong in this hall?
Its candlelight cannot be seen against all this brilliance.
No, Heiblok, I shall stay away from this court:
A merchant should stay among merchants.
– Joannes Six van Chandelier[1]

The social standing of the druggist

The meanings of 'merchant' and 'druggist' were ambiguous concepts in the early modern Republic. 'Op quaade tongen' ('On Evil Tongues') (J229) delves directly into this reality. The text says a lot about the reception of Six's poems among his contemporaries, and will therefore form the starting point for the theme of this chapter: the social prestige of the druggist-poet Joannes Six van Chandelier. This poem shows that readers assessed the quality of Six's poems on the basis of the social origin of the poet. I shall quote the short poem in its entirety:

Men seit: hy is een koopman, een droogist,
Een kraamer van droogh kruid, voor een Kymist,
En Arts: hy heeft noch konst, noch weetenschap,
Wat kan syn rym meer zyn dan ydle klap?
Dit volk, van zulk vooroordeel ingenoomen,
Strykt oordeel, uit een schaapenbreins schapraai,
Als blinden van de kleuren van karsaai.
Ik staa veel toe, aan die quaadaardge Momen:
Nochtans ik klap niet, als een paapegaai.
Een tuinboer plukt wel spreuken, van de boomen.

They say he is a merchant, a druggist,
A pedlar of dry spices for a Chemist
And a Doctor: he has neither art nor knowledge,
What can his rhyme be, then, but mere idle chatter?
These people, filled with such prejudice,
Make judgments with brains no bigger than that of a sheep,
As blind people might judge the colours of woollen fabric.
I'll grant a lot to these ill-natured men of Momus:
However, I won't chatter away, like some parrot.
A garden farmer in fact picks aphorisms from trees.

1 (J626), Six's contribution to *Liber amicorum* of Jacobus Heyblocq (1623–1690).

Critics point to three different aspects of the profession of druggist: first, the druggist's trade; second, the nature of the merchandise, dried spices; and third, the training involved. In the view of these critics, Six 'has neither art nor knowledge'. They therefore ask, 'What can his rhyme be, then, but mere idle chatter?' He is merely a supplier of 'dry' medicines to chemists and doctors, who, unlike him, have a university degree.[2] According to the critics, the poems of the merchant-druggist are like 'the chatter of parrots'. But Six defends himself: they judge his poems without having read them; a 'garden farmer' can in fact make 'aphorisms' – meaningful poetry. 'Garden farmer' is likely a euphemism here for 'druggist': 'farmer' could refer to another term of abuse used by the elite, while 'garden' refers to the botanical origin of the trader in herbs and spices.

In this chapter I will examine these aspects in more detail. The theme is therefore the social position of the druggist among other professional medical groups on the one hand, and the nature of the druggist's 'dry spices' on the other. In contrast to the view of Six's profession in literary history, as an everyday activity based on which Six works away tirelessly at his down-to-earth, realistic view of life, I want to show that the merchant-druggist trade in fact gave cause for concern to readers of his poems who were concerned about their morality.

The druggist's trade

Six uses a variety of words to describe his profession – 'apothecary', 'grocer, and 'merchant' – but the central concept is 'druggist'. For a precise explanation of these concepts, we have to refer to the historiography of pharmaceutics. Unfortunately, there is no modern authoritative study on the early modern grocery store – several researchers have pointed out that there has been little interest in the place of the merchant-druggist in the history of pharmaceutics in the Netherlands – but there are a number of minor works that can help us here.[3] According to D.A. Wittop Koning, a historian of pharmaceutics, in the seventeenth century there was no great distinction between *drogist*, 'druggist', and *kruidenier*, 'spice merchant' or

2 The verses two and three can be explained in two ways: in the opinion of 'a chemist and a doctor', Six has 'neither art nor knowledge', or: Six is a 'pedlar of dried spices' who supplies 'a chemist and a doctor'. I would like to thank Helmer Helmers for drawing attention to this difference in meaning. The latter is the more plausible interpretation. But as I want to show in this chapter, much of the criticism of druggists came from doctors and chemists.

3 D.A. Wittop Koning, *Compendium voor de Geschiedenis van de Pharmacie van Nederland*, 1986; C.D. Jongman, 'De historische ontwikkeling van het kruideniersbedrijf in Nederland', in: F.L. van Muiswinkel & J.C. Berk, *Het kruideniersbedrijf*, 1951, pp. 3–15.

'grocer'.[4] Both the druggist and the grocer were suppliers to the pharmacist, and both names were thus used interchangeably for one and the same person.[5] Initially, a grocer (in Middle English 'spicer') was the same as an apothecary, but the grocery trade changed under the influence of the great immigration from the Spanish Netherlands in the sixteenth century. This grocery trade that came to Amsterdam, and that entailed overseas trade with distant regions, melded with the local druggist profession that in the meantime had gone from being a retailer to being a 'wholesaler of spices, drugs and dyes' – this is thus the early modern definition of the druggist. Unlike the medieval spice merchant, the early modern grocer was no longer allowed to prepare medicines, but had to specialise in the purchase and sale of simple medicines (*simplicia*) on a large scale, so that they could also be a supplier to the pharmacist.[6] Wittop Koning goes on to say that the grocery profession 'would also give the professions of sugar refiner, tobacco merchant and chemist a higher profile, thus further differentiating the profession'. This division caused a further redefinition of the druggist's trade, which took place after Six van Chandelier's time: retailers of personal-care products as we know them today.[7] The distinction was not absolute: there were all kinds of combinations in the early modern period, such as the 'apothecary-grocer', and the development of the relationship between the apothecary and the grocer varied from city to city. In 'Op quaade tongen', we saw that Six's profession was referred to derisively as 'peddling', as well as 'trading'. It is possible that his family business was engaged in retailing in addition to their main activity, wholesaling. The correct historical name for Six's profession is thus *koopman-kruidenier*, 'merchant-grocer', or *koopman-drogist*, 'merchant-druggist'. Because I discuss Six's poetry in connection with the pharmaceutical practice in this study, I will also use the term 'druggist-poet'.

4 *Cf.* the translation of *kruydenier* in Hendrick Hexham, *A large Netherdutch and English Dictionarie; Composed out of the best Netherdutch Authours*, 1658, unpaginated: 'One that sells all sorts of Spice, or a Grosser'.

5 D.A. Wittop Koning, *De handel in geneesmiddelen te Amsterdam tot omstreeks 1637*, 1942, pp. 60–64. The seventeenth-century sense of 'grocer': 'a spice merchant who handled larger or wholesale quantities (thus dealing in "gross amounts")', Paul Freedman, *Out of the East: Spices and the Medieval Imagination*, 2008, p. 116.

6 Wittop Koning, 1942, p. 22. See also the definition of 'drogist' in Sijbrand Feitama, *Uitbeeldingen van Staaten, Ambagten en Neeringen*, 1685, p. 29. As noted above, Six's family consisted of immigrants from the Spanish Netherlands. We do not know whether they were involved with the international trade in drugs and spices, but the Jeheu family were registered as apothecaries in Brussels. My thanks to Wim Heijnen for this information.

7 Wittop Koning, 1942, pp. 60 and 61. Jongman (1951, pp. 48 and 49) assumes that the *kruidenier-koopman* combination existed for just a short intermediate period. The wholesalers probably lost the first part of the name, *kruidenier*, towards the end of the early modern period. Sebastien A.C. Dudok van Heel speaks of a 'development from grocery to drugstore' (in '"De Gapert" van de kruidenier Hendrick Anthonisz Wissel: Damrak No. 50', *Amstelodamum*, 1976, p. 2).

Following on from the historical development of the profession of druggist, I will discuss the merchant-grocer here in more detail in relation to the development of other medical professions. In the seventeenth century there was a delineation of various medical professions. In 1637, for example, apothecaries and physicians in Amsterdam became more closely connected through a collaboration between the newly established *Collegium Medicum* and the apothecaries' guild. These institutions began to regulate the activities of doctors and apothecaries in Amsterdam more systematically, for example by supervising pharmacies and registering new *medicinae doctores* and apothecaries. A diploma was required of doctors from the medical faculty of a university or college, and a masterpiece – a piece of work by a craftsman accepted as qualification for membership of a guild as an acknowledged master[8] – was required of apothecaries as proof that they were proficient in preparing medicines. The druggists stayed behind in the pedlars' guild from which the apothecaries had detached themselves, thus losing much of their prestige in relation to their former fellow guild members.[9]

The reorganisation of the medical landscape took on greater proportions in the mid-seventeenth century, thus creating a separation between the pharmacy business, which was increasingly regarded as a science because the preparation of medicines was becoming more specialised, and the druggist's trade, which was becoming more and more the hallmark of commerce. This reorganisation took place not only in Amsterdam, but also in other Dutch cities. Paragraph 22 of the Middelburg Ordinance of 1624 is typical of the new relationship between the pharmacist and the druggist. It says, in part:

> From now on, no Grocers, Druggists and pedlars, or others who do not completely understand the art of Apothecary, may make or sell any medicines, Laxatives or Vomitives, or any other compositions related to the art of Pharmacy [...][10]

This development was also to be seen in other European countries. In her study on perfume in early modern England, Holly Dugan shows how the apothecaries' tenuous relationship with grocers had existed almost as long as their trade.[11] A deterioration

8 Definition from the Oxford English Dictionary.

9 Annet Mooij, *De polsslag van de stad. 350 jaar academische geneeskunde in Amsterdam*, 1999, pp. 36–40; Cook, 2008, 133–163. See also R. Bijlsma, 'Oud-Rotterdamsche "Cruydenierie"', *Rotterdamsch Jaarboekje*, 1912, pp. 91–99.

10 'Hier voortaen geen Cruydeniers, Drogisten en kraamers ofte andere, hun d'Apothecarye niet volcomentlyck verstaende, eenige medicynen, Laxativen ofte Vomitiven ofte eenige andere compositien de Pharmacie aengaende, moogen maecken of verkoopen [...]', Willem Stoeder, *Geschiedenis der pharmacie in Nederland*, 1891, p. 60.

11 Holly Dugan, *The Ephemeral History of Perfume. Scent and Sense in Early Modern England*, 2011, pp. 135–142.

of the relationship must be understood in the light of the creation of the gentlemanly codes in scientific circles in Europe, where characteristics such as refinement and trustworthiness were brought into play as the bases for scientific work. The ideal of the seventeenth-century scholar was the truth-loving scientist – a social category that was directly opposed to that of the common liar or idle prattler. In this context, concepts such as 'quack' and 'merchant' took on negative connotations. They were used figuratively by gentlemen scientists as an insult for people who had no *entree* to their community. These codes were particularly visible in England, where the Royal Society emerged from an aristocratic culture, but they also took place in the more bourgeois Netherlands.[12] A Dutch example of this can be found in the writings of the doctor and chemist Franciscus de le Boë Sylvius (1614–1672). From 1641 to 1658 he lived in Amsterdam, where his medical practice enjoyed great prestige. In 1651 he was elected 'supervisor' of the *Collegium Medicum*. Then, in 1658, he was appointed Professor of Medicine at the University of Leiden. There he built what seems to be the first university chemical laboratory. In his inaugural speech there, *Oratio inauguralis de hominis cognitione* (*An Inaugural Address on Human Cognition*) (1658), Sylvius mentions self-knowledge, sobriety and rationality as guiding principles for disinterested scientists. These ideals can be interpreted as an expression of the gentlemanly codes in the Republic. They can be traced back to neo-stoicism, which emphasises virtues such as *apatheia* (imperturbability) and *constantia* (constancy). Sylvius's art collection contained many scenes of quacks and mountebanks surrounded by greedy, rapacious customers. Pamela H. Smith, who has examined the collection, relates these motifs to Sylvius's status as a learned physician. The depiction in these paintings of quacks as comic individuals serves to underline class differences within medicine.[13]

A member of *Collegium Medicum* is mentioned in Six's poetry: Bonaventura Coegelen van Dortmont (1633–1710). Even though he was a student of medicine when he was in contact with Six, it is likely that, at that time, he wanted to be seen as a representative of the ideals of the disinterested scientist. Coegelen van Dortmont is mentioned in three poems in *Poësy*:[14] From the content of these texts

12 Stephen Shapin, *A Social History of Truth: Civility and Science in Seventeenth-Century England*, 1994, pp. 94 and 95. For the process of aristocratisation in Dutch scientific culture, see: Klaas van Berkel, *In het voetspoor van Stevin: Geschiedenis van de natuurwetenschap in Nederland 1580–1940*, 1985, p. 35.

13 Pamela H. Smith, *The Body of the Artisan*, 2004, pp. 183–204 and 229–232. This does not mean, however, that Sylvius was critical of Six: Sylvius was in touch with the preacher Johannes Hoornbeeck, a friend and cousin of Six's. Hoornbeeck was married to a niece of Franciscus de le Boë Sylvius. Many of Sylvius's books were in Hoornbeeck's library, see E.D. Baumann, *Francois dele Boë Sylvius*, 1949, pp. 47 and 48. Sylvius also had Hoornbeeck as a patient. See T. Briemen, *Johannes Hoornbeeck (1617–1666): eminent geleerde en pastoraal theoloog*, 2008, p. 83.

14 'Op de reedenstryd, van de lydinge des krunkeldarms, door Bonaventura Koegelen van Dortmond, alvooren hy, t'Uitrecht, geneesheer weird' ('On the Disputation on Sufferers of Colic, to Bonaventura

it appears that he cured a skin rash on one of Six's hands, and that Six wanted to express his gratitude with a precious gift: an exclusive cutlery set decorated with bloodstone. According to 'Op versmaade erkentenisse voor het geneesen mynes hands, door Bonaventura Koegelen van Dortmond, aan den selven ('On the Gift That Was Refused, for Curing my Hands, to Bonaventura Coegelen of Dortmond') (J448), the student refuses the fancy gift from his patient. Coegelen van Dortmont thus shows that he is cautious about further strengthening his contacts with Six. But why? The exchange of gifts takes place in a society in which the social distance between druggists and doctors is growing.

The response that came from 'Op quaade tongen' did not just come out of the blue. The druggist is only a supplier of medical raw materials 'for a chemist and a doctor'. The criticism was that they themselves were not familiar with medical and scientific matters, and that their approach to materials was characterised by unbridled desires, not by distance and rationality. The *herbalist* Six – according to the first meaning of the *kruidenier* in the *Woordenboek der Nederlandsche Taal*, the word is a direct translation of the Latin *herbarius* – protests against his exclusion from a community in which druggists and apothecaries had previously operated under the same conditions.[15] Through the composition of poetry, the occupation of the early modern learned gentleman, Six tries to maintain the image of the druggist as an erudite botanist, a learned gentleman. He thus wanted 'Op quaade tongen' to serve as testament to his status as a self-confident individual. In his famous oration at the inauguration of the *Illustere School* in Amsterdam in 1632, the aforementioned Casparus Barlaeus, had, after all, introduced the *Mercator sapiens* or the ideal of the wise merchant – someone who combined commercial activities with classical learning. Moreover, Six belonged to a family with ambitions. The location of the family business, 'The Gilded Unicorn', next to the Town Hall on Dam Square reflects both the wealth and the trade network of the family. Even though the poet's father, Jacob Six, was not a part of the patriciate, he certainly belonged to the well-to-do citizenry of Amsterdam (Plate 2).[16] On the basis of the semantic

Coegelen of Dortmond, after He Was Made Physician, in Utrecht') (J443); 'Dank, aan Bonaventura Koegelen van Dortmond, geneesheer, voor het geneesen mynes hands' ('Acknowledgment for Curing my hands, to Bonaventura Coegelen of Dortmond') (J444); 'Op versmaade erkentenisse voor het geneesen mynes hands, door Bonaventura Koegelen van Dortmond, aan den selven ('On the Gift That Was Refused, for Curing my Hands, to Bonavontura Coegelen of Dortmond') (J448).

15 In 'Steetuinkroon aan Joannes Snippendal' ('Crown of the City Garden to Joannes Snippendaal') (J146), Six addresses the botanist Snippendaal as a *kruidenier* (l. 29). See my analysis of the poem in Chapter 4, pp. 135–136.

16 The family was one of the thousand richest in the city. This estimate is based on the tax that Jacob Six paid on his wealth in 1631, see J.G. Frederiks & P.J. Frederiks, *Kohier van den tweehonderdsten penning voor Amsterdam en onderhoorige plaatsen over 1631*, 1890. According to the 1630 census, Amsterdam had 115,000 inhabitants. In 1691, the City of Amsterdam estimated Joannes Six van Chandelier's wealth to be

instability of the concepts that I have covered here, we must pay attention to how Six uses 'kruidenier' and 'drogist' in his self-portrayal as a merchant-poet. What meaning do these terms have for Six's poetics? I shall come back to this presently.

Dry versus green spices

Six's unique approach to materials is central to the research that has been done on him, but little attention has been paid to what his goods consisted of; they are described by literature scholars only as 'medicinal herbs'. Six himself uses the now-obsolete term 'droogery', 'drugs', to refer to his goods. Just as the meaning of the term 'druggist' was influenced by a redefinition from the world of the medical profession, 'drugs' was, in early modern times, an increasingly ambiguous concept. The key term in this debate is 'dry spices', as Six calls his merchandise in 'Op quaade tongen'. But first, a more precise explanation of 'drugs': we find this in the historiography of pharmaceutics. A list of 'medicines used' gives us an impression of the assortment of items in the early modern pharmacy.[17] In addition to once-exotic but nowadays everyday kitchen spices such as cinnamon, pepper, nutmeg and ginger, we find all sorts of unusual commodities. Typically classical medicinal herbs such as aloe, rhubarb, lavender and oleander are included alongside fabulous wonder drugs such as devil's dung (asafoetida) and mandragora. We also find, classed as medicines, products that these days we would not regard as medicines at all, such as lemons, raisins and dates, gems, metals such as gold and silver, bloodstone, myrrh, incense, and opium – a narcotic. Musk and ivory are also on the list, as well as poisons such as arsenic and even strange items such as lion meat, crocodile and the so-called *mumia*: pulverised Egyptian mummy.[18] In short, this list contains not only substances of plant origin, but also substances of mineral and animal origin. *Specerij* and *kruid*, both meaning 'spice', were broader concepts in the seventeenth century than they are today. Seventeenth-century pharmaceutics does not draw sharp semantic lines between the concepts 'spices' and 'drugs'.[19] These are *simplicia* – simples, as they were called – all of which come from 'the three realms of nature'. In early modern pharmacopoeias – the standardised, official pharmaceutical recipe books – the

40,380 guilders, and asked him to pay 200 guilders in tax. Six protested and specified that his wealth was 13,559 guilders. See the list of notarial deeds in Appendix II.

17 Wittop Koning 1942, pp. 8–10.

18 *Cf.* also the list of early modern grocery items included in Jongman, 1951, pp. 6 and 7.

19 According to meanings 7 and 9 in the WNT, 'kruid' is synonymous with concepts such as *specerij*, 'spice', *kruiderij*, 'seasonings', and *poeder*, 'powder'. See also the definition in Ria Jansen-Sieben, 'Van drogen, kruiden en specerijen', in: Albert Deman & Christian Cannuyer (eds.), *Specerijkelijk. De specerijenroutes*, 1992, pp. 32–41.

materia medica thus consisted not only of *vegetabilia* but also of *animalia* and *mineralia*.[20] Besides these *simplicia,* there were also *composita,* compound medicines that were made from components of all three aforementioned categories.

In addition to these three realms, there was a fourth: chemical medicines from the 'kymist', who was mentioned in Six's poems. These remedies can be connected to new medical theories from Paracelsus, which had many adherents in Europe, and to the iatrochemist, or *chymist,* who was in an intermediate position between the alchemist and the modern chemist.[21] The main goal of Dutch iatrochemists was to make medicines, but the search for the philosopher's stone and the ability to make gold (chrysopoeia) was not forgotten. The seventeenth century was in many ways a heyday for the alchemists, although many seventeenth-century chemists distanced themselves from them. The iatrochemists rejected organic medicines, and opted for chemical remedies. But that did not mean that they rejected spices – far from it. According to the notarial inventory of Sylvius's house, his laboratory included 'a box full of all kinds of spices'. They were probably used by Sylvius when he made his tinctures, essences and oils.[22] Moreover, the dividing lines between the old and new medicines were not that strict. Official pharmacopoeias included recipes of both Galenic and iatrochemical origin. A well-known physician-poet, Daniël Jonctys (1611–1654), to whom Six refers on two occasions, combined an iatrochemical way of thinking with Galenic principles, thus following the example of the German iatrochemist Daniel Sennert (1572–1637), who was popular in the Netherlands. This middle ground seems to have been widespread in medical circles in the Netherlands, even among orthodox Calvinists with a pronounced anti-Cartesian bent. And Six's poetry also contains chemical terms and concepts such as purification, fermentation, and transformation. I will come back to these later. And many of the druggist's products that are to be found in Six's poems are chemical substances. But at the same time he uses the term 'Galenus'/'Galeen' when referring specifically to doctors.[23]

As a result of the ambivalence about 'grocers' discussed above, it will be useful to take a look at the pharmaceutical concepts at Six. What terms does he use himself? A cursory investigation shows that *kruid,* both 'herb' and 'spice' in English, is the

20 See also A.M.G. Rutten, *Blue Ships: Dutch Ocean Crossing with Multifunctional Drugs and Spices in the Eighteenth Century*, 2008.

21 H.A.M. Snelders, *De geschiedenis van de scheikunde in Nederland*, 1993, pp. 11–36; Wittop Koning 1954, pp. 1–5; Lawrence M. Principe, *The Secrets of Alchemy*, 2013.

22 'Casge met alderley cruyden', Th.H. Lunsingh Scheurleer, C. Willemijn Fock & A.J. van Dissel (eds.), *Rapenburg. Geschiedenis van een Leidse gracht*, part IIIa, 1988, p. 342.

23 *Cf.* 'Ter eere van de fonteine Nieuwe Geronster of Klein Tonneken' ('In Honour of the Spring at Géronstère or small Tonnelet') (J107), l. 9, and 'Lange mantel, achter het lyk van Jan Bikker burgemeester' ('Long Cloak behind the Body of the Burgomaster Jan Bicker') (J347), l. 33.

most frequent term in Six's *oeuvre*.[24] It occurs about thirty times. In some cases, it is used in the widespread early modern meaning of the word discussed above. In 'Leeven te Spa' ('The Life at Spa'; J101, l. 39), for instance, Six refers to theriac and mithridate – drugs from antiquity that were popular in the Renaissance – as 'spices'. These were *composita* – that is, compound medicines – consisting of vegetable, animal and mineral ingredients. *Speceryen/specerye* – spices – also occurs, but less frequently. When he is referring explicitly to his company, Six means trading in 'droogery' or 'droogen' – drugs. 'Speceryen' and 'droogery' each occur only three or four times in Six's work. The latter concept calls for a bit more attention. 'Drogerij' is a rare word in contemporary Dutch, but on the basis of the etymological meaning of the term and our merchant-poet's poetics, this concept is more interesting than the more frequent *kruid*. Just like 'kruiderij' and 'specerij', 'drogerij' was originally a collective noun, and that is how Six van Chandelier uses it, in addition to the even rarer 'droge' (plural 'drogen'). 'Droge' comes from the French *drogue*. 'Drogue' is in turn a derivation from the Middle Dutch, from 'droghe' in collocations as 'droge waere' ('dry goods') and 'droghe vaten' ('dry barrels'), which was mistakenly understood as 'barrels for dry goods', so that 'droghe' also began to mean 'dry goods'.[25] The Old French 'drogue' is also the origin of the English 'drug'. 'Drogerij' makes it clearer than 'kruid' does that it is a matter of imported merchandise that is not fresh. The term thus refers to the practice of drying herbs and other materials, and that implies that they are intended for long-distance transport. Incidentally, 'drogerijen' should be understood as 'conserved' rather than as 'dry' raw materials, because in the early modern period they were found in both dry and wet form: compare the formulation 'natte en drooge Droogen' – 'wet and dry drugs' used by the druggist-poet Sijbrand Feitama.[26] As mentioned above, the seventeenth-century merchant-druggist also traded in liquid formulae such as tinctures, jams, essences and oils – the chemicals of the *chymist*. After the medieval discovery of distillation technology, alcohol solutions, among other things, became important. This group seems to have built up a large part of its retail stock, as evidenced by a trade petition sent to the King of Spain by Six and other merchant-druggists: the document mentions 'quintessence of chimica, salts, oils, spirit, extracts'.[27] We see this illustrated in pictures of alchemists and *chymists*

24 *Cf.* the translation of *kruydt* in Hexham, 1658, unpaginated: 'an Hearbe of the Garden or Field, also Spice'. *Cf.* also the modern Dutch word *kruidnagel*, clove.

25 See the lemma in M. Philippa *et al.* (eds.), *Etymologisch Woordenboek van het Nederlands*, 2003–2009. Some other reference works say the word originated from the Arabic: The word 'drug' derives from the Arabic *dowâ* – remedy – and then passed as *doga, droga* into the Romance and from there into the Germanic languages': Schmidt 1924, p. 1. However, more recent etymological dictionaries reject this idea.

26 Sijbrand Feitama, *Christelijke en stigtelijke rymoeffeningen*, 1684, p. 260.

27 For this information: Appendix II; Dudok van Heel, 1976, pp. 1–11.

in Dutch art from the early modern period, such as 'An Alchemist in His Study' by Egbert van Heemskerk (Plate 3). In the foreground, on the tables and on the floor, there are many different jars: small ones containing dyes and pigments, and a larger earthenware one, probably containing *simplicia.* The globe in the middle of the picture symbolises the exotic origin of drugs; the same goes for the turban, which the man at the writing desk seems to be wearing. The sword hanging from the ceiling – the Sword of Damocles – represents the moral dangers associated with alchemical transformation.[28]

'Drogerij' produces more diverse associations than does 'specerij' or 'kruid'. On the one hand, the exotic origin of drugs has positive connotations, such as 'new' and 'mysterious', and on the other, negative ones, such as 'strange' and 'unreliable'. The dryness (*droogheid*) of various druggist's products evokes other negative properties, such as 'withered' and 'inanimate', while, paradoxically, they are actually medicines and aromatics. Even Cornelis Kiliaan's well-known dictionary, to which Six himself refers in *Poësy*, adds a warning to his definition of the word: 'Pharmaca enim violenter corpus exiccant & extergunt, alimenti verò adferunt nihil' ('Drugs plunder and dry out the body, but add nothing to food').[29] So there is a crucial difference between herbs that came from local herb gardens, and exotic spices that came to the West in preserved form, often unrecognisable. In early modern medical writings, the phrase 'drooge ende groene kruyden' ('dry and green spices'), is used.[30] In the Middle Ages, these 'dry' spices and drugs passed through many middlemen before arriving in the West. Knowledge of the origin and effects of the substances was obscured and distorted in the process. The great distance between the producing and consuming countries meant that exotica were subject to mystification and illusion.

Against the backdrop of these negative connotations and the aforementioned changes in the medical professions, it is not difficult to understand other complaints against druggists. Both the druggist and the new chemical medicines were sniped at in the pamphlet *Den Desolaten Boedel der Medicijne deses Tijdts* (*The Insolvent Estate of Present-Day Medicine*) from 1677. Written in the form of a conversation between a physician and an apothecary, the pamphlet discusses the competition among the various groups of medical practitioners. The druggists are hauled over the coals: We read that they are known for their deceitfulness – that they sell small ampoules of distilled medicines from their

28 See other paintings with similar symbols: Elisabeth Berry Drago, *Printed Alchemists: Early Modern Artistry and Experiment in the Work of Thomas Wijck*, pp. 133 and 177.

29 See the lemma at C. Kiliaan: dbnl.org/tekst/kilioo1etymo1_01/kilioo1etymo1_01_0001.php

30 See the 1637 request by apothecaries from Amsterdam, addressed to the Board of the city, in: Stoeder 1891, p. 94.

East Indian boxes at prices that are far too high, and that they are doing great harm to the apothecaries:

> They play the brave quacks by selling Medicaments and lure the customers away from the Apothecaries. They keep the profits for themselves, and they fool and cheat people with laxatives, sweat cures [...] They sell Chemicals, of which they have no understanding, all to the detriment of the human body.[31]

This reality was at the root of the criticism in 'Op quaade tongen'. I will return to the negative associations of drugs in Chapter 3, where I will delve deeper into the scientific discussion of the distinction between Six's indigenous and exotic medicines. As we shall see, the terms 'withered', 'strange' and 'unreliable' were key to arguments in this debate.

Drugs as a panacea

There is more to say about early modern 'drugs'. As we have seen, in earlier literary analyses of Six, 'drogerijen' was thought to mean 'medicinal materials'. But according to Wittop Koning, in the seventeenth century drugs were 'not yet entirely intended for pharmaceutical use. Several items were used primarily in other businesses, such as dyers, while others, were more significant as scents for churches and as kitchen herbs than as medicines'.[32] This is confirmed in recent studies on the history of pharmaceutics. On the basis of the data on drugs in the archives of the East and West India Company (the VOC and the WIC) and in seventeenth- and eighteenth-century pharmacopoeias, which attest to a rather varied use of the merchandise the VOC and the WIC were trading in, A.M.G. Rutten introduces the term 'multifunctional drugs' as a definition of early modern druggist's products.[33] This opens the door to a completely different perception of the merchant druggist in the Dutch Republic, especially as regards their social status.

31 'Sy speelen dapper den Quacksalver met verscheyde Medicamenten te verkoopen, om de luiden van de Apothekers te trekken, daer sy haar profijt van de selvige hebben, en de menschen veel wijs maken en bedriegen, met purgatien, sweetingen [...] sy verkoopen Chimicalia, daer sy voor al geen kennis hebben, tot schade van het menselicke lichaem', *Remedie voor den desolaten boedel. Der Medicijne deses Tijds; Uytgesproken van Doctor Over het Pesthuis, en Apoteker in het Gasthuis*, 1677, pp. 10, 17–18. According to Luuc Kooijmans, the pamphlet was written by members of literary society Nil Volentibus Arduum, by the lawyer Andries Pels and the physicians Lodewijk Meijer and Johannes Bouwmeester, see Luuc Kooijmans, *De doodskunstenaar. De anatomische lessen van Frederik Ruysch*, 2004, pp. 133–135.

32 Wittop Koning, 1942, p. 24.

33 Rutten, 2008, pp. 17 and 32–33. The 'multifunctional drugs' discussed in Rutten's study are categorised as 'cosmetic', 'spice', 'perfume', 'lubricant', 'dye', 'fumigant' and 'insecticide' (p. 33).

A good illustration of the multifunctionality of an early modern herb in Six's work can be found in a praise poem dedicated to hemp, 'Kennep' (J19). I will quote the poem, a sonnet, it in its entirety:

Verachtlik needrigh kruid, op 't veld noch staande in blaaren,
Maar wat ontveinst uw groente al wonders in haar schacht?
De koopman, als ghy weikt, riekt muskeljaat en lacht.
De Dief, foei duivelsdrek, bleekt sonder te bedaaren.
De Lynbaan draaide u niet tot bint en kaabelgaaren,
Of ghy beteert beklomt het top van pyngeslacht.
De Weever had den draad van 't Web niet uitgewracht,
Of ghy vlooght in de locht, met bergen langs de baaren.
Wat is de voorschoot van die wispeltuurge vrouw,
En strooijeres van schat, uit alle werrelds oorden
Dan Kennep toebereidt tot seil en kaabeltouw?
De winden plaagen 't bosch, maar niet op Amstels boorden,
Hy steltse strax aan 't stuur. Zoo werd de zee een schouw.
Zoo bintmen oost aan west, en suiden vast aan noorden.

Wretched, lowly drug, still in leaf in the fields,
But such wonders as your stem conceals! –
The merchant, when you are soaking, smells musk and laughs.
The Thief, asafoetida – for shame! – turns pale and does not recover.
Hardly had the Rope-walk turned you into ropes for tying and cabling,
Than, tarred, you climbed to the top of the family of pines.
Hardly had the Weaver laid the last thread on the Web,
Than you flew in the air, with mountains along the waves.
What is the apron of fickle Lady Luck,
And distributor of treasure, from all corners of the world,
Than hemp prepared for sail and cable rope?
The winds sweep through the woods, but not on the banks of the Amstel.
It [the hemp] immediately leads them away. So the sea becomes a ferry.
And thus we bind East to West, and South to North.

This sonnet is typical of Six's work, with its mannerist language, combined with the sensory description of the druggist's wares. Hemp that is soaked (as part of the production process), so that the bark comes loose from the stem, emits a fragrance that the trader likes, but that the thief fears. This contradictory olfactory sensation reflects the multifunctionality of hemp rope. On the one hand, it is used as cable to moor ships in the merchant fleet and, on the other, as rope for nooses. The rest of the sonnet examines the first use in more detail, in complex, baroque visual language. The metaphors 'the family of pines', 'mountains' and 'woods' all refer to merchant ships, while 'the apron of fickle Lady Luck' alludes to the capricious Fortuna, the goddess of luck, whose loose clothing is depicted as a sail bulging in the wind. Six artfully transforms something 'wretched, lowly' – an insignificant plant that does not flower – into a symbol of divine prosperity, and he puts all of this on conspicuous display. The seam in Fortuna's garb (her 'apron') is made of hemp fibres. Thanks to hemp, various continents are connected to each other. To understand these metaphors, we must remember that Fortuna was also seen as the goddess of trade and shipping, and that ships were often named after her.[34] Thanks to hemp, people can travel the ocean and reach foreign kingdoms. The multifunctional utility of hemp also manifests itself on a higher social level. Its use in nooses underlines its importance in maintaining public order, while its use in making ropes for shipping shows that it promotes Dutch trade and prosperity. It is therefore tempting to ask whether 'lowly drug' serves as a self-image for the 'lowly' merchant. In *Poësy*, Six identifies himself more often with the goods he trades in. I will discuss other examples of this later on. So the merchant portrays himself as a socially useful person. The poem presents the profession as the driving force behind the economic, social and cultural prosperity of the Republic, as a vehicle for international contacts and exchange.

Thus far, then, everything is clear. But there are certain uses of hemp that are not discussed in the poem. The Latin name for it – the term used in the pharmaceutical profession – is cannabis. It evokes very different associations – far from the *lowliness* that this poem attributes to the herb. Because as early as the seventeenth century it was known that cannabis makes you *high*. It is therefore a drug in the sense not only of a 'medicine', but also of a 'stimulant' and an 'addictive and hallucinating narcotic', in keeping with the modern English meaning of 'drug'. Cannabis as an intoxicant is mentioned in the botanical standard work from Six's time, *Herbarius of Cruydt-boeck* (1644) by Rembertus Dodonaeus (Rembert Dodoens), who tells how roasted hemp seed was used as a dessert in banquets in classical Greece. Hemp seed, we read:

> It is what you eat at the end of the meal, to excite cheerfulness and to give the drinks taste. It warms quite a lot: therefore, if you have enjoyed a bit too much of it, it climbs to the head and sends many hard and spice-like vapours and fluids upwards, and it often tends to arouse quite some pain, dizziness and melancholy in the head.[35]

34 In allegorical images, Fortuna is often at the helm of a ship with a ship's sail above her head. See Cesare Ripa, *Iconologia of Uytbeeldinghen des Verstants*, 1644, p. 131. *Fortuna* was, for instance, the name of a ship carrying opium to Marocco for Six's father, see Appendix II.

35 '[I]s't ghene dat men in't laetste van de maltijden eet om vroligheydt te verwercken / en smaeck in den dranck te doen krijgen. Het verwarmt seer veel: daerom een weynigsken te veel daer van genoten / klimt

Interestingly in this connection, Dodonaeus also mentions the intoxicating effect of hemp in relation to the production of rope (Fig. 2.1). He warns against the water in which the herb is put during the process of soaking, because the water 'acquires and keeps such a bad and poisonous power that those who drink from it are almost not to be healed, but usually die from it'.[36] Interestingly, in Six's time, the term 'drugs' was also used in the sense of 'intoxication' – that is, in the derivation 'droggig', 'druggy'. This is clear from a Dutch translation of a work by the German occult writer Heinrich Cornelius Agrippa von Nettesheim, *Van de onzekerheid en ydelheid der wetenschapen en konsten* (*On the Uncertainty and Vanity of Science and Arts*) (1650). In a chapter on 'giftmengende magia' ('magic mixed with poison'), the author speaks of 'natuurlijke Magia, dienze de vergiftende of *droggige* noemen, die door dranken, en minnepappen en veelderleije kruidmiddelen der giftmengers te werk gesteld word' ('the natural magic, which they call toxic or *druggy*, which are prepared in drinks, love elixirs and multiple drug mixtures of the poisoners'). Six van Chandelier, who was quite erudite, was undoubtedly aware of the intoxicating effect of drugs. He refers to Dodonaeus in *Poësy*, but, perhaps not surprisingly, in 'Kennep' he makes no mention of the function of the plant as a stimulant and a luxury item. He only mentions the functions of hemp that are useful for society. In this choice, Six follows D.V. Coornhert's ethical guidelines for the Christian, prudent merchant in *De Coopman* (*The Merchant*). Coornhert criticises those who consume 'medical drinks' 'not for health, but the delicacy of taste'.[37]

This miraculous pharmacology gave drugs an appeal that transcended the realm of pharmaceutics. The mythical origins of exotic drugs gave them an aura of chic refinement. In contrast to medicines put out by the pharmaceutical industry today, which have a short lifespan (pills are generally taken right after they are bought), many early modern medicines were not intended for consumption at all. They were regarded as long-term preventatives. Jewellery containing gold and precious stones thus had the function of amulets, and bezoar stones, as they were called – hollowed out stones from the stomachs of Asian goats, covered in precious metal and intended as drinking cups – were said to be antidotes to poisons. Such medicinal showpieces make clear the non-pharmaceutical applications of early modern drugs. Herbs served as exhibition pieces, status symbols, decorative items

nae 't hooft / ende seyndt veele herte ende specerijachtighe dompen ende wasdommen nae bovenwaerts; ende pleeght soo dickwijls eenige pijne / draeyinghe ende swaerigheydt in't hooft te verwercken', Rembertus Dodonaeus, *Herbarius oft Cruydt-boeck*, 1644, p. 856.

36 'Soo quade ende vergiftighe kracht krijght ende behoudt / dat de ghene die daer van drincken/bijnae met gheen hulp te ghenesen en zijn, maer ghemeynlijck daer van moeten sterven', p. 857.

37 'Medicinale drancken', 'niet om zyn ghesontheyts, maer om des smaecx leckerheyts', D.V. Coornhert, *De Coopman*, [1580] 1969, p. 14.

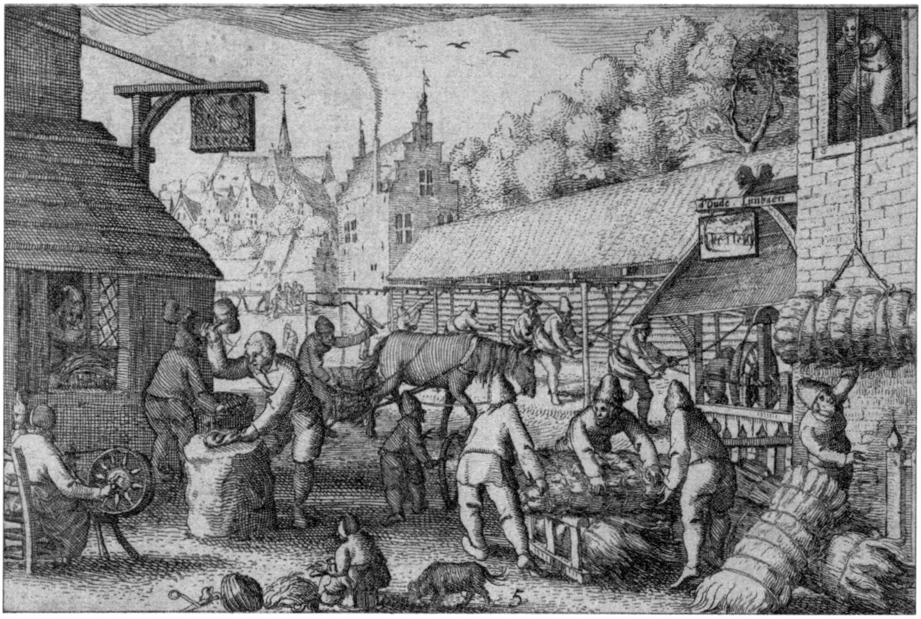

Fig. 2.1: Claes Jansz. Visscher, *Flax and hemp industry.* In the background a ropework can be seen. 1608. Etching. (© Rijksmuseum, Amsterdam).

and gifts. These drugs were not stowed in medicine chests, but were meant to be shown off. Writing praise poems about exotica is a typical example of this kind of showy display of medicinal delights.[38]

The sober druggist

In 'Kennep', Six profiles himself as a 'humble' merchant, and he emphasises the socially utility of herbs. It is against this background that I turn now to texts in which Six discusses the concepts of 'druggist' and 'dry' in order to investigate how he constructs his public persona. We have already touched on the negative word plays in Dutch on 'drogist' ('druggist'), whereby a 'droog' ('dry') or 'uitgedroogd' ('dried out') individual is said to lack a certain vitality. In Kiliaan's dictionary,

38 Mario Braakman, 'Pronken met geleend licht. De Westeuropese geneesmiddelencultuur in de 16de en 17de eeuw', *Medische Antropologie*, 1990, pp. 25–39; Wolfgang Schivelbusch, *Das Paradies, der Geschmack und die Vernunft. Eine Geschichte der Genussmittel*, 1990. And *cf.* William Eamon's discussion of 'secrets' in *Science and the Secrets of Nature: Books of Secrets in Medieval and Early Modern Culture*, 1994: 'virtuosi gathered "secrets" not because they found them useful but because they gathered them as pleasant diversions and as ornaments of gentility' (p. 306).

which I mentioned above, 'drooghaerd' is defined, with a reference to the Roman playwright Terence, as 'homo aridus' ('dry man'), and 'valde auarus' ('very greedy'). This is the classic description of the miser.[39] In this sense, Bredero uses the word in the play *Angeniet* (1618): 'een Drooghist, waar uyt men nau sou parsen / Een droppel nats of twee; 't is al vervrosen stijf, / En hy en heeft gheen lust noch leven in sijn lijf' ('a Druggist from whom you could hardly squeeze a drop of liquid, who already is frozen and stiff, and whose body has neither lust nor life').[40] We also find examples of this in Six himself. In 'Antwoord aan Gerrit Brand den iongen' ('Answer to Geeraert Brandt the Younger') (J18, l. 8), he says, self-mockingly, that he is not suitable for love, and ironically calls himself a 'koel drogist' ('cool druggist'). The concept of humoral types figures in this self-portrayal. According to Galen, each humoral temperament consists of a combination of two of the four basic qualities: dry, moist, cold and warm. 'Dry' dominates two types of personality: the warm-dry *cholericus,* or 'hothead', and the cold-dry *melancholicus*. In this case, the 'drogaard' is the *melancholicus*. But, although 'droog' evokes connotations such as 'avaricious' and 'joyless', it could equally refer to more positive properties – 'sober' and 'subdued' – in contrast to the widespread image of the Dutch merchant in the early modern period as an ignorant, uninterested phlegmatic.[41]

This interpretation seems to form the basis for several of Six's texts. I will begin by discussing 'Het boek, aan den leeser' ('The Book, to the Reader') (J119), an important metapoem in Six's *oeuvre.* I will cite the first eight lines again:

Ik ben een boschmaagd, kind van zoo een droogen geest,
Meer doende, in droogery, dan boeken ooit geweest.
O Amstelvliet, uw druk gebuurende aan het Spaaren,
De vindster van die konst, was vroevrouw van dees blaaren.
Haar reed gerief, dat min, dan ouders pennen, kost,
Queekt werlden van papier, in schaapenleer gedost.
Haar kosten zyn zoo klein [...]

39 See the connotations 'drogist' in the WNT. Kiliaan's dictionary: dbnl.org/tekst/kilioo1etym01_01/kilioo1etym01_01_0001.php

40 G.A. Bredero, *Angeniet*, 1982, p. 179. *Cf.* also the judgment of the poet Jeremias de Decker as a 'simple *kruidenier*' in the reception of his poetry, Jeremias de Decker, *Goede vrydag ofte Het lijden onses heeren Jesy Christi*, 1978, pp. 6–7.

41 For the doctrine of temperaments in the early modern period, see Nancy G. Siraisi, *Medieval and Early Renaissance Medicine: An Introduction to Knowledge and Practice*, 1990. See also a reference book from Six's own time: Johan van Beverwijck, *Schat der gesontheyt*, 1656, pp. 1–78, especially pp. 13–24. On the representation of the Dutch as phlegmatics, see Dorothee Sturkenboom, 'Understanding Emotional Identities. The Dutch Phlegmatic Temperament as Historical Case Study', *BMGN*, 2014, pp. 163–191.

I am a virgin of the forest, the child of a dry spirit,
Devoted more to trading drugs than to books.
O flood of Amstel, your printing works near Spaarnestad,
The inventor of the art was a midwife of these pages.
The ease of her printer's art, which costs less than what our parents spent on pens,
Creates worlds of paper, dressed in parchment.
Her costs are just as small [...]

Six's collection of poems – his 'children' – is a printed work on the book market. He portrays his mental work as a material product. The print shop is described as a 'midwife' of the bundle. She 'creates worlds of paper' and 'her costs are just as small'. Six presents diligence and economy as the values on which the production of literature must be based: they are borne of a 'dry spirit'. And if we read a little farther, we find a list of questions that Six expects his poems to raise among readers from Amsterdam, and that go back to his profession as a merchant-druggist (l. 45–54):

Wie of die Six mach zyn? 't Is immers geen droogist?
Hoe is het meug'lik, dat die kaarle zoo veel wist?
Hy moet wis meer, dan ik, deurleesen, en deursoeken.
Hy weet wat meer dan ik. Maakt hy zoo heele boeken?
Wat mach er beeter zyn, of Vondels werk, of dat?
Wat heeft ons Amsterdam al geesten in de stad?
Men roept zoo van Homeer die in 't Latyn van Trooijen
Zoo deftigh schryven zou, men durft zoo veel uitstrooijen
Van Metteformis van Ovidius gemaakt,
Ik wed heur werk by dat noch hand noch vinger raakt.

Who could this Six be? Isn't he a druggist?
How is it possible that this chap could know so much?
He should certainly have read and searched through things more than I have.
He knows more than I do. Does he make many books?
Which ones are the best – Vondel's or his?
Do we have so many wise people here in this city of ours, Amsterdam?
People can talk as much as they want about Homer, who so beautifully
Wrote about Troy in Latin, and people may talk
About Ovid's *Metteformis*,
But I bet their works are nothing compared Six's.

We see here the same prejudices that Six tackled in 'Op quaade tongen': First, how can a merchant-druggist know so much? Second, does he want to compare himself to a celebrity such as Vondel or to great figures of the classical period? Six explains that a druggist is capable of writing learned texts, but he does not want to have anything to do with exalted praise. He rejects these prejudices by showing in quite some detail the lack of knowledge on the part of this lout ('kinkel') (l. 56), who speaks in dialect: Homer's epics were of course written in Greek, not Latin, and the correct name for Ovid's work is *Metamorphoses*. Vondel represents, as do Homer and Ovid, an elevated poetic style to which Six does not want his to be compared. The message is that poetry must be judged by a different yardstick. 'Ik traghte ook na geen lof' ('Nor do I seek fame'), writes the merchant-poet emphatically (l. 39). He opposes the expectations that Dutch readers have of poetry as something exalted and exclusive.

This self-portrayal as 'humble' or 'low' is explored in depth in two subsequent metapoems: 'Afscheid aan myn rymen' ('Farewell to my Rhymes', J120), where Six, following the example of the classical satirist Persius, describes his verses as deformed and deficient creatures – 'Wat haanen zyn dit sonder kammen, / Gebulten, scheelen, manken, lammen?' ('What kinds of roosters are these, without combs, humpbacked, squinting, limping, lame?') (l. 25–26) – poems that will generate criticism; and 'Begin met God' ('Beginning with God', J121), in which Six shows his Calvinistic background. To quote the first lines of the latter: 'De mensch behoort niets aan te raaken, / Eer hy den stuurman aller saaken, / Om raad, vraaght, needrigh van gemoed' ('No one should touch anything before humbly asking the helmsman of all things for advice') (l. 1–3). We recognise again D.V. Coornhert's ethical guidelines in these poems. In his *De Coopman*, Coornhert writes that, 'in order to be a good merchant, one must be a good Christian', and that the upstanding Christian merchant is a person that loves 'humility' and 'moderate sobriety'.[42] And in each of these poems we also find elements that were likely borrowed from the poem we mentioned in the introduction: 'Coornherts rymerien aenden rymlievenden leser': As with Six, in Coornhert the poems themselves speak. They tell of how they came into being, call the author 'their father', and present themselves as rhymes that are 'slecht ende recht, ruydt en grof' ('sincere and simple, plain and rough') and 'geensins verciert' ('not adorned at all') and that have nothing in common with the elevated, mythological 'Poeteryen' of contemporary writers, because Coornhert produces 'ware saken' ('true things') in Dutch, and distances himself 'vande hoge Parnasser spraken' ('the language of the high Parnassus').[43] But, unlike in Coornhert's poem, the self-critical attitude sometimes seems to turn into self-loathing. In another metapoem, 'Raad aan den geenen, die myn rymen mishaagen' ('Advice to Those who Dislike my Rhymes') (J393), Six writes that the paper on which they are written

42 'Dat om een goet coopman te zyn, een goet Christen moet wesen', 'hy bemint ende soekt die nederheyt [...] matige soberheyt', D.V. Coornhert, *De Coopman*, [1580] 1969, pp. 11 and 22.

43 D.V. Coornhert, *Het roerspel en de comedies van Coornhert*, 1955, pp. 156–159.

can be used as 'peeperhuisjes' (literally 'pepper houses', that is 'paper cones'), or, worse, as toilet paper. Aside from being an imitation of Horace, this must again be seen in the context of Calvinism. According to Susan Karant-Nunn, Calvinists must abase themselves before God.[44] In Horace, and especially in Persius, Six has apparently found a model for poetic self-abasement. I will return later to Six's *imitatio* of Persius.

Six's poetics of 'dryness' in the sense of 'sobriety' is also found in other texts. His self-image as a 'dry mind' is echoed in the expression 'myn drooge pluim' ('my dry quill') (in 'Myn antwoord, aan den selven', J258) – a reaction to a poem by Six's poet friend Reyer Anslo; in this text Six also presents himself as a 'bad poet', unable to write complete poems. He tells us his rhymes are 'only sketches' (l. 50 and 61). In giving his own interpretation of 'druggist' and 'dry', he is keen to fend off prejudices that readers might have based on his social background. This research into the social context of the early modern trade in drugs thus serves as a corrective to how Six has been presented in literary history. According to M.A. Schenkeveld-van der Dussen, Six's self-image as a rhymester is based on his professional background: a realistic bourgeois position that is closer to 'reality' than the 'universalism' of poets such as Vondel. However, in this chapter I have shown that this is also a construction. Six redefined his professional name in opposition to elements of his profession with which he did not want to be identified: uncontrolled passions, strangeness, and opulence.

This reading is also a corrective to the perception of Six as an idiosyncratic poet in literary history. In fact, he was not the only merchant-druggist who wrote poems and who consciously profiled himself as a grocer-poet. The collection by Six's fellow Amsterdammer and druggist, Sijbrand Feitama (1620–1701), *Christelijke en stigtelijke rymoeffeningen* (*Christian and Edifying Rhyme Exercises*) (1684), has several surprises in store. Not only is there a poem in the collection dedicated to Six van Chandelier, in which Feitama thanks him for his Psalms of David – there was thus contact between these two druggist-poets – but the book also contains texts in which a poetic programme is set out that has interesting parallels with Six's. In the foreword to the volume, the publishers of Feitama's poetry tell us that Feitama distanced himself from the great names of poetry: in the theme of his collection, 'die het Stigtelijke en Geestelijke raakt, is het geoorlofd verder van de hoogdraavendheid der hoog-geleerden af te wyken' ('which touches the Serene and Spiritual, it is permissible to move farther away from the grandiloquence of the learned'). And the opening poem shows interesting similarities to 'Het boek, aan den leeser'. I will quote from the beginning of the piece:

44 See Susan Karant-Nunn, *The Reformation of Feeling: Shaping the Religious Emotions in Early Modern Germany*, 2010, p. 252. See also Herman Roodenburg, 'The Body in the Reformation', in Ulinka Rublack (ed.), *The Oxford Handbook of the Protestant Reformations*, 2017, pp. 643–666. For 'Raad aan den geenen', see Jacobs, 1991 II, pp. 685–686.

Ziet hier een Mengel-moes gedicht
Van Rymen, door een Oud Drogist
Op 't Waater in de Gulde Bril;
Doorzing, of lees ze luid of stil.
't Zyn Psalmen, Lied'ren, en Gebêen,
En overzettingen, by een
Gebragt door Lieden zeer Geleerd,
Die deezen Rymer hoog waardeert.

Look at this, a mishmash of a book
of Rhymes by an Old Druggist
From ''t Waater in de Gulde Bril' [Feitama's address in Amsterdam].
Sing the poems, or read them aloud or quietly.
There are Psalms, Songs and Prayers,
And translations, Gathered together
By Learned Friends
Who greatly appreciate this Rhymester.

In spite of this humble presentation of Feitama as a poet, the publishers of his book include poems in his collection that contain references to exotica and stimulants.[45] But it should also be said that Feitama's poetry is not at the same literary level as that of Six's. Feitama's text is simpler in terms of its language and style.

The interpretation of the druggist as a socially responsible person in Six's poetry is clear in 'Mildicheit, aan Tomas Alein, Sjerif, Van Londen' ('Courtesy to Thomas Alleyn, Sheriff, in London') (J436). The text is addressed to an English grocer who had been apprenticed to a certain 'vanden Bergh' (l. 14) in Amsterdam, but who had now made a career in administrative circles in London.[46] Six likely wrote this text as a result of a reception given by this London sheriff in the summer of 1655, when Six was on a commercial trip to England.[47] '[D]ie pottebakkers soon, / Geklommen, op een kooninghs throon' ('That son of a potter, who climbed onto a royal throne', l. 21–22), Six calls him – referring to King Agathocles of ancient Syracuse, who was

45 *Cf.* titles such as 'Vraage op de Tabak ('Question on Tobacco') and 'Op een Quikzilver Dief' ('On a Quicksilver Thief'). See also Chapter 5, note 19. *Cf.* also the self-presentation in D.P. Pers, *Suyp-Stad, of Dronckaerts Leven* (*Guzzle City, or a Drunkard's Life*), 1978, pp. 89–90: 'mijn verdorde penn' and 'mijn drooge sangh' ('my dried-up pen') and ('my dry song'). The druggist should not be confused with his grandson and namesake who was also a poet, Sijbrand Feitama (1694–1758).

46 On the early modern English grocer: Jon Stobart, *Sugar and Spice: Grocers and Groceries in Provincial England, 1650–1830*, 2012; on Thomas Alleyn: John Benjamin Heath, *Some Account of the Worshipful Company of Grocers of the City of London*, 1854, pp. 274–276.

47 Jacobs, 1991 II, p. 748.

proud of his potter's origins. In the text, Six invokes their common social origin. He writes that they both belong to the 'droogh geslacht' ('dry family') (l. 19). And he argues that one can go quite far with such a background. When Six was invited to eat with him, Thomas Alleyn was a 'sjerif' in London. Six predicts that he will climb higher up the administrative ladder and become Mayor of London – 'drogisten roem dan, op dat hoofd, / Dat u een groot faam belooft' ('druggists will then praise you, whom a great fame is promised', l. 77–78). In 1659 or 1660, Alleyn did indeed become mayor of London. When King Charles II returned to England in 1660, he was welcomed by Alleyn, who was elevated to the rank of knight and baronet soon afterwards. The text expresses not only Six's gratitude to his host, but apparently his own aspirations: he wants to show his Dutch readers that druggists are reliable and virtuous, and that they can well be entrusted with leadership positions. In the sixteenth century and the beginning of the seventeenth, grocers did indeed sit on Dutch city councils, but starting in the mid-seventeenth century the possibilities for social mobility seemed to lessen. Six expresses the wish that he himself can have such a career.

Conclusion

In the end, Six was never made a regent or a burgomaster. In later texts there seems to be a certain disappointment with his social status: in his contribution to Jacobus Heyblocq's famous *album amicorum* (which I quoted in the beginning of this chapter), Six expresses embarrassment at having had his name recorded in an album full of distinguished names: 'A merchant should stay among merchants'. The same is true of 'Erkentenisse, aan den eedelen heer Joan Six, heer van Vromaade, oudscheepen, voor synen Muiderberg' ('Acknowledgement, to the Noble Sir Joan Six, Lord of Vromade, Alderman, for his Poem "Muiderberg"') (J625), which appeared in 1676 in pamphlet form, addressed to the famous Jan Six (1618–1700), the namesake of our druggist-poet. It is one of the last verses we know by Six van Chandelier. In it, the poet recalls a remark from his schooldays: he was called the Small Six; Six van Vromade, the Great Six. Now that verdict is truer than ever, Six observes, pointing to the contrast between their social careers: 'Ik ben nergens toe bequaam, / Dan om koopmanschap te dryven' ('I am fit for nothing but conducting business') (l. 51–52). While the 'beroemde weetenschappen, / En onkreukelik gemoed' ('renowned knowledge in many fields and unimpeachable mind') will bring the aforementioned 'van top tot top, / In eerampten, heerlik op' ('to ever greater heights, gloriously, in high office') (l. 57–62). A few years after the publication of this pamphlet, in 1679, he was given a seat on the city council, and in 1691 he became burgomaster. The leadership career of his namesake seemed to be a desirable, but no longer achievable, goal for Six van Chandelier.

Although Six van Chandelier could never have become a Six van Vromade, there are examples of people from the same social background who managed to gain status and prestige. One of them was Jan Commelin (1629–1692). From his shop 'In de Crocodil' on the Kalverstraat – the same street in which Six's 'De Vergulde Eenhoorn' was located – this Commelin supplied pharmacists and hospitals with 'dry spices' that he had purchased from the VOC and the WIC. He used the wealth that he amassed through this trade to make his career. Commelin moved from the Kalverstraat to the Herengracht, held honourable positions such as the regent of the Spinning House, and was personally selected by Stadtholder William III to sit as adviser to the city council of Amsterdam. In 1682, together with Johan Huydecoper, he founded the new Hortus Botanicus of Amsterdam, to which he was appointed as supervisory board member and botanist. In this position, he wrote and compiled important botanical works, such as the first flora of the Netherlands, which I mentioned above.[48] Although Commelin did not get to be burgomaster, his career was impressive. When the new Hortus was founded, the painter Gerard Hoet portrayed him as a learned gentleman in a study full of flowers, plants and botanical books – perhaps specimens from his own Dutch flora – and with a stylish environment in the background – perhaps a reference to his country estate, Zuyderhout, in Haarlem, which he had bought in 1676 with money from his wife, Belia Vinck, who was quite rich (Plate 4).[49] His past as a merchant-grocer of 'In de Crocodil' had been completely erased. Although he did not have any medical training, he was – in the words of Luuc Kooijmans – a 'self-made botanist'.[50] Commelin's career is a further example of the theme of this chapter: the difficulties associated with having a social profile as a merchant-druggist in the early modern Republic. The terms 'druggist' and 'drugs' did not represent a sense of reality, in

48 This new hortus is not to be confused with the first hortus of the city, founded in 1638 – see my discussion of 'Steetuinkroon aan Joannes Snippendal' ('Crown of the City Garden to Joannes Snippendaal') (J146), Chapter 4, pp. 135–136.

49 Commelin's first wife was Digna van Wissel, who came from the family of one of the first merchants to start a grocery business in Amsterdam, after the centre of world trade had shifted from Antwerp to Amsterdam (Dudok van Heel, 1976, pp. 1–11).

50 D.O. Wijnands, *The botany of the Commelins*, 1983, pp. 6–9; Luuc Kooijmans, *De doodskunstenaar. De anatomische lessen van Frederik Ruysch*, 2004, pp. 155–160. Although Commelin was in practice the manager of the Hortus Amsterdam, he never became a professor at the institution. That position was held by Frederik Ruysch. For the paradoxical career of Commelin, first as a trader in exotics and then as a collector of native plants, see Alix Cooper, *Inventing the indigenous: Local Knowledge and Natural History in Early Modern Europe*, 2007, pp. 46–47. For the portrait of Jan Commelin, see N. Middelkoop (ed.), *Kopstukken: Amsterdammers geportretteerd 1600–1800*, 2002, pp. 164–165. I will return to Commelin in Chapter 4. *Cf.* the career change of the family Breyne in Danzig, from 'materialists' to scientists: Jos Kuijlen, 'De Danziger botanicus en koopman Jacob Breyne (1637-1697) en zijn betekenis voor de Hollandse plantkunde', *Tijdschrift voor de Geschiedenis der Geneeskunde, Natuurwetenschappen, Wiskunde en Techniek*, 1977, pp. 116–118.

line with the view of Six's professional background in literary history. They were terms that, on the contrary, generated negative associations – in terms not only of the traditional flaws associated with commerce, such as avarice and uncontrolled passions, but also of outlandishness and opulence, and even the miraculous. Six's poetry transcends the paradigm of realism.

I have also shown that Six's case was not isolated. Merchants based their self-presentation on a collective feeling, according to which they endowed their profession with positive qualities. The appeal to a common descent in 'Mildicheit, aan Tomas Alein' testifies to this. The question is, of course, whether other merchants to whom Six wrote poems were willing to be portrayed as druggists. There are no references to Six in Jan Commelin's work (although we know they were in contact with each other). But as we have seen, Six was not the only merchant to profile himself publicly as a sober druggist-poet. Friends of Sijbrand Feitama published a collection of his poems, where he is presented as a humble druggist, just like Six. Feitama must have admired the poetry of his famous fellow druggist. It is possible that the publishers of Feitama's book were familiar with this affinity he felt. They may, indeed, have used Six as a source of inspiration when writing the introduction to the book. Like Six, Feitama is presented here as an honest and humble druggist-poet.

3. Drugs in the Wunderkammer

Abstract

Chapter 3 is devoted to a non-medical use of drugs: as collector's items and objects of research in the Wunderkammer, which was popular in the early modern period. I argue that Joannes Six van Chandelier sees the wondrous nature of exotic collectibles as sources not only of sensory pleasure and of insights into nature, but also of moral danger, especially the vices avarice and *curiositas*, an immoderate and un-Christian thirst for knowledge. In poems on rarities such as bezoar stone, tulips, and human and animal bones, Six develops literary strategies that present himself as a learned merchant who recognises these dangers and has them well in hand.

Keywords: Cabinet of curiosities, senses, avarice, curiosity, bezoar stone, tulips

Ziet Sijbrand Feitama hier uitgebeeld na 't Leeven,
Zijn Geest wort daagelijks weetgierig omgedreeven
In Prenten na de Konst, in Vreemde Droogerij,
In wond're Raarigheen, alsook in Poësy.

See Sijbrand Feitama, here portrayed after Life,
His Spirit dwells everyday curiously
Around Art prints, around Foreign Drugs,
Around marvellous Rarities, but also around Poetry.
– Jan Norel[1]

1 Caption on a portrait of the 65-year-old druggist-poet Sijbrand Feitama. The caption reads, 'In Amsterdam, 1685', written by the poet and mathematician Jan Norel. The portrait is a parchment drawing made by Jan van Somer. See Ellinoor Bergvelt & Reneé Kistemaker (eds.), *De wereld binnen handbereik. Nederlandse kunst- en rariteitenverzamelingen, 1585–1735*, 1992, II, pp. 83–84.

Spaans, R., *Dangerous Drugs: The Self-Presentation of the Merchant-Poet Joannes Six van Chandelier (1620–1695)*. Taylor & Francis Group, 2020
DOI 10.5117/9789462983543_CH03

Cabinets of curiosities

An interest in rarities played a central role in the early modern intellectual world. Since the Middle Ages, monarchs and aristocrats had had collections of curiosities that were well known throughout Europe and that were must-see stopping-off points for scientists and scholars travelling abroad. This practice of building up a collection of works of art and natural materials spread to other social strata in the Renaissance:

> Closely connected with this new surge of interest in natural wonders was the emergence of collecting as an activity not just of patricians and princes, as in the High and Later Middle Ages, but of scholars and medical men as well. Unlike princely collectors, who continued to prize precious materials and elaborate workmanship, physicians and apothecaries collected mainly *naturalia*, which reflected their own interests in therapeutics and were relatively affordable.[2]

This trend was particularly pronounced in the Dutch Republic. The collectors were usually physicians, apothecaries and merchants from the upper middle class. Noteworthy examples include the famous collections of Bernardus Paludanus, a doctor, and Jan Jacobsz Swammerdam, an apothecary and the father of the famous researcher.[3] But they were not the only ones: there were also a good number of smaller cabinets in the Netherlands. As can be seen from the lines by the poet Jan Norel quoted above in his portrait of Sijbrand Feitama, one of Six's fellow druggists, whom we discussed in the preceding chapter, Feitama was able to present himself as a collector of 'Foreign Drugs' and 'Marvellous Rarities' (Fig. 3.1). The shop of the merchant-apothecary Joan Breyne – the Breyne family were among Six's trade connections – also contained an *exoticotamia*, a cabinet of exotic objects, in which not only *naturalia* but also *artificialia* – works of art from foreign cultures – were on display.[4]

The merchant-druggists were thus an important group within the collectors of *curiosa*, and their cabinets had a somewhat broader function. On the one hand,

2 Daston & Park, 1998, p. 149.

3 See the standard work on collections of curiosities in the early modern Netherlands: Ellinoor Bergvelt & Renée Kistemaker (eds.), *De wereld binnen handbereik. Nederlandse kunst- en rariteitenverzamelingen, 1585–1735*, I and II (exhibition catalogue), 1992; and Ellinoor Bergvelt *et al.* (eds.), *Collection: from the Cabinet of Curiosities to the Art Museum*, 1993. And see Eric Jorink, *Reading the Book of Nature in the Dutch Golden Age, 1575–1715*, 2010, pp. 257–344.

4 The English doctor and philosopher John Locke describes Joan Breyne's collection as 'a very great collection of natural and artificial rarities most brought from the East Indies'. See Bergvelt & Kistemaker, 1992, pp. 274, 310. And see item numbers 114, 120 and 126 in Bergvelt & Kistemaker, 1992, II. Breyne (1634–1693), who lived on the Singel, was a nephew of the aforementioned Danziger merchant-druggist Jacob Breyne. Joan Breyne had done his training as a druggist at 'Sara Juliaens', Six's family business (Bergvelt & Kistemaker, 1992, p. 315), as had Jacob Breyne the Elder and the Younger.

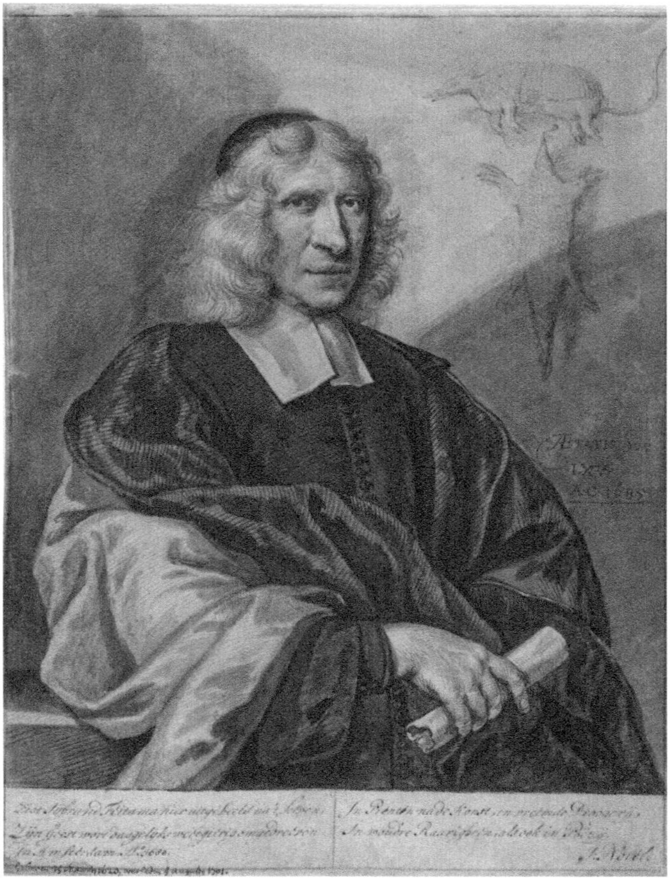

Fig. 3.1: Jan van Somer, *Sijbrand Feitama*, 1685. Parchment drawing. (© Amsterdam Historical Museum).

the collectibles served the purposes of scientific research, and on the other they were part of their stock of medical supplies. The curiosities being exhibited could thus be turned into medicines for sale without a problem. But to what extent these traders in exotic wares were willing to sell the exotica they had on display is another matter. They seemed to be adept at exploiting the impressive character of their cabinets. This is evident from Sijbrand Feitama's answer to Jan Norel, the author of the verses in his portrait, as to why he was collecting exotic, fearsome animals:

Het Versje, Vriend Norel, door u my opgedraagen
Vereist myn antwoord, op het geen gy my komt vraagen,
Als met verwondering; hoe dat het kan geschiên,
Dat zoo veel Monsters in myn Winkel zyn te zien?

Daar gy my oordeelt van natuure meedelydig,
En vreede-lievend, dog dit schynt daar teegen strydig;
Dat zulke dieren, van een overwreeden aard,
Door een meedoogend mensch met lusten zyn vergaard.
Ik gaf u groot gelyk, indien dezelfde leefden,
Maar wyl ze dood zyn, agt ik daar voor beesten
Onnoozel. Dog ik weet, dat gy maar met my speelt,
Dies d'eerste en tweede vraag van u my niet verveelt;
Zy dienen tot vermaak, wanneer de Kooplui wachten.
Geloof my hier vry in, 'k heb anders geen gedagten.
't Zyn dog meest vreemdigheên, die in myn winkel zijn.
Daar ieder een voor vreest, al is 't hem medicyn.

The verse, my friend Norel dedicated to me,
Demands my answer, on the thing you ask me,
With astonishment: How is it possible
That there are so many Monsters to see in my Shop?
The fact that you judge me to be a sympathetic
And peace-loving person, makes this a contradiction:
That such animals, of a cruel nature,
Are desirously gathered together by a compassionate man.
I would completely agree with you, if these animals lived,
But as they are dead, I consider them to be harmless beasts.
Anyway, I understand that you are jesting with me.
Therefore, the first and second questions from you do not bore me:
They serve for entertainment for the waiting Merchants.
Trust me in what I say: I have no other thoughts.
It is mostly strange things that are in my shop.
Everybody fears them, as though they were their medicines.[5]

Roelof van Gelder has gone into more detail about the motives people had for collecting curiosities. One was the sensory pleasure that a collection aroused. He writes that shells, precious stones, and the skins and armour of animals unknown in Europe had a stimulating effect on the visitor's sense of smell, their hearing, their vision, and their taste. According to the theories of Daston and Park, beholding wonders was an

5 'Aan Johannes Norel' – 'Aan den Zelven', Feitama, 1684, pp. 267–268. On the contact between Norel and Feitama, see B.J. Broos, 'Notitie der Teekeningen van Sybrand Feitama: de boekhouding van drie generaties verzamelaars van oude Nederlandse tekenkunst', *Oud Holland*, 1984, pp. 15–17. The fear of medicines, because of their nasty taste, was a *topos* in the early modern period.

emotionally unsettling experience. They believed it astonished, enchanted or even frightened the beholder. At the same time, the feeling of wonderment was a cognitive act: the beholder could get new insights from it.[6] When the French physician Charles Patin visited the house of one member of the Witsen family, who were known for their collections of curiosities, he wrote that it seemed to be built not so much for living in as to please the eye. An example of the latter is the poem 'Dankbaerheid aen Johan Volkaertsz. / Konst-yveraer, en Lief-hebber der Vreemdigheden, / Over het mild vertoonen syner seldsaemheden' ('Gratitude to Johan Volkaertsz. Advocate of Art, and Lover of Strange Things, for the Generous Display of his Rarities') by Joachim Oudaen, a poem of praise for the cloth merchant Jan Volckertsz's collection of *naturalia*. At the sight of the collection of curiosities, the glittering carbuncles, mother-of-pearl, and so on, Oudaen senses that ''t vernuft word stom, en reikt niet veer genoug' ('reason falls silent, and does not reach far enough [to understand the phenomena]'), because a 'gansche Eeuw sou't alles niet verhalen' ('whole century would not be enough to explain all this'); 'Weg Plinien, Albarten, Aristotelen' ('Away with you, disciples of Pliny, Albertus Magnus, and Aristotle'), he continues. For Oudaen, the sight of this is a transcendent cognitive experience.[7]

Although Feitama does not use such strong words as Oudaen, the same effect is attributed to Feitama's collection. Other than as medicines for sale, Feitama's exotic animals served as sensual entertainment for waiting customers. In spite of the modest description, a certain pride in his possessions can be read between the lines. In the background of the portrait of Feitama mentioned above, two of his 'monsters' are depicted: a stuffed armadillo and a stuffed Javanese pangolin – possibly the showpieces from his medical supply/collection of *naturalia*.[8] As we shall see, the sensory effect played an important role in the treatment of rarities in Six's poetry.

Possessing a cabinet of curiosities must therefore be seen in the light of the gentlemen's codes. Such a cabinet was testament to its owner's scientific interest

6 See Roelof van Gelder, 'Noordnederlandse verzamelingen in de zeventiende eeuw', in: Ellinoor Bergvelt *et al.* (eds.), *Verzamelen: van rariteitenkabinet tot kunstmuseum,* 1993, p. 138; and Daston & Park, 1998. And *cf.* 'sinnelickheden' ('sensual things') the word for curiosities used by the pharmacist Christiaen Porret – see Claudia Swan, 'Collecting *Naturalia* in the Shadow of Early Modern Dutch Trade', in: Londa Schiebinger & Claudia Swan (eds.), *Colonial Botany: Science, Commerce, and Politics in the Early Modern World*, 2005, p. 230.

7 Joachim Oudaen, *Poëzy, verdeeld in drie deelen* (*Poetry, Divided into Three Parts*), 1712, part I, pp. 138–140; see also Bergvelt & Kistemaker, 1992, p. 331.

8 On Feitama's collection, see Bergvelt & Kistemaker, 1992, p. 318. On apothecaries and merchant-druggists as collectors, see Jaap van der Veen: 'Dit klain Vertrek bevat een Weereld vol gewoel. Negentig Amsterdammers en hun kabinetten', in: Bergvelt & Kistemaker, 1992, pp. 242–243. See also Claudia Swan's discussion of the *naturalia* that were exhibited in the *hortus* of Leiden University and that were considered to be *materia medica:* 'They were clearly appreciated for their exoticism, their foreignness, rather than for their medical application', Swan, 2005, p. 226.

and worldliness. Let us look again at Jan Norel's lines of verse on Feitama's portrait: they tell us that his spirit is characterised by a curiosity for art prints, poetry, foreign drugs and wondrous rarities. As a merchant-druggist, Feitama will have been satisfied with the verse, which presents him as a *gentleman-virtuoso*.[9] Crucial to our understanding of the verses is the term 'curious', which in the early modern era was undergoing redefinition: At the end of period, 'curiosity' was less closely associated with desire, unhealthy knowledge, instinct and pride – the meanings Augustine gives to *curiositas* in his *Confessions* – and regarded more and more as something positive, as the hallmark of the selfless 'connoisseur' or *curieux*. But in the seventeenth century the term had still not lost its negative association, as I will show in this chapter.[10]

Bezoar stone

Jan Norel's lines of poetry might just as well have been put under a portrait of Six van Chandelier. In view of the close connection between trade and the collection of *exotica*, it is likely that the Six van Chandelier family's shop and showroom also served as a cabinet of curiosities. The name of their shop in Kalverstraat, 'De Vergulde Eenhoorn' ('The Gilded Unicorn'), itself testifies to a longing for the wondrous and the rare. The German student Christian Knorr von Rosenroth, who visited various cabinets in Amsterdam in 1663, writes in a report of his travels that he had seen a walrus tusk in 'Den Eenhoorn in Kalverstraat'.[11] He probably means Six van Chandelier's shop. In Six's poetry there are many examples of an interest in *artificialia* – some poems are dedicated to precious and wonderful art objects and paintings[12] – but also, of course, to *naturalia* such as 'veders paapegaais op

9 For the interest *virtuosi* had in exotics and curiosities, see Brian Cowan, *The Social Life of Coffee: The Emergence of the British Coffeehouse*, 2005; William Eamon, *Science and the Secrets of Nature: Books of Secrets in Medieval and Early Modern Culture*, 1994, pp. 221–229.

10 For the change in the meaning of the term, see Daston & Park, 1998, pp. 122–123, 303–310, and 434, note 7.

11 R. Fuchs & J.C. Breen, 'Aus dem "Itinerarium" des Christian Knorr von Rosenroth', *Jaarboek Amstelodamum*, 1916, p. 221. The English translation is as follows: 'A tooth of a manatee, curved like a ram's horn. I have seen one like it, only much larger, in the Kalverstraat in The Unicorn, whose lower cross-section is one-and-a-half feet in height.' Since manatees do not have large teeth, this must have been a walrus tusk (in the Latin text, Knorr speaks of 'Dens Mannati').

12 For example, 'Liefdes voorbeeld, afgebeeldt door Rubbens' (J380). Rubens was a much-sought-after artist in early modern art cabinets. Rubens was in fact a distant relative of Six. My thanks to Wim Heijnen for this information. And *cf.* the silver *tazza* with a bacchanalian scene in 'Aan Jan van Mansdale' (J371); and rare guides on antique and modern monuments in Rome in 'Gelúk op reis, aan Antoni Duivelaar' (J302).

d'Indiaan' ('parrot feathers on the Indian') and the bones of what was said to be a giant from Basel, which were famous in the seventeenth century.[13] In 'Aan Arnoud van Someren' (J166), Six praises the transformation of *naturalia* into *artificialia*. Six expresses his admiration for how van Someren has turned raw rosewood, a material that Six had previously given to him, into two knives with handles, which Six now receives as gifts. And in a poem we find a bizarre comparison: Six calls his favourite poet, Horace, a bird of paradise – the wondrous bird from the Far East that was the highlight of many cabinets of curiosities.[14] In this chapter I will discuss four poems in which Six treats materials as *curiosities*. I will show how Six sees the wondrous nature of exotic collectibles not only as a source of sensory pleasure and of insights into nature's mysteries, but also as a source of social and moral dangers. What I am interested in here is the literary strategies that Six develops in these poems in order to establish himself as a learned, down-to-earth merchant who recognises these dangers and has them well in hand.

That the merchandise Six had in stock served more or less as a cabinet of curiosities is evident from 'Dank, aan Isaak de Bra, voor een besoarsteen, van Rio de Plata meegebracht, en my vereert' ('Thanks to Isaak de Bra for a Bezoar Stone Brought from Río de la Plata and Presented to Me') (J467). The text is a tribute to the merchant Isaak de Bra, who gave Six this rarity from the West Indies, l. 21–28:

Hoe langh ik dees robyn,
Erfvyand van fenyn,
Aan anderen vertoon, of in myn kas sie leggen,
Zoo zal myn dankbaar hart verplicht goedaardigh seggen:
Dit is dat duur juweel,
Uit 's werrelds vierde deel,
De silvervliet, op groot gevaar van schip, en leeven,
Onthandelt, door de Bra, my onverdient gegeeven.

As long as I show this ruby,
This arch-enemy of venom,
To other people, or put it on display on my cabinet,
My grateful heart will be obliged to say good-naturedly:
This is the expensive jewel
From the fourth corner of the world,
Which was, unwarrantedly, handed to me by De Bra,
At great risk to his ship and his life.

13 'Hangelroede [Fishing rod], aan Arnoud van Someren' (J336), r. 12; 'Schetse van Venecie' (J97), l. 71–72.
14 See Chapter 8, pp. 280–281.

Like Feitama, Six mentions that he will not sell this drug to his customers, but will store and exhibit it in his shop as 'an expensive jewel, / out of the fourth corner of the world'. Notice the *topos* of the heroic merchant in this poem. Six himself confesses that he is 'geen Merkuur op wegh' (l. 7) – not a commercial traveller in the East or West Indies – but says that Isaac de Bra was. Six praises Bra for the great risks he has taken to obtain these *exotica*.[15] He calls the bezoar a 'ruby' and a 'jewel' in the quotation – but just what is a bezoar? The most common kind, *lapis bezoar orientalis*, came from bezoar goats living in Persia, but *lapis bezoar occidentalis*, which came from llamas and vicuñas from Peru, was also popular, as we can see from this poem. A bezoar is a petrifaction found in the gallbladder or stomach of these animals (Fig. 3.2). In the Middle Ages, this rare item was considered to be a medicine as fabulous and mystical as the horn of a unicorn. It was seen as an antidote to all kinds of poisons.[16] Johan van Beverwijck writes that a bezoar works 'through special and hidden properties against poison and poisonous bites, malignancy caused by fevers, and other diseases'; and is so popular that it is subject to 'many forgeries'.[17] Its exclusivity is also evident from the fact that the stone was preserved in golden frames and holders, and that it occupied a prominent place in cabinets of curiosities. If we bear this in mind, Six's enthusiasm is understandable. At another point in the text, the Calvinist even links the 'wondrous power' of the stone to the 'heilig oliesel' ('holy unction'), the sacrament for the dying in the Catholic Church (l. 17–19). This expression of thanks in poetic form also points to another non-medical characteristic that is attributed to this medicine. It serves as proof of the strong friendship, and the positive trading relationship, between De Bra and Six, and thus also as proof of Six's well-established position as a trader.

Tulips versus shells

In *Poësy*, however, there is also some ambivalence regarding the collection and exhibition of *exotica*. I will discuss three poems that reflect this uncertainty. First, there is 'Val van Haarlems Flora' ('Fall of the Flora of Haarlem') (J163), a text about the tulip mania of 1637. According to Anne Goldgar, collecting tulips should not be seen as a separate phenomenon, but as part of a broader fascination with the

15 For the notion of the heroic merchant, see Laura Caroline Stevenson, *Praise and Paradox: Merchants and Craftsmen in Elizabethan Popular Literature*, 2002.

16 Lemery, 1743, pp. 101–102; Bergvelt & Kistemaker, 1992, p. 243; Van Andel 1928, pp. 95–110.

17 'Uyt sonderlinge, ende verborgen eygenschap tegen vergif, ende vergiftige beten, Quaataardigheydt in Koortsen, ende andere sieckten [...] menigvuldigh vervalschen', *Schat der ongesontheydt* (*Treasure of Ill-Health*), 1656, p. 46.

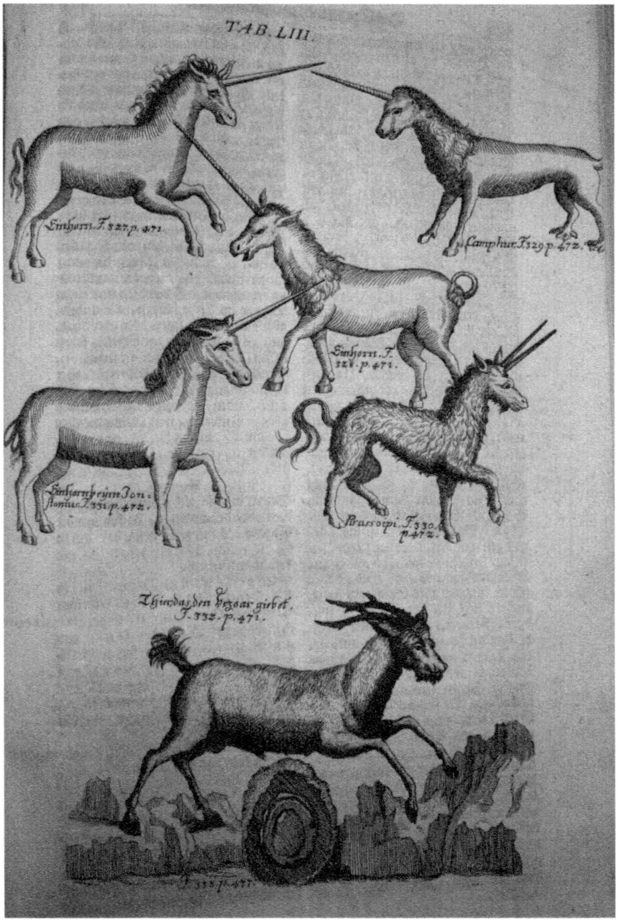

Fig. 3.2: Illustration of unicorns and a bezoar goat with a bezoar stone in Pierre Pomet, *Der aufrichtige Materialist und Specereÿ-Händler* […], 1717. (© University Library of Oslo).

strange and the mysterious.[18] When tulips first arrived in the Low Countries, it was even ascribed healing powers.[19] Six himself emphasises its exotic origin. In the poem he calls it a 'kappadooker bloem' (l. 7). Cappadocia is a region in Turkey.[20]

'Val van Haarlems Flora' is in the form of a literary still life. The tulips depicted are accompanied by the typical attributes of this motif in painting: various types of

18 For example, together with various exotic products, Tulips figure in a personification of Asia in the decoration of the Amsterdam Town Hall. Asia is presented as a woman in exotic clothing, accompanied by her three children, each of whom offers a gift from the Far East: incense, spices and tulips. See Anne Goldgar, *Tulipmania: Money, Honor, and Knowledge in the Dutch Golden Age*, 2007, p. 11.

19 Goldgar, 2007, pp. 20–61.

20 Jacobs, 1991 II, p. 287.

shells, horns and insects (Plate 5). The role of the shells deserves special attention, since they are used as a contrast to the tulips. In a comparison between these two types of collector's items, Six discusses which is more valuable from a moral standpoint. The shells come out on top: they are imperishable, unlike the tulips, which are 'reckless, despicable and brittle' (l. 5–6). By contrast, neither winter frost nor summer vermin damage the shells (l. 25–32):

> Maar de geestge schelpen derven,
> Op heur onvergaande verven,
>   Niet vergaande voor de stof,
>   Stoffen met gewisser lof.
> Sy verachten soomerplaagen,
> En die 's winters 't land deurjaagen.
>   Al het snood gewurmte mydt,
>   Dat het, op dat harde, byt.

> But the artful shells,
> With their imperishable colours,
> Which do not perish before all other things perish,
> May [therefore] brag with more certain fame.
> They evade the plagues of the summer,
> And those that drive through the land in the winter.
> All the pernicious worms avoid
> Biting on these hard shells.

Six uses the durability of shells as an image for reliability and steadfastness, while presenting the transience of tulips as a symbol of fickleness – a quality with which tulips were indeed associated at the time, as evidenced by the title of the text. In the end, the significant price increase and the subsequent collapse of the tulip trade and its social consequences are outlined (l. 45–69): Six concludes that the tulip trade reflects the fickle 'handel' ('trade', but also 'behaviour') of the flower itself (l. 69): it grows, withers and falls.

Myth has it that people from all social strata of the population were swept up by tulip mania, but in her study on the tulip trade, Anne Goldgar tells us that the phenomenon was limited to a smaller group – mainly traders and craftsmen from the middle class, such as pharmacists and merchant druggists.[21] This reality was apparently palpable to Six: the poet's father came from Haarlem, his uncle Abraham went bankrupt in Haarlem, and another relative, the Haarlem merchant Hans Baert,

21 See Chapter 3, 'Florists', in Goldgar, 2007.

appears in historical presentations on tulipmania. Baert was involved in conflicts with Amsterdammers to whom he had sold tulips, but who had refused to accept the bulbs and pay the purchase price. This Baert is in all probability the same 'Hans Baard', a merchant colleague and a cousin of the poet, to whom Six addresses a series of poems in *Poësy*.[22] In a contest between the two commodities, the merchant-poet shows that he chooses the more morally defensible product, and is keen to show that he knows the difference between reputable and disreputable trade.

Bones of animals and humans

A completely different kind of *curiosa* is discussed in another 'literary still life' by Six. 'Op doodshoofden, en geraamten van beesten, ten huise van Jan Gerritsen Indies heelmeester. Aan den selves' ('On human heads and skeletons of beasts, in the house of Jan Gerritsen Indies, Surgeon. To the same person') (J125). Indies was a cousin of Six van Chandelier's. As the title shows, the poem is about a collection of human heads and animal skeletons that Six has been allowed to study at the surgeon's home. Six may have seen the collection when he was delivering medicinal spices, and wrote this text as a token of gratitude both for the purchase the surgeon had made and for the opportunity to view the collection. Commercial and family interests coincided in the early modern period. The emphasis on bones as a collector's item is logical in view of Gerritsen Indies's profession: anatomical knowledge was important to the practice of surgery.[23]

The poem expresses both a fascination for and a fear of the collection. Six tells us that thoughts of death, which is in store for every human being, come to the fore for the viewer (l. 5–12):

  Aansie, zoo dringht dat stomme been
  Een stem, door bei myn nieren, heen.
Geen duistre brandklok kan zoo baaren,
Als deesen myn gedacht vervaaren.

22 Mike Dash, *Tulipomania: The Story of the World's Most Coveted Flower & the Extraordinary Passions It Aroused*, 2000, pp. 190–191; and Chapter 4, 'Grieving Money', in: Goldgar, 2007. Six's two poems to Hans Baard, 'Letter to Hans Baard in Haarlem' (J211) and 'Fooi' (J212), will be discussed in Chapter 8. Tulips are not mentioned in the document on Abraham Six's bankruptcy – see Appendix II. The bankruptcy could also have been a consequence of Abraham's enterprise in Ingria – see Chapter 1, p. 50.

23 Jan Gerritsen Indies was married to Catharina Kemp, daughter of Catharina Juliens, Six's maternal aunt – see Appendix II. The father of Jan, Gerrit Indies was a barber-surgeon in de Sint Jansstraat in Amsterdam – see Jacobs, 1991 II, p. 235. Gerrit Indies can be seen in 'Anatomical Lesson by Dr. Sebastiaen Egbertsz. de Vrij' (1563-1621), attributed to Nicolaes Eliasz. Pickenoy, dated 1619, exhibited at Amsterdam Museum.

Hier pronkt een langhgehalsde swaan,
En daar een kluchtge baaviaan,
En aan de syden staan dry koppen
Van menschen, schrikkelyke poppen.

Look at us – thus those dumb bones
Make a voice permeate both of my kidneys.
No horrible fire bell causes fright
As much as these bones alarm my thought.
Here, a long-necked swan preens,
And there, a funny baboon,
And on the sides, there are three heads
Of human beings, terrifying dolls.

Especially the sight of the three human heads is terrifying. Six experiences this fear physically: a voice with a dangerous message that penetrates the kidneys.[24] The heads were probably the highlight of Gerritsen Indies's anatomical collection. By 'dolls' Six presumably means shrunken heads – that is, human heads that had been reduced and preserved after a cumbersome process (the removal of skull, fat and eyes, and subsequently the cooking and drying of the head). This custom was still followed in the early modern period in New Guinea and in the Amazon region, where the shrunken heads were used for ritual purposes. The three heads referred to probably came from one of these areas (Fig. 3.3). We read in the following passage that their appearance not only arouses fear of the barbaric practices of foreign peoples, but also raises dangerous questions about the afterlife. Six writes that the heads prompt us to distort religious truths (l. 23–30):

Hoor daar des Sadduceers schimp:
Daar praalen nu die braave geesten,
Vermengelt met geraamt der beesten.
O menschen kind, wat zyt ghe trots?
Dit been, wiens vleisch nu wat verrots,
Leert u bemerken 't broose leeven,
Van syn bewooners opgegeeven [...]

Hear the mockery of the Sadducees:
There, the noble people are parading about,

24 *Cf.* the *Statenvertaling* comment on Proverbs 23:16, where the kidneys are described as the 'inwendichste krachten der ziele' ('innermost forces of the soul').

Among skeletons of beasts.
O human child, why so proud?
This bone, whose flesh is now rotten away,
Teaches you the fragility of life,
Which has been abandoned by its residents [...]

'The mockery of the Sadducees' refers to the ridicule of the Sadducees, a religious group within Judaism that questioned the Christian resurrection.[25] The sight of such a mixture of human and animal bones – and worse still, of the shrunken heads, which imply tampering with corporeal remains – puts the spectator on a dangerous path: how can the resurrection take place on Judgment Day when the bones of the dead have been disturbed?[26] But Six prefers an alternative explanation, and informs the reader that another interpretation of the collection of bones is possible. The bones remind the viewer of the transience of earthly things, and help them understand themselves so they are ready for death. Nobody can escape death: before you know it, your skull and your worm-eaten bones will be up on a shelf, on display by a surgeon or an apothecary (l. 29–36):

  Leer u die eindlik sterven zult,
  Al sterven, eer de tyd vervult.
Eer, niemand is doch vry, of seeker,
By een Barbier, of Apoteeker,
  Uw doodshoofd, en doorknaaghde schonk,
  Mee, op een berd, zal staan te pronk.
Leer, menschen, van dees beengewelven,
Apolloos spreuke, kent u selven.

Teach yourself, you who shall die once,
To die, before the times comes.
Before – nobody is excused or secure –
Your skull and shank, gnawed through,
Will also be displayed on a shelf
At a barber's or an apothecary's.
Teach yourself, mankind, from these chambers of bones,
Apollo's saying: Know thyself.

25 Matthew 22:23 and Acts 23:8; Jacobs, 1991 II, p. 236.
26 *Cf.* Six's fear of what would happen to his own body if he were to die in a foreign country: 'Bussekruid vervloekt. Aan myn moeder' ('Accursed Gunpowder. To My Mother') (J383), l. 29–30.

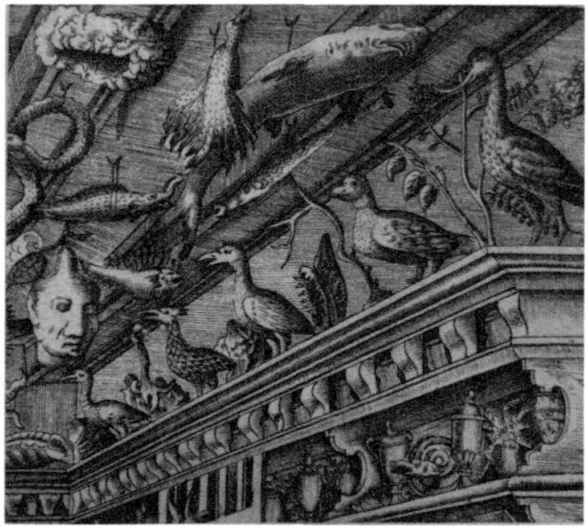

Fig. 3.3: Human heads were also found in other early modern cabinets of curiosities. Here an illustration from Benedicto Ceruti and Andrea Chiocco, *Musaeum Franc. Calceolarii jun. Veronensis*, 1622. (© University Library of Oslo).

Six may have had many reasons for writing this poem. Both he and his cousin, Jan Gerritsen Indies, would have benefited from mentioning the collection. The fame of a collection, and thus the renown of its owner, depended on its regular inclusion in art and poetry. Both men, who were from the 'lower medical professions', were able to present themselves as distinguished, learned gentlemen. As recent research has shown, the seeds of new scientific practices were being sown in the early modern knowledge networks of craftsmen, artists and traders.[27] That brings us to another important point: Six's argument is echoed in the scholarly philosophical debates of his time about the boundary between legitimised and unlegitimised knowledge. The central theme of the text is the danger posed by a *curiositas,* a dangerous inquisitiveness. Many Protestant theologians opposed forms of science that brought people into contact with the inexplicable and the enigmatic aspects of existence. In Augustine's *Confessions*, the Church Father calls the fascination with human corpses and other curiosities a 'disease of curiosity'. At best, he thought, such curiosity was perverse and useless. At worst, it could lead people away from God and salvation. As a Calvinist, Six was influenced by Augustine. This is evident from 'Verdorventheit der Natuure' ('Corruption of [Human] Nature') (J340), where Six refers to Augustine and emphasises original sin. Augustine saw curiosity as amongst

27 Pamela H. Smith & Paula Findlen (eds.), *Merchants and Marvels: Commerce, Science, and Art in Early Modern Europe* (2002); Smith, 2004; *cf.* also Deborah Harkness, *The Jewel House: Elizabethan London and the Scientific Revolution*, 2007.

sins of the first rank, and linked it to the original sin of Adam and Eve. Writing in the early modern Netherlands in the tradition of Augustine, D.V. Coornhert described the 'schadelijcke Weetsuchtigheyt' ('harmful thirst for knowledge') as a useless vice and an unhealthy yearning – as opposed to the curiosity that aims for self-awareness. Six takes the same view of *curiositas* in 'Op doodshoofden, en geraamten van beesten', where the *curiosa* in question could set malleable individuals on the wrong path.[28]

However, by demonstrating the dangerous effect of the collection, Six shows that he is aware of this. In order to justify his interest in natural history, he shifts attention from the materials to his own person – to the ethical appeals of *nosce te ipsum*, 'know thyself', and *memento mori*, 'remember you will die'. He warns against a perception of the objects based on an uncontrolled passion such as pride (l. 26). The poem thus provides a moral legitimisation of the collection of such enigmatic *naturalia*. The merchant-druggist informs the reader that he is aware of the dangers associated with collecting and examining *exotica*. Given a choice between two interpretive possibilities, he chooses the one that corresponds to the ideal of the virtuous gentleman: He approaches the materials with the help of virtues such as *ratio* and *apatheia*.

Madam Miserly's cabinet of horrors

The last poem that I will discuss in this chapter is 'Gierigheits wooninge en gestaltenisse' ('The Residence and Shape of Avarice') (J99). Already in the first lines, the wondrous features as a theme. The text places Six in the vicinity of the Italian city of Cumae, west of Naples. This area was famous for its many caves and, according to Virgil's *Aeneid*, it is here that the entrance to the underworld could be found. In l. 1–6, our traveller enters one of these caves and experiences something incredible:

> Het wonderlykste, op reis gesien,
> Vertellens waardigh, aan de liên,
> Die nimmer zyn van huis geweest,

28 See D.V. Coornhert, *Hert-spiegel. Godlijcker schrifturen* (*Heart Mirror, Theological Writings*), 1632, p. 149; D.V. Coornhert, 'Tweede Boeck. V. Hoofdstuck. Van kennisse en wetenschap' in: *Zedekunst, dat is wellevenskunste* (*Ethics, or the Art of Living Well*) [1586] (1942), pp. 123-133. And *cf.* my discussion of 'Verrukkinge van sinnen' ('Rapture from the Senses') (J401) in Chapter 8. For discussions on Augustine, curiosity and science in the early modern period, see Peter Harrison, *The Fall of Man and the Foundation of Science*, 2007. Another example is the diplomat Coenraad van Beuningen, who collected curiosities but then suffered a mental breakdown. In 1665 he said that he no longer felt like gathering knowledge and curiosities, because they increased his spiritual anguish: C.W. Roldanus, *Coenraad van Beuningen. Staatsman en libertijn*, 1931, p. 162. This reference I have from Kooijmans, 2004, p. 464.

Dan in de Boeken met den geest,
Was gierigheits gestaltenis,
En waar, en hoe haar wooningh is.

The most wonderful thing seen while travelling,
Worth recounting to people
Who have never been away from home,
Except in books, in their minds,
Was the shape of avarice,
And where and how her dwelling is.

The cave is presented as the home of the personification of *avaritia*, one of the seven deadly sins, but also a figure popular in the Middle Ages and the Renaissance, and especially in the early modern Dutch iconology in which she was known as 'Vrouw Gierigheid' – 'Madam Miserly'.[29]

Six allows his imagination to run free in the poem. Madam Miserly – a 'vrekke, en nimmer satte tesch' ('miserly and never-satisfied wench') (l. 18) – is, in accordance with the depiction of avarice in iconographic works, presented as the daughter of Pluto, the god of both earthly riches and the underworld (Fig. 3.4). And in keeping with the myths connected with Cumae, once a centre of ancient culture, she is also depicted as a priestess of the Apollonian cult there. In Cumae there was a 'steene tempel' ('stone temple') in honour of Apollo, with an adjoining cave in which the Cumaean Sibyl, one of the most famous oracles of classical antiquity, made her predictions (see l. 7–16). The stingy woman thus has a double identity. Six presents her on the one hand as a personification of avarice – 'Madam Miserly' – and on the other as a remnant of pagan faith from antiquity.[30] Finally, a third label could apply to her: as an Apollonian priestess, 'voorseggende [...] versierde waarheit' ('predicting an invented truth' – that is, lies) (l. 13–14), she emerges as a poet-prophet.[31]

29 Schama, 2004, pp. 323–343; De Vries, 2004, p. 142.

30 For the iconological depictions of *avaritia* with respect to this poem: Cesare Ripa, *Iconologia of Uytbeeldinghen des Verstants*, 1644, pp. 168–171; Jacobs, 1991 II, pp. 153–154. *Cf.* also *Lof der Geldsucht* (*In Praise of the Desire for Gold*) by Jeremias de Decker, where, just as in Six's poem above, Madam Miserly appears as a goddess with her own cult.

31 In his explanation of the elevated conception of poetry in antiquity, Theodore Rodenburgh emphasises the relationship between the Roman *vates* (the poet-prophet) and the holy Sibyls: 'aangezien beyde de oraclen van Delphos, en vande voorzegginghe der Sybillen in vaersen verwitticht waeren, en in maetighe voet-ghedichten, zoo aerdichlijck verzaemt, en met zo rijcken en milden vernuft ghepoëtiseert, datter scheen een Hemelsche kracht in te berusten' ('Since both the oracle of Delphi and the predictions of the Sibyls were expressed in verses, and on metrical foot, so nicely gathered, and with such a richly and generous reason poetized, so that a Celestial force seemed to reside in it.'): Theodore Rodenburgh, *Eglentiers*

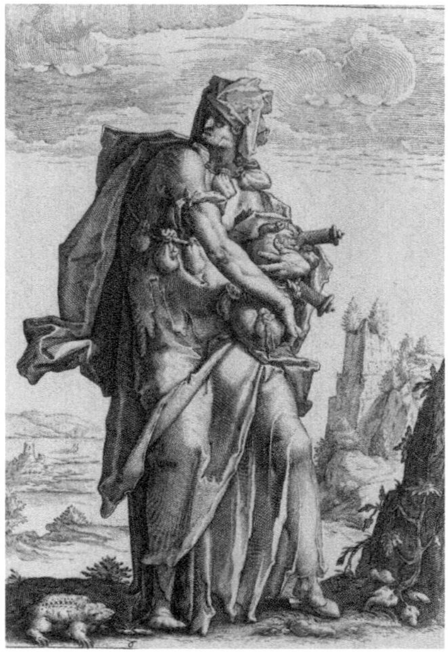

Fig. 3.4: Jacob Matham (attributed to), after Hendrick Goltzius, *Avarice*, c. 1585–1589. Engraving. (© Rijksmuseum, Amsterdam).

This long poem has a narrative structure: a local guide takes the travelling merchant-poet to the home of Madam Miserly in the innermost part of the cave, where she lets him in and then takes on the role of guide. Here we see an interesting parallel with classical literature. Although Six does not actually mention Virgil, the cave dweller in 'Gierigheits woninge en gestaltenisse' appears to play the same role as the Cumaean Sibyl in the sixth book of the *Aeneid*. In that epic, she appears as a guide and offers Aeneas advice on how to find the shade of his dead father in the underworld. But her guiding role is different in Six's poem. To the Calvinist merchant-poet, she does not offer a path to a good, Christian world, but to an evil, heathen one. She guides – or rather, lures – Six towards his own nightmare.[32]

poëtens borst-weringh (*The Battlement of the Eglentier's Poets*), 1638, pp. 5–6. Caverns were also regarded as the abode of poetic and prophetic madness: Gerardus Vossius, *Poeticae Institutiones*, 2010, II, p. 1901.

32 There is indeed a cave of Sibyl – *Antro della Sibilla* – near the 'Avernus lak' (l. 7), the Lago d'Averno, a crater lake, but it was not discovered until 1932. In early modern travel guides, however, there is also a cave called 'het Hol van Sybilla'. Could Six have visited it? The area was a tourist attraction in the seventeenth century. Travel guides of the time say of this cave 'dat onsen Salighmaecker daer ter Hellen is gedaelt' ('where our Saviour descended to hell') (Lambert van den Bos, *Wegh-wyser door Italien*, 1661, p. 473; Anna Frank-van Westrienen, *De groote tour. Tekening van de educatiereis der Nederlanders in de zeventiende eeuw*, 1983, p. 298). We do not know whether such local Catholic myths had any significance for Six, but

Pluto's daughter shows the surprised Dutchman the rooms containing her most precious possessions. The cave is full of treasure chests with money in them. The money was obtained unfairly: Madam Miserly presents herself as the mother of all the evil deeds that are committed in the world for the sake of economic gain (l. 132–140):

Haar kinders heeten Argelist,
Bedrieger, Loogen, Meineed, Twist,
Haat, Moordenaar, Nyd, Woekeraar
Muntbootser, Schrooijer, Dobbelaar,
Maatkorter, Tweederhandeschaal,
Kymist, en Myner van metaal,
Die sy beslaapen van haar man,
Haar eigen vaar, in droom gewan.

Her children are called Malice,
Deceiver, Lies, Perjury, Contention,
Hate, Murderer, Envy, Usurer,
Counterfeiter, Coin-Clipper, Gambler,
Shortener of Measures, Weigher with Two Scales,
Chemist, and Mine digger,
Whom she begot in a dream,
When sleeping with her husband, her own father.

According to the quotation, her children were conceived in a nightmare with her own father, the devil. Madam Miserly promises that, if Six ever honours her children, she will fulfil his deepest desires. The relationship the merchant-poet has to the wealth that has been gathered can be characterised throughout the poem in terms of a critical distance, but no sooner has this tempting proposal been made than his detachment turns into desire (l. 313–322):

O bestemoeder, ryke vrouw,
Zyn al die koffers geld, ik trouw,
Geen mensch op aarden is zoo ryk,
Noch in vernoegingh uws gelyk,
Dus bad ik: lieve, laat myn oogh,

an identification with Christ is common in his poetry. The treasures with which Six is seduced in this 'woestyn' ('wilderness') (l. 23) are also reminiscent of Jesus' temptation by the devil (Matthew 4:8–10). According to tradition, this temptation of Christ also took place in a cave in the wilderness.

Plaisieren, in dat ryk vertoogh,
Van zoo veel kostelyk metaal,
Op dat ik t'huis wat vremds verhaal,
En elken reiser, naa dees kust,
Voor al, te reisen, maak belust.

O grandmother, rich woman,
If all these coffers are filled with gold, then I assume
That no person on earth is as rich,
Or as satisfied, as you.
Thus, I asked: Dear, let my eye
Enjoy this rich display
Of so much precious metal,
So that I may tell those at home
Of these strange things,
And make each traveller
Desire to visit this coast.

The text is thus more than a satire on *avaritia*. In order to understand the poem properly, we should also take Six's social background into account. He sets up a confrontation with the vices of his profession, all of which stemmed from the main sin of avarice. By placing himself in the underworld of Pluto, the god of wealth, the trader exposes the great moral risks involved in his profession. The role he assigns to his senses in this connection is striking. As can be seen from the quotation, it is mainly the eyes that are running a risk when confronted with 'so much precious metal'. Vision was seen as the sense with the greatest influence on people – as the path along which lust and desire arise. In 'Goudsucht' ('Desire for Gold') (J279), which I will discuss in Chapter 4, Six shows how the 'pleasant rays' of gold enchant our eyes and afflict our bodies with obsessions. The physician Johan van Beverwijck thus regards *avaritia* as an illness that, just like other desires, can be treated medically: 'This intemperate desire is like gangrene'; it devours 'our natural affection and fills us with bad humours'.[33]

'Gierigheits wooninge en gestaltenisse' is one of the most fascinating texts in *Poësy*. The extremely dramatic and imaginative effect – caused by the unpleasant animals at the entrance to the cave and the barking of the witch's dog, for instance

33 'Dese onmatighe begeerlijckheyt is als het kout vyer'; it devours 'onse natuerlijcke genegentheydt, ende vervult ons met quade humeuren', Johan van Beverwijck, *Schat der gesontheyt* (*Treasure of Health*) 1656, p. 49. For a further discussion of lust as an illness, see Chapter 4. *Cf.* Eric Jan Sluijter, *De 'heydensche fabulen' in de schilderkunst van de Gouden Eeuw. Verhalen uit de klassieke mythologie in de Noordelijke Nederlanden, circa 1590–1670*, 2000, p. 160.

– is reminiscent of the grotesque, imaginative paintings by Hieronymus Bosch, Pieter Bruegel the Elder and David Teniers the Younger. Recent research has pointed to the central role that exotics and the culture of the cabinets of curiosities play in the paintings of Bruegel.[34] This brings us to an important point in the text: the interest in the miraculous is visible not only in the sumptuous treasures, but also in the detailed descriptions of the home of Madam Miserly and of the 'stature' of her person. Six goes into all sorts of detail regarding her study, her kitchen, and her sleeping quarters, as well as her appearance and her attire. I shall examine these details more closely here, focusing on the theme of this chapter.

The greed of Madam Miserly is reflected in a surprisingly large number of exotica: precious and rare, but also terrifying, objects that amaze the eyes of our Dutch visitor. As I mentioned above, Six describes her clothing in considerable detail (l. 115–130):

Wanneer men op heur kleeren let,
Het booven lyf is slordigh net,
Gelascht van wolven tot een jak.
De mouwen van een panthers sak.
De rokwol, van gemengde kleur,
Daar sietmen bloote billen deur.
De sleutelriem, om 't lyf gehaakt,
Zyn haaviksklaauwen saam gemaakt.
Te rechter weeght daar aan een tasch
Genaait, van 't stroopsel van een dasch.
De schorteldoek is bontsinkleer,
Om stryt met geuren van goor smeer.
Den hals pronkt met een vosse staart,
Gekraaght, en voor de kou bewaart,
De toffels draaghtse van geen os,
Maar van een wree rhinoceros.

If you pay attention to her attire,
Her upper body is a sloppy, tattered smock,
Patched together from wolfskins into a jacket.
The sleeves are made of panther skins.
The wool of the shirt, of mixed colours:

34 See Tine L. Meganck, *Pieter Bruegel the Elder: Fall of the Rebel Angels: Art, Knowledge and Politics on the Eve of the Dutch revolt*, 2014. *Cf.* David Teniers the Younger, 'The Rich Man Being Led to Hell', National Gallery. *Cf.* also the genre 'sottobosco', and Karin Leonhard, *Bildfelder. Stilleben und Naturstücke des 17. Jahrhunderts*, 2013, which also discusses the pharmaceutical significance of *naturalia* in portraiture.

Through them you see her bare buttocks.
On her key-belt, hooked around the waist,
Hawks' claws are attached to each other.
On the right side, there hangs a bag,
Sewn together from the flayed skin of a badger.
The apron is of polecat leather,
With odours that compete with those of rancid fat.
The neck flaunts the collar
Of a foxtail, which also protects against the cold.
The slippers she wears come, not from
An ox, but from a brutal rhinoceros.

The various hides, skins and claws that make up her clothes come from all sorts of exotic animals: wolves, panthers, hawks and rhinoceroses. In keeping with the theme of the poem, these animals provide samples of the 'wonderlykste' Six has seen on his travels. What is remarkable in this passage is the humour Six displays. The cave dweller is wearing 'slippers' 'from a brutal rhinoceros', and her 'bare buttocks' can be seen through her skirt. It is not only her clothes that are wondrous, but Madam Miserly herself turns out to be a miraculous being. Six describes her elsewhere in the text as a fabulous 'harpy' (l. 175).

That these terrifying objects were classified as pharmaceutical goods is evident from early modern pharmacopoeias.[35] The French apothecary Nicolas Lemery writes of the hawk that 'its flesh, its fat and its stool are praised as eye medicines and remedies to help women in childbirth', and that the badger is a 'timid and fearful animal' that has 'a lot of oil and volatile salt in its body', which, he says, are effective against diarrhoea and tuberculosis, among other things. And of the rhinoceros he writes: 'The horns, nails, and blood, are all used in medicine [...] The dose [of horns] is one to two scruples, as either an infusion or powder, which, when drunk in wine, purifies the blood and is a good preservative against infectious air'.[36] It is not clear, however, to what extent these recipes were actually used. We remember Feitama's verses about the fearful animals in his shop, which he describes as exhibits rather than actual drugs. Paintings of the shop interiors of early modern pharmacists and druggists, where stuffed exotic animals such as crocodiles served as ceiling decorations, speak the same sort of language. The crocodile, by the way, is mentioned a few lines later in the section of the poem

35 See also the horns of exotic animal species that are discussed in 'Uitroep om hoornafsetters' (244), which is discussed in Chapter 4, pp. 155–163.

36 Lemery, 1743, pp. 5, 600 and 610; *A Compleat History of Drugs, written in French by Monsieur POMET* [...] *To which is added what is further observable on the same subject, from mess. LEMERY*, 1737, Book 1, p. 250.

depicting 'Madam Miserly': 'Om hoogh, daar hanght een paaviljoen, / Van 't welfsel weegende, aan een koord, / Van Krokodils te saam geboordt' ('Up there, there is a canopy, hanging by a cord from the ceiling, made of crocodiles that are sewn together') (l. 186–188).[37]

And there is more to be said on this listing of macabre medical *curiosa* in the description of Madam Miserly's study, 'het binnenhof' (l. 200), where her office is and where she keeps her accounts. That alone is 'bekykens waard' ('worth looking at') (l. 201). We read (l. 209–232):

Op taafel leit het reekenboek,
Deur vingren, op het reeknen, kloek
Niet half volreekent, van heur schat,
In schuld, en diese reeds besat.
Hier neeven heeft se schryfpapier,
Gemerkt met sperwers, en een mier:
Een seegel als een griffioen,
In staal, om brieven toe te doen:
Doorteert harpuis, in plaats van lak:
Een pen mes dat haar broer doorstak:
Een hoornige bekladde kom,
Met gallen, seik, alluin, en gom:
Schryfpennen uit een Arends arm:
Sand uit Charibdis waaterswarm:
Kryt van het bloedich Britsche strand:
En sponsen van de selve rand,
Van mossigh steenigh zeegeberght,
Gelijk die Kristus heeft geterght.
Ook kleeft daar by tot ondersoek,
Van geldswaardye, meenigh boek.
Noch kryghtmen toetsteen, goudgewicht,
Ballans, en schrooischaar in 't gesicht.
Een koopere uur, die konstnaars tart,
Hoe kon die koop die pry van 't hart?

37 *Cf.* the *curiosa* that were discussed in Joan Breyne's cabinet of curiosities: 'elantsklauw', 'leeuwskoppen', 'cabinet, met schilpadt ingeleyt', 'witte zee-spons', 'slakjes', and a 'glas met hagedissen, slangen en duysent-been' ('elk claw, lion heads, cabinet inlaid with turtle, white sea sponge, snails and a glas with lizards, snakes and millipedes'): *Catalogus van een groote partij extraordinaire curieuse Rariteyten* [...] *Joan Breyne*, 1693, pp. 4, 9 and 28. And *cf.* 'Het naturaliën-kabinet van de Delftse apotheker Jan van der Meer', in: Bosma-Jelgersma, *Vijf eeuwen Delftse apothekers*, 1979, pp. 121–127.

On the table is the account book,
By fingers, which are ready to calculate,
Not yet half-counted, of her
Outstanding debts and of property
Which she has already got.
Next to her, she has writing paper
With a watermark in the form of a sparrowhawk and an ant:
An iron seal with a griffin,
Used to close letters:
Resin mixed with tar, instead of lacquer:
A penknife which [she used] to kill her brother.
An inkwell made of horns,
With gall, urine, alum and gum:
Writing pens made of the feather of an eagle:
Crayon from the bloody shores of Britain:
And sponges from the same reef
– Of a mossy, rocky seascape, –
As the one that tormented Christ.
Next to her there are also sticky books
To determine the value of various coins.
You also catch sight of touchstone, gold weight,
A balance, and scissors for clipping coins.
A brass clock, which defies instrument makers,
How could that monster find it in her heart to buy the clock?

If we compare the description of Madam Miserly's office with the actual office of an early modern merchant, some interesting similarities stand out. A nice description of such a space is given by the historian G.D.J. Schotel.[38] The 'sturdy oak pultrums and office chairs covered with leather', the 'leaden inkwells', the 'sand and wafer boxes', the 'goose-feather quills', the 'pencils and rulers' and the bell that Schotel speaks of – all have their equivalents in Madam Miserly's abode. Instead of a 'goose-feather quill', she uses an eagle feather; instead of a leaden inkwell, she uses a 'an inkwell made of horns, / with gall, urine, alum and gum'. Her letters are sealed, not with lacquer, but with 'resin mixed with tar'. She not only uses her penknife to sharpen the pen, with which she writes off outstanding debts; she has even used it as a murder weapon. That the writer is a man with pharmaceutical expertise can be seen from this passage. The substances gall and gum can be recognised from the bitter galnut ink, to which urine and alum

38 G.D.J. Schotel, *Het Maatschappelijk Leven onzer Vaderen in de Zeventiende Eeuw*, 1905, pp. 223–224.

have been added. This last compound is alumina sulfuric acid, a substance used in dyeing, medicine and for other purposes.[39] Sometimes, according to Schotel, a merchant family's study was connected to the living room. Also the sleeping place of Madam Miserly is connected with her office: her bed consists of bedding from a 'ruige beer' ('shaggy bear'), her pillows are 'tigerdier / Gevult met pluimen van een gier. / Het deksel is een luiparts vacht / Met soomen van een slangh, omwracht' ('tiger skin filled with feathers of a vulture. The blanket is a leopard rug, with a hem made of snake skin') (l. 247–252): The description of her workspace is therefore based on a premises from Six's time, with a retail space that has a curiosity cabinet in it, as well as an office and a living room.[40] Once again, the frightening objects refer to the combination of in-store stock and a collection of the merchant-druggist's curiosities.

The distinction between the *exotica* in an early modern drugstore and those in the cave of Madam Miserly is clear: in 'Gierigheits wooninge en gestaltenisse', emphasis is put on the origin of the hides, skins and horns that are mentioned: they come from wild animals in non-Christian countries. Six thus puts an ethical spin on the collection of exotic medicines. As we noted above, the cave dweller has a dual identity: she is also a Sibyl. Indeed, when she turns directly to Six at the end of the tour she gives him, she sounds like a priestess of some heathen cult, a guardian of a temple full of frightening fetishes – and she also acts as a mouthpiece for atheism (l. 303–308):

Nu sie myn schaamel hof voorts om,
Dit ruil ik, voor geen Keiserdom:
Dit zyn de Gooden, die ik eer,
Om welke ik 't Heemelsch Hof afsweer,
Indien 'er Heemel is, of Hel,
Waar mee ik mynen geest niet quel:

Now when I gaze further at my poor court,
I would not exchange this for any Empire,
These are the Gods whom I honour:
For which I renounce the heavenly court,
Whether there exists a heaven or hell,
[A question with which] I do not trouble my mind.

39 See 'aluin'[1] in the WNT, and Lemery, 1743, pp. 25–26.

40 Another poem by Six discusses various activities he carries out himself in his home, including bookkeeping for his drug business: ''s Amsterdammers winter' (J96), l. 803.

Collecting earthly materials thus arouses pride in the collector, which is incompatible with the grace of God. Objects from barbaric countries tempt the collector to question Christian doctrines, such as in 'Op doodshoofden, en geraamten van beesten'. Six describes not only trade based on immoral conduct, but also the act of collecting dangerous *exotica,* as occupations pursued by the daughter of Pluto, the god of the underworld.

And there is more to say about the text. One of the frightening objects from this horror cabinet deserves further research. Among Madam Miserly's writing utensils is a '[k]ryt van het bloedich Britsche strand' ('chalk from the bloody British shore') (l. 223). This chalk is not a fantasy product – it was actually found in early modern pharmacopoeias. Under the keyword 'Blood-Stone', Lemery describes a type of crayon from England:

> There is another sort of blood-stone brought from England, called the bastard hæmatitis [...] it is afringent, and is call'd hæmatitis, from ἆιμα, blood, because, being powder'd, it is of the Colour Blood, and stops bleeding.[41]

But Six has another explanation for the hue of this substance: 'the bloody shores' allude to the decapitation of Charles I – the blood from 'Rariteiten te koop'. The possession of this kind of material sheds more light on the dangerous desire the poem is about: *avaritia*. Madam Miserly is as bloodthirsty as the English republicans, the 'assassins of the king'. Her bookkeeping is done with blood-red ink. The lines that follow elaborate on this. The same applies to the sponge Madam Miserly uses in her bookkeeping. It comes from the same 'rocky seascape' as the sponge that was soaked in vinegar to torment Jesus as he hung on the cross.[42] Neither Madam Miserly nor Cromwell shuns treachery to satisfy such devilish lusts. As noted above, her children are called 'Deceiver, Lies, Perjury' and 'Murderer'. The double reference to the murder of King Charles and that of Christ links avarice to the worst of the seven deadly sins, *Superia*, pride, from which all other sins derive.[43]

41 *A Compleat History of Drugs, Written in French by Monsieur POMET* [...] *To which is added what is further observable on the same subject, from mess. LEMERY*, 1737, Book 3, p. 366.

42 'Steenigh zeegeberght' could also refer to the 'bloedich Britsche strand'. In that case Six is relying once again on Pliny the Elder. In his *Naturalis Historia*, he treats sponges that are dyed as luxury items, some dyed even with the exclusive purple from the purple snail (Pliny XXI, 123).

43 *Cf.* the paintings of Bruegel, especially 'Fall of the Rebel Angels', that both express a moral warning against the excess of unbounded collecting, and warnings against hubris and pride, see Meganck, 2014, pp. 107, 131 and 163.

Conclusion

This chapter examined the multifaceted reality of 'drugs' and 'druggists' in early modern times – something one would not expect, given the characteristics of the 'druggist' as an unimaginative 'bore' ('droogaard'). As we have seen, the miraculous and the fabulous were an inseparable part of the world of the seventeenth-century spice merchant. The texts we have looked at show how Six problematises this aspect, in accordance with the poetics of the learned merchant-druggist: his self-portrayal as the dry, in the sense of sober, herbalist. As a sober merchant, Six shows his awareness of the distinction between transitory and imperishable collectibles in 'Val van Haarlems Flora', and between lawful and unlawful knowledge, as in the discussion of the various epistemological interpretive possibilities we find in 'Op doodshoofden, en geraamten van beesten'. A misapprehension of these objects, which encompasses an uncontrolled sensory perception of materials, would involve the creation of dangerous desires: greed, pride and idolatry. In the eyes of the merchant-druggist, these desires are to be understood as physical illnesses. I will return to this presently.

And as a sober merchant, Six also demonstrates that he is able to distinguish between reality and fantasy. There is, in fact, still a conclusion to be drawn from the special 'chalk from the bloody British shore' in 'Gierigheits wooninge en gestaltenisse': the hue of Madam Miserly's chalk refers to the fictional nature of the entire text. Of course, the colour of English chalk does not come from Charles I's blood. Six deliberately mingles fantasy with reality in order to address prejudices associated with his profession as druggist. That applies to the whole poem and to everything it describes. The last lines are a repetition of the opening phrase (l. 325–328):

> Dit 's 't wonderlykste op reis gesien,
> Vertellens waardigh, aan de liên,
> Die nimmer zyn van huys geweest,
> Dan, in de boeken, met den geest.

There is an ironic undertone to these lines. A yearning for the miraculous was, as I have shown in this chapter, a characteristic of early modern society, and the druggist in particular was viewed as an exponent of the miraculous. But Six ridicules this expectation. What is most wondrous manifests itself 'in books, in the mind', and not through the senses of the merchant-druggist travelling abroad. The desire for the wondrous among people in Amsterdam, who would have read this poem, would be satisfied thanks to Six's imaginative writing, and not to the mysterious ingredients in his drugstore. Neither Six's trips for trading purposes to foreign climes, nor his exotic medicines that he has on display satisfy this desire.

4. Drugs as remedies

Abstract
This chapter discusses the use of exotic plants and spices as medicines and foodstuffs, as presented in the poetry of Joannes Six van Chandelier. An apology for indigenous herbs at the expense of exotic drugs written by the physician Johan van Beverwijck plays a large role here. I argue that Six attributes the illness in his spleen to his exposure to exotic drugs and spices. In my analysis of poems Six wrote on his illness and his medical treatment, I show how the wholesaler of luxury goods portrays himself as an ascetic on a strict diet consisting of local herbs, as a self-conscious Batavian who avoids luxury food, and as a patient who undergoes severe bloodletting treatments to clean his body and his mind of 'fiery' elements.

Keywords: Johan van Beverwijck, debate on indigenous versus exotic drugs, botanical gardens, ambergris, gold, exotics horns

't Schijnt het wert dan eerst bequaem,
Als men 't geeft een vreemde naem;
't Schijnt het krijgt dan eerst sijn prijs,
Als men dees en geen maeckt wijs
Dattet van het Moren-lant,
Of den Barbarysche strant,
Dattet van den Indiaen
Herwaerts komt dreven aen:
't Dunckt de slechte Luyden best,
Wat ons geeft een vremt gewest.

It seems that it first becomes effective
When one gives it a foreign name:
It seems it first gets its price,
When one lets the man in the street know
That it came from the land of Moors,
Or from Barbarian shores,
That it came drifting hither

Spaans, R., *Dangerous Drugs: The Self-Presentation of the Merchant-Poet Joannes Six van Chandelier (1620–1695)*. Taylor & Francis Group, 2020
DOI 10.5117/9789462983543_CH04

From the Indians:
That which seems to please the crowd best,
Is what a foreign region gives us.
– Jacob Cats[1]

The doctrine of humours

'Tell me what you eat and I'll tell you who you are', goes a well-known aphorism.[2] In early modern times, this would have been taken literally. Joannes Six van Chandelier, who paid a lot of attention to how his public persona was perceived, would certainly have taken it seriously, because food was an important part of his identity when it came to his role, not only as a supplier of drugs and spices, a merchant-druggist, but also as a consumer of medicines, a patient. Six had an ailment of the spleen, and in his poetry he devoted a great deal of attention to its course and its treatment. Both identities will be discussed in this chapter.

The reason for the close link between food and identity can be found in the physiological and medical theories of Six's day. I will summarise here the most important of these. This brings us to the Galenic theories about the six *res non-naturales, i.e.* the 'non-natural' health issues. In addition to the four *res naturales*, which can be considered part of the inner or fixed nature of a human being, our health is influenced by six external factors: climate, effort, sleep, bowel movement, food and passions (*i.e.* emotional well-being).[3] In particular, the influence of food should not be underestimated. According to Galenic medicine, what was ingested had an effect on an individual's physical and psychological state. Not only medicines from pharmacies, but also ordinary foodstuffs influenced one's health. It is worth noting in this connection that the Dutch word 'recept' means both *recipe* and *medical prescription*. The boundary between the culinary and the pharmaceutical was quite porous in the seventeenth century. Food and medicine had a clear goal: to restore a balanced *krasis* in the organism. The *diet* (of Greek word borrowed into Latin as *diaeta*, a term that originally means 'way of life', in both the medical and moral sense) therefore played a central role in Renaissance medicine.[4] Research on

1 Johan van Beverwijck, *Inleydinge tot de Hollandtsche Genees-middelen* (*Introduction to Dutch Medicines*), 1656, p. 6.

2 'Dis-moi ce que tu manges, je te dirai qui tu es', in : Jean Anthelme Brillat-Savarin, *Physiologie du goût*, 1986, p. 9.

3 Johan van Beverwijck, *Schat der gesontheyt*, 1656, pp. 17–19.

4 For the role of diet in Galenic medicine, see Ken Albala, *Eating Right in the Renaissance*, 2002, and Marleen Willebrands, *De verstandige kok. De rijke keuken van de Gouden Eeuw*, 2006. For Galenic dietetics in early modern poetry, see Schoenfeldt 1999.

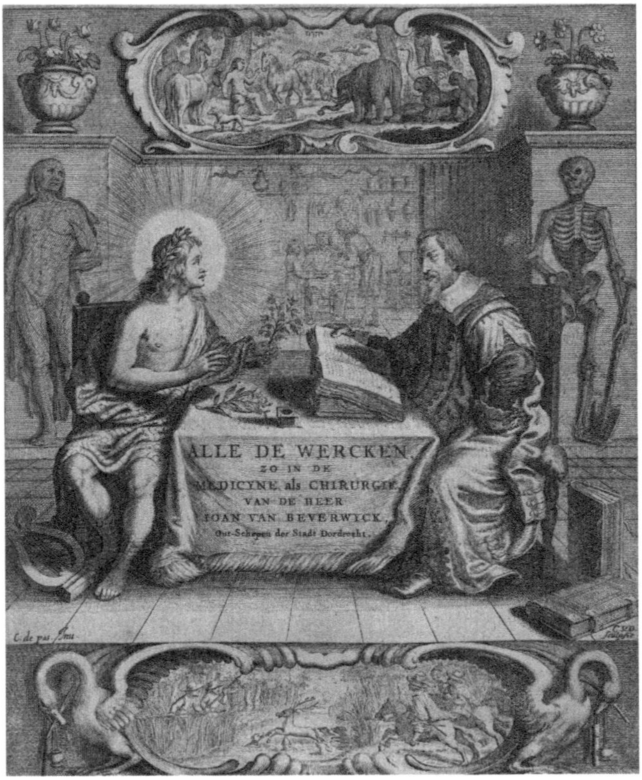

Fig. 4.1: Illustration of Cornelis van Dalen (I) & Crispijn van de Passe (II), the title page of Johan van Beverwijck, *Alle de wercken, zo in de medicyne als chirurgie*, 1656. (© Rijksmuseum, Amsterdam).

early modern spices is therefore impossible without taking into account the Galenic properties attributed to them. Just like humans, food and medicine were divided according to their different qualities, based on the element that predominated in the substance: a medicine was therefore hot, cold, humid or dry, and each of these qualities was classified into four different degrees. A melancholic type was thus advised to follow a 'wet' diet. Many of the tropical spices were seen as dry and hot to the third or fourth degree, so Six speaks in a poem of 'heete speceryen / als peeper, naagels, look, en gember' ('hot spices such as pepper, cloves, garlic, and ginger').[5]

The physician and writer Johan van Beverwijck was a highly influential figure in medicine in the Dutch Republic. Lia van Gemert calls him the 'institution' of the Golden Age. This is a position he obtained thanks to the three medical reference works he published in Dutch, *Schat der gesontheyt, Schat der ongesontheyt, ofte*

5 'Leeven te Spa' (J101), l. 262–268.

Geneeskonste van de sieckten, and *Heel-konste* (*Treasure of Health, Treasure of Ill-Health, or Medicine of Sick People,* and *Surgery*), which were published between 1636 and 1645 (Fig. 4.1). New editions of these works appeared throughout the seventeenth century.[6] In his discussion of drugs in *Schat der ongesontheyt,* Johan van Beverwijck mentions – besides this concept of Galenic qualities – two other properties of medicines: the second has to do with such categories as thickening, purifying, and opening up. 'Thin' medications spread more easily in the body than 'thick' ones. The third property refers to 'a hidden property in the whole essence of the medicine' – it can have either a dispelling or a changing effect. The dispelling traits draw something to themselves with which they correspond, while the changing ones have a hidden property that is diametrically opposed to the poison in our bodies and change it in such a way that it can no longer harm us.[7] We also find these two properties in Six's work: in a poem of praise for Spa water, 'Leeven te Spa' (J101), he refers to the mysterious power of the classic miracle cures theriac and mithridate to explain the healing power of the mineral water (l. 39–41):

> Gelyk Triakel, ende Mitridaat, van kruiden
> Ook hinderlyk van aard, nochtans veel sieke luiden,
> Vreemd helpen, op de been, zoo heilen deese wellen
> veel siekten, waar de konst geen reede af kan vertellen.

> Like Theriac, and Mithridate, [composed] of spices
> Which [separately] also are harmful, but nevertheless help sick people
> In a strange way; in the same manner, these springs heal
> Sick people, in a way that medicine cannot explain.

'Dry' thus appears once again as a central concept in the argument. Besides these theories, this chapter will discuss the negative connotations of 'dry drugs' mentioned earlier: 'obscure', 'strange' and 'unreliable'. These concepts are discussed in the polemic *Inleydinge tot de Hollandtsche Genees-middelen* (*Introduction to Dutch Medicines*) by Johan van Beverwijck, which will have a central place in this chapter. These are thus medications that, paradoxically enough, were considered to be pathogenic substances.

I will argue that Six was influenced by Van Beverwijck or by the same theories as Van Beverwijck, referring to texts in which Six makes a distinction between indigenous and exotic drugs. I will also turn to Six's ailment, and look at whether he presents his

6 Lia van Gemert, 'Johan van Beverwijck als "instituut"', *De zeventiende eeuw*, 1992, pp. 99–206; Lia van Gemert, afterword, in: Joh. van Beverwijck, *De schat der gezondheid*, 1992, pp. 164–182.

7 'Een verborgen eygenschap van het geheele Wesen der Genees-middelen', Van Beverwijck, *Schat der ongesontheyt*, p. 27. *Cf.* also Six's mention of the so-called weapon salve ('wapenzalf') in P.E.L. Verkuyl, 'Een dichterlijk pamflet naar aanleiding van de komeet van 1664', *Tijdschrift voor Nederlandsche taal- en letterkunde*, 1996, pp. 30–43.

merchandise as a cause of his own illness. In other words, did Six consider himself to be a 'dealer in poisons'? But first, I will look again at the relationship between realism and imagination when it comes to food and medicine. The concept of 'reality' is also an important point of orientation in early modern discussions on the trade in exotic drugs.

Literary feasts

The exotic, unknown origin of spices determined their identity. That is why foreign drugs and spices were so appealing as culinary and medicinal goods. It is often said that, in addition to their function as preservatives, spices were used mainly to mask the foul taste of old and spoiled food. But more recent research refutes this myth. Their use was based more on the hint of mystery and imagination with which they were surrounded than on their real nutritional value or beneficial effect. They functioned as gastronomic decorations on the dining table, as a means to distinguish oneself socially.[8] The fact that exotic food was associated with riches and wealth is particularly evident in what are known as the showpiece still-life paintings of the seventeenth-century, which portrayed meals full of exotic fruits and spices, such as the still lifes of Willem Kalf and Pieter Gallis (Plate 6).[9] Only the richest people could afford such feasts. The lower classes had to settle for indigenous alternatives to precious spices. This applied to spices used either for medicinal purposes or in the kitchen. But the aura of exclusivity around spices in the Middle Ages was disappearing in the early modern period. The discovery of the sea routes to ''s werrelds kruidighst deel' ('the spiciest part of the world') – as Six calls the East Indies in 'Voorwind, naa nieuw Batavie, aan 't Schip de Paarle [...]' ('Tailwind, to the New Batavia, for the Ship "De Paarle" [...]') (J374, l. 4) – had made it easier to get supplies, and lowered their prices. But even though exotic drugs became accessible to the wealthy bourgeoisie, their aura of mysticism and exaltation still remained largely intact.

There are many examples in *Poësy* of the appeal exerted by exotic delicacies. The festive poems and poems of thanks that Six wrote to business associates are full of references to refined aromas. This is illustrated, for example, by 'Vischmaal, aan Manuel Spranger' ('Fish Meal, to Manuel Spranger') (J174). Cheerful outbursts such as '[d]e visch bemint het vocht, en wil wel drymaal swemmen: / In waater eerst, daar naa in sausse, en dan in wyn. De wyn is oorsaak van een lustigh saamenkoomen' ('the fish loves moisture, and will swim three times: first in water, thereafter in sauce, and then in wine. The wine is the cause of a cheerful meeting') (l. 24–26) set the tone in this group of texts. In the early modern period, sauce was different

8 Schivelbusch, 1990; Smith, 2001; Freedman, 2008.

9 See for example Julie Berger Hochstrasser's research into the depiction of pepper, lemons and other luxury goods in painting in the early modern Netherlands, *Still Life and Trade in the Dutch Golden Age*, 2007.

from what we think of these days when we think of sauce. Moralists regarded it as adding only colour and flavour, as gastronomic cosmetics.[10] Wine also evoked different associations in the early modern period. In the eyes of the moralists, wine was an un-Dutch luxury. When Six writes an *imitatio* of Horace's address to a wine jug (Ode III, 11), he replaces the jug with its Northern European equivalent: 'Aan het bierglas' ('To the beer glass') (J398). But at the same time, the wine trade was one of the pillars of the Dutch commodities market, and merchants and grocers were also involved in it; and it is possible that Six himself was among them.[11]

Another example is 'Dank voor een gerookten salm, aan Pieter Loones' ('Thanks for a smoked salmon, to Pieter Loones') (J357). Once again the representation of the heroic trader is at the heart of Six's text. The setting is the First Anglo-Dutch War (1652–1654). Pieter Loones is a hero, Six exclaims, because this merchant, trading with Russia, has circumvented the English blockade with the sole aim of supplying Six with a culinary delicacy: smoked salmon from Moscow (l. 40–48):

Ghy had my geen salm gegeeven.
  Nu heeft my dees lekkerny
Heusch verbonden, aan uw gunste,
Heb daar voor des rymers kunste,
  Bastaard van de poësy.
Minnaar van het rymend galmen,
  Lees myn rym, met zulk vermaak,
  Als my geeft de lekkre smaak,
Van uw onverdiende salmen.

You did not give me any salmon [also: psalm].
This delicacy has, in a courtly way,
Connected me to your favour,
I give you therefore the art of the rhymester,
Bastard of poetry.
Lover of the rhyming resonance,
Read my rhyme, with the same pleasure
As the delicious taste I get
From your undeserved salmons [also: psalms].

10 Joan Thirsk, *Food in Early Modern England: Phases, Fads, Fashions, 1500–1760*, 2007, pp. 247, 323.

11 Jongman, 1951, p. 45; M.R. Bijlsma, '*Oud-Rotterdamsche "Cruydenierie"*', *Rotterdamsch Jaarboekje*, 1912, pp. 91–99. Compare Six's positive poems about wine: 'Welkomste in Rome' ('Welcome to Rome') (J263) and 'Scheepskroon, voor Marten Harpertse Tromp, ridder, L. admiraal van Holland en Zeeland' ('Ship's Crown, for Marten Harpertse Tromp, Knight, L. Admiral of Holland and Zeeland') (J342). For early modern views on wine and drunkenness, see D.P. Pers, *Suyp-stad of Dronkaerts leven*, 1978, pp. 24–55.

Six calls himself a 'bastard of poetry'. We have already learned to not always take literally this rhetorical modesty, which is so typical of Six. This example of self-deprecation must be read in the light of the daring language play with 'salmon' in the passage cited. Six felt humbled in the face of such a gift of 'divine' origin. The taste of these Northern exotica is as exalted as a biblical psalm. His thanks for them, in the form of this poem, are, by contrast, merely rhymes. And he would, he says, seek refuge in the monastery of the Carthusians, who are known for their strictly eremitic monastic life and frequent fasting, if their diet consisted of smoked salmon (l. 21–24). We recognise this playfulness with Catholic references from 'Dank, aan Isaak de Bra, voor een besoarsteen' (J467).[12]

Another delicacy, also from Moscow, is mentioned in 'Dank, aan Manuel Spranger. Voor kaaviaar' ('Thanks to Manuel Spranger, for Caviar') (J135). This time, too, Spranger has brought a valuable commodity.[13] In this poem, too, we recognise Six's rhetorical modesty. He confesses in jest how unworthy he feels to be receiving this gift. Caviar is simply dangerous to him: 'Dit's peeper, in het neusgat van den stier' ('This is pepper, in the nostril of the bull') (l. 23), he writes, referring to his status as a young bachelor. According to the Galenic system, pepper is hot in the fourth degree. At the end of the poem, the poet rejects the gift, because such a hot substance brings him 'te dicht ontrent den gloed' ('too close to the glow') (l. 38). It could also be that he rejects it because he has an ailment of the spleen. However, although his relationship status and health mean that eating caviar is not advisable for him personally, that does not mean that he disapproves of caviar as a commercial product for his drugstore. Just as it is today, in the early modern period Russian caviar was a luxury commodity. Once again, then, I regard the use of the topos of modesty in the text as an expression of gratitude to one of his business associates.[14]

Even more daring erotic allusions are made in the literary description of another delicacy. The peaches in 'Dank aan Hendrik Laurents Spiegel, voor een mandeken met Persen' ('Thanks to Hendrik Laurents Spiegel, for a basket with Peaches') (J15) are so tempting that a virgin would like to exchange the 'gulde vlies van haar juweel' ('gilded fleece of her jewel') (hymen) for it (l. 6–8). Six also says they are 'nectersoet' ('sweet as nectar') (l. 6) – and similar to 'Tyrisch purper' ('Tyrian purple') (l. 7),

12 *Cf.* 'Zielmisse, aan Pieter van Alteren Fiskal der Admiraaliteit' ('Soul Misse, to Pieter van Alteren, Fiscal of the Admiralty') (J335), where Six approaches an old friend, a high tax official, with flattering words, asking him to get some drugs loose from the customs officers that had ended up there because of mislabelling. Here Six also plays with Catholic references.

13 Manuel Spranger also appears in a third text: 'Een stuk van een meloen aan Manuel Spranger' ('A Piece of Melon for Manuel Spranger') (J273). See Chapter 8, p. 264. For biographical details on Manuel Spranger, see http://research.frick.org/montias/browserecord.php?-action=browse&-recid=2351 (consulted 17 May 2019).

14 *Cf.* also Nigel Smith's discussion of another poetic luxury meal of Six, 'Oesters te Kolchester' ('Oysters in Colchester') (J450): Nigel Smith, 'Cross-Channel Cavaliers', *The Seventeenth Century*, 2017, pp. 446–447.

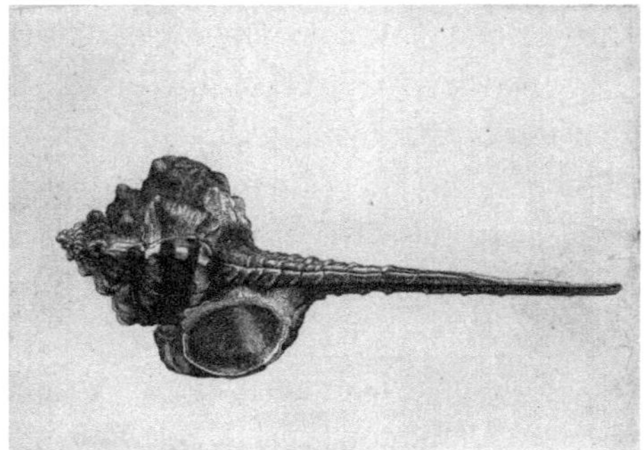

Fig. 4.2: Wenceslaus Hollar, *Murey snail*. A snail from the same family as the purple snail, c. 1644–1652. Etching. (© Rijksmuseum, Amsterdam).

the exclusive dye obtained from the purple snail (Fig. 4.2). As I mentioned in the introduction, this dye was considered the most precious in the ancient world, and was reserved for kings and other high-ranking persons. The comparisons show how highly this Persian product was valued. Lemery writes about the peach: 'Its flesh is marrowish, winish, and very pleasant to taste', and therapeutically it is good, among other things, 'at relieving the serum in the brain'.[15]

The merchants mentioned in the poems cited here probably belonged to Six's trading network. Many of these literary feasts would therefore have taken place after the signing of a contract of sale – indeed 'Vischmaal, aan Manuel Spranger' emphasises that the festive meal takes place 'naa [een bezoek aan] de beurs' ('after a visit to the stock exchange') (l. 9). In my opinion, both the texts themselves and the exotica mentioned in them should be seen against this background. They are intended to strengthen the links among the merchants concerned. The trade agreement may even have covered parties to the goods described in the poem.[16] The caviar trade between Amsterdam and Russia is proof of this. According to Eric Henk Wijnroks, this trade was very profitable:

> High profits stood to be earned from the caviar trade. In Russia, one barrel of caviar could fetch 15 to 20 Flemish pounds, while in Italy prices were sometimes 10 or even

15 'Haer vleesch is mergachtig, wynig, sappig, en van smaek zeer aangenaem','om de weivochten der hersenen te ontlasten', Lemery, 1743, p. 538.

16 In the urban culture of the early modern Republic, there was a great fondness for feasts and toasts, often combined with poetry reading. These festivities were characterised by a lot of formal and ceremonial display. On all kinds of occasions, from official holidays to weddings, engagement and farewell parties where people would go on long journeys, there would be banquets with refreshments. See Schama, 2004, pp. 178–188. See also the chapter 'Drinking Like a Man', in: Roberts, 2012, pp. 75–97.

> 20 times higher. As a link between the Italian and Russian markets, Amsterdam was the only Western European port where there was a lively trade in caviar.[17]

In Wijnroks's overview, Spranger is mentioned as a trader who did business in Russia. We already know that Six travelled to Italy as a merchant. It is possible that he bought Russian caviar from Spranger with a view to selling it to his business associates in Southern Europe.

The 'literary still-life paintings' discussed above are celebrations full of joy and a zest for life. In literary history, many of these verses are considered to be not only among the most beautiful and best poems in Six's *oeuvre*, but also among the highlights of literature from the Dutch Golden Age.[18] Their realism is indeed striking. But 'reality' and 'everyday character' are elastic concepts in this context. I would not go so far as to say they are examples of unpretentious everyday life. They are too strongly coloured by the aristocratic aspirations of elite culture. They are far from the idea of the Netherlands as a society characterised by honesty and simplicity. If we are looking for the kind of food that expresses austerity and modesty, that would be the primeval Dutch herring, cheese and stew – products that have a greater cultural and social symbolic value, and that served as the socio-religious hallmarks of the united and righteous Batavians – as the Dutch called themselves, referring to the myth of the heroic Germanic tribe, in their struggle against the tyrannical Spanish.[19] Willem Frijhoff and Marijke Spies emphasise that, in the middle of the seventeenth century, when Six was writing his poems, the rebellion against Spain had already reached mythical proportions. By contrast, Six's time was not dominated by the war of freedom against an oppressive country, but by the trade wars with England and by the struggle for power on the world's high seas and for the routes to colonial riches. At the same time, this period was marked by domestic disputes and the promulgation of laws on opulence, which proscribed excess and luxury. In the poetry of a wealthy spice merchant, we expect to find exotic delicacies on the menu, but as we shall see, Six also includes his diet in his self-portrayal as a sober druggist.[20]

17 Eric Henk Wijnroks, *Handel tussen Rusland en de Nederlanden, 1560–1640*, 2003, p. 342. For Amsterdam as a link between markets in Italy and in Eastern Europe, see Wätjen 1909, pp. 333–346. See also Israel, 1989, p. 47.

18 See, for example, the choice of text in G.A. van Es, *Poësy van J. Six van Chandelier: bloemlezing uit zijn dichtwerk*, 1953; M.A. Schenkeveld-van der Dussen, *Dutch Literature in the Age of Rembrandt: Themes and Ideas*, 1991.

19 On the myth of de Batavians, see: H. Kampinga, *De opvattingen over onze oudere vaderlandsche geschiedenis bij de Hollandsche historici der XVIe en XVIIe eeuw*, 1917; Hugo Grotius, *The Antiquity of the Batavian Republic*, with notes by Petrus Scriverius, 2000.

20 Willem Frijhoff & Marijke Spies, *1650. Hard-Won Unity*, 2004, pp. 36–39. *Cf.* ''t Lof van den Pekelharingh', 'Praise to the Salted Herring' by Jacob Westerbaen (the text is a translation of a Latin poem by an otherwise

Introduction to Dutch Medicines

Moralistic warnings against the excessive use of drugs and spices were common in the art and literature of the Republic. But there were also moralists who opted for more punitive measures and categorically rejected non-native medicines. *Inleydinge tot de Hollandtsche Genees-middelen: Ofte Kort bericht, dat elck landt ghenoegh heeft tot onderhoudt van het leven, ende de gesondtheydt der inwoonders* (*Introduction to Dutch Medicines: or Brief Message, That Every Country Has Enough to Support Life, and the Health of Its Inhabitants*) (1642) by Johan van Beverwijck is important in this connection. Van Beverwijck advocates the use of indigenous herbs rather than imported spices. It was not only in the Republic that his book would become influential. And two years later, he wrote a Latin translation of the book, *Autarkeia Bataviae, sive introductio ad medicinam indigenam*.[21]

According to Van Beverwijck, God provided every country with the medicines it needs to treat the diseases and ailments that are found there. In this view he was supported by numerous classical and contemporary authorities, from Pliny the Elder to Jacob Cats. He warned that the supply of medicines in his day was unsustainable. Patients now had to turn to 'several incomprehensible mishmashes' from Arabia and India, and 'for a small ulcer, a remedy must be obtained from the Red Sea'. These medicines benefit, not the patient, but others: 'Strange and far-fetched drugs [...] that serve more to make pharmacists rich than to make the sick healthy'. Van Beverwijck's plea does not imply that he considers European products superior to those from other countries. He holds that, just as tropical products are harmful to Europeans, European food – cabbage and onion – is unhealthy for Asians.[22]

The doctor's position is based on several arguments. However, one explanatory model gets particular attention – the humoral-climatic theories of classical authorities: the idea that people in northern countries should use plants grown under the same climatic conditions as they live in. This explanatory model is based on an analogy between microcosms and macrocosms: our bodies are related to the

unknown Laurens). Salted herring is 'goede medicyn; / Thrijakel kan niet zijn / Zoo waardigh om te loven' ('good medicine; Theriac cannot be worthy of the same praise.') Does the person who eats herring not live more healthily than 'die met / uijtghelesen / En dert'le leckerny sijn darmen / gulsigh vult?' ('the one who fills his intestines, greedy with superior and luscious delicacy?'), asks the poet rhetorically at the end. See also Gregor J.M. Weber, ''t Lof van den Pekelharingh. Von alltäglichen und absonderlichen Heringsstilleben', *Oud Holland*, 1987, pp. 126–140, quote on p. 127. For the classic miracle cure theriac, see Chapter 8, pp. 237–240.

21 For the influence that this polemic had on doctors in the Netherlands and abroad, see Cooper, 2007, pp. 41–50. But Van Beverwijck was not the first to take this stand in the early modern period. *Cf.* the writings of the German physician Ulrich von Hutten and the English moralist Timothy Bright: Freedman, 2008, pp. 147–149; Johnson, 2008, pp. 123–165.

22 'Verscheyde, en onbegrijpelijcke Mengel-moessen [...] voor een kleyne sweringe moet een heel-middel uyt de Roode-zee ghehaelt werden'; 'vremden en ver-gehaelde Drooghen [...] die meerder streckten om de Apothekers rijck, dan om de Krancken ghesont te maken', pp. 6 and 9.

climate of the country in which we grew up. The temperature and quality of native plants and herbs thus correspond to those of our body and mind, 'since the foreign and outlandish ones are utterly strange to us, since they originate and subsist under another sky, in another air, from another earth, and water.' In other words, 'cold' Europeans should be careful with spices and herbs from 'hot countries', which disrupt their physical nature and cause illness. The pathologising effect of strange drugs therefore also applies to our feelings and thoughts. This was also evident from Van Beverwijck's argument: 'Each country has its air, earth, and temperance, from which we in different ways derive the shape of our bodies and minds'. He emphasises 'that foreign drugs have no more in common with our bodies than strange manners have with our spirits and minds'.[23] The humanist physician derived these ideas from those of classical writers. Pliny, in his *Naturalis Historia*, considered a number of times what he saw as the dangerous influence of the decadent East on the simple, honest character of the Roman people. The same view is expressed in the literary ideals of Six, Persius and Horace.[24]

Van Beverwijck then puts forward four other arguments against the use of foreign medicines. I have already mentioned this in my analysis of the concept of 'drogerijen', but I will discuss it in more detail here.[25] The first argument concerns the originality of medicines – that it is uncertain whether the imported drugs correspond to the remedies described in classical works. We can

> not be assured that Drugs that are brought from afar are the same as those we find in the books of Physicians of old, because of the variety in their names, and because we frequently find their characteristics austere [in classical works]; those who describe these drugs therefore fall of necessity into discord and differences of opinion.[26]

He gives a few examples: anyone who can show the horn of a unicorn and prove that it comes from a real unicorn, and 'no one yet knows what ambergris is'.[27]

23 'Daer de Vremde, en Uytheemsche daer van gantsch vervremt zijn, als die onder eenen anderen Hemel, in andere Lucht, uyt andere Aerde, en Water hare oorspronk, en onderhoudt getrocken hebben'; 'elck landt heeft sijne lucht, aert, en gematigheyt, waer van wy verscheydelijck ontleenen de gestaltenis van onse lichamen en geesten'; 'dat de vremde droogen niet meerder met ons lichaem over een en komen, als de vremde manieren van onsen Geest en Gemoet', pp. 3 and 7.

24 For example, Pliny XXII, 118. For the Roman reception of exotic commodities, see: Grant Parker, 'Ex Oriente Luxuria: Indian Commodities and Roman Experience,' *Journal of Economic and Social History of the Orient*, 2002, pp. 40–95. See, *e.g.,* Persius' Satires 5 and 6, and Horace's Epistle II and Ode I. 38 and II.15.

25 See Chapter 2.

26 'Ons niet versekert houden, dat de Droogen, die van soo verre gebracht werden, alle deselvige zijn, die wy vinden in de boecken van de oude Genees-meesters, aengesien de verscheydenheyt van haer benamingen, en dat wy haer ken-teyckenen dikwils so sober beschreven vinden, daer daerom de nieuwe Kruyt-beschrijvers nootsakelijck in verschil, en oneenigheyt vervallen', p. 7.

27 'Het is noch niemant bekent wat Ambergrijs is', p. 7.

The second point concerns the freshness and strength of medicines: if foreign drugs are the same as those described by the classical authorities, storing them for a long time will spoil them and nullify their effects:

> For the Druggists who get them [the medicines] first, even though they stored them for many years, expect their buyers, and when they are purchased, they often remain for a long time still in the Pharmacy boxes, so that they eventually become mouldy (as you can see on long Pepper, Chinese root, and everything that carries an excess of moisture) and become maggoty; and therefore, when their freshness is gone, they also lose their healing power.[28]

The third argument concerns the common practice of falsification in the trade in, and preparation of, medicinal products. Even though exotic goods arrive fresh in the Republic, 'we cannot be assured that they are pure and unadulterated'. This is because of their unknown origin and the fact that these imported commodities pass through intermediaries before reaching European consumers. According to Van Beverwijck, it is important in this respect who these middlemen are: 'Moors, Turks, and Jews, who think they do a favour to God if they deceive the Christians'. The doctor then gives examples of expensive medicines that are subject to fakery, such as bezoar, saffron, aloe and opium.[29]

The fourth point concerns the prices of foreign medicines, and contains a social argument: foreign drugs cost 'often so much that the common man, who cannot recoup the expenses, is forced to wait', thus causing a lot of pain and even death. The high price then becomes a value in itself. He emphasises that the wisdom of the poor is no less than that of the rich, after which he speaks out against the use of exotic medicines as status symbols. This use of foreign medicines is discussed on a number of occasions in *Inleydinge tot de Hollandtsche Genees-middelen.* The author sees two reasons for the phenomenon. Referring to Cicero, he points to the 'disgust we feel at our own things' and to the appeal of 'Seldenheyt' ('Rarity'), which makes exotic products more expensive than local ones. But Van Beverwijck has it that, just as Indian products in the Netherlands are seen as embodying 'strangeness, rarity, and expensiveness', Dutch products such as cabbage and parsley would be seen in the

28 'Want de Droogisten, diese eerst krijghen, al hielden sy deselve noch veel jaren, verwachten haren koopman, en die al gevonden zijnde, blijven dickwils noch lange in de Apothekers doosen waer sy ten laetsten vermolmen (ghelijckmen veel siet aen de lange Peper, wortel China, en al dat wat overtollige vochtigheyt by hem heeft) en wormstekigh werden, en so met de verssigheydt oock haer kracht verliesen', p. 7.

29 'Wy en konnen ons niet versekeren, datse suyver en onvervalst zijn'; 'Moren, Turcken, en Ioden, die Godt een dienst meenen te doen, als sy de Christenen bedrieghen', p. 7. Adulterated goods were also something that the Six family had to deal with. In a notarial deed from 1652, Six reported on receiving a precious medicine: a load of bottles of so-called Balsam of Peru, delivered from Venice, that turned out to be 'counterfeit goods'. See Appendix II.

same way in India.[30] In other words, it is not a question of the natural characteristics of the commodity itself, but of socio-economic mechanisms, of the whims of the market and of merchants who are able to exploit the appeal of the unknown. It is not the goods themselves that determine prices, but the imagination with which they are associated and the status they have acquired in Western countries. In Van Beverwijck's view, it is not foreign products that are the problem, but their importers.[31]

Johan van Beverwijck's discussion of exotic drugs is in line with a discourse on luxury in which themes such as 'race' and 'ethnicity' play a role. The title of the Latin translation of his book, *Autarkeia Bataviae*, makes it clear that Van Beverwijck's radical argument is not only a plea for indigenous products, but also a formulation of a specifically Dutch character. He tells us that luxury medicines are incompatible with the morals and customs of the Batavian people, whose main characteristics are equality, solidarity and humility.[32] Van Beverwijck argues that there is a connection between indigenousness, austerity and health on the one hand, and strangeness, luxury and disease on the other. The bodies of the Dutch are at stake: their Dutchness is threatened by transformative foreign forces. Dangerous stimulants arouse barbaric passions in 'cold' Northerners, as well as dangerous drives such as greed, lust and pride – vices that, in the eyes of Protestant moralists, were typical of aristocratic, decadent Southern Europe. What is important in Van Beverwijck's argument is that the Batavians are defined not so much on the basis of external characteristics such as skin colour as on the basis of an inner, physical condition which in turn is related to the diet and lifestyle of the people. This explanation is in line with the concept of *geohumoralism,* which I discussed in the Introduction: in early modern times, 'race' was still a pliable concept, and a change in diet, for instance, could bring about a radical change in identity.[33]

The Greek *autarkeia* (autarky) means an attempt to achieve full economic independence. In addition to rejecting 'hot' medicines on the grounds of their humoral incompatibility with European people's bodies, Van Beverwijck's argument therefore recognises classical economic arguments against international trade: the high prices of 'kostelijcke droogen' undermine the domestic economy (p. 6). But what is interesting to us is the medical theories that suggest a pathologisation of international trade. In Van Beverwijck's opinion, the import of exotic spices into the Republic is no less objectionable than the slave trade and the exploitation of innocent peoples in the colonies.

30 'Dickwils soo veel, dat de ghemeene man, die de onkosten niet en kan vergelden, gedwongen is te verwachten'; 'walging van onze eigen dingen'; 'vremdigheydt, seldenheyt, en dierte', p. 9. See Cicero, *On Ends*, 1931, book 1. 10, p. 13.

31 Van Beverwijck's argument is illustrated in a poem by Jacob Cats that is included in the polemic, 'Geestige Herdersklachte' ('A Spiritual Complaint of the Shepherd') (p. 6), which appears at the beginning of this chapter.

32 *Cf.* Frijhoff & Spies, 2004, pp. 36–39.

33 *Cf.* Meijer Drees, 1997; Rebecca Earle, *The Body of the Conquistador: Food, Race and the Colonial Experience in Spanish America, 1492–1700*, 2012.

The issue is what the consequences of the polemic were, because, as we know, there was, of course, no abrupt end to the colonial power to trade with distant parts of the world, the Dutch Republic in fact dominated the world trade in this period.[34] Moreover, Van Beverwijck's inconsistencies are striking; after all, his other medical books, as we have seen, contain a great deal of praise for the beneficial powers of foreign drugs and spices, and they incorporate foreign plants into the Western humoral system. Researchers such as Lia van Gemert and Julie Berger Hochstrasser argue that we should therefore take his polemic with a grain of salt. According to Van Gemert, Van Beverwijck argues that 'one should use the power of every available medicine, as long as one does not want to have it no matter the costs, and as long as one keeps in mind that one's own product is preferable.'[35] However, as I noted in my introduction, other researchers claim that the work had moral, cultural and scientific consequences. Alix Cooper argues that an interest in native plants was by no means a self-evident process, but that it was embedded in the struggle between the foreign and the indigenous. She mentions in this connection the first extensive native work on the flora of the Netherlands, *Catalogus plantarum indigenarum Hollandiae* (1683) by Jan Commelin. A look at other important medical works in the Republic confirms her observation. In his foreword to *De Nederlandtse Herbarius of Kruydt-boeck* (1670) (Fig. 4.3), the Amsterdam doctor Petrus Nylandt writes that the book includes Dutch plants that he has gathered, 'so that it is unnecessary to search for or import, with great curiosity, and at even greater expense, other foreign Spices and Plants from faraway Countries whose Climate is quite different from ours'.[36]

Instead of economic consequences, one would then speak of the influence that the discourse of indigenous versus foreign plants had on the cultural, scientific and social life of the Dutch Republic, because the dangers of exotic and expensive drugs from the city apothecary is a *topos* in praise poems on rural life. For example, Jacob Westerbaen speaks, in his praise poem on his Ockenburgh estate, of 'Drogien' ('drugs') that 'have long been desiccated, mouldy and rotten', while Constantijn Huygens argues in his *Dagh-werck* that 'what we consume from our own drugstore should be less nauseous than what is brought from abroad'.[37] Below I will argue that

34 See Israel, 1989.

35 Hochstrasser, 2007; Lia van Gemert, '"U Kunst gelt over-al": een Dordtse arts tussen West en Oost', *Literatuur: Tijdschrift over Nederlandse letterkunde*, 1993, p. 16–22, quote on p. 19.

36 'Soo dat het onnoodigh is, andere vreemde Kruyden en Gewassen in ver geleden, en seer van onsen Climaet verscheyden Landen met groote curieusheyt, en noch meerder onkosten op te soecken ofte over te brengen'. See the unpaginated introduction by Petrus Nylandt, *De Nederlandtse Herbarius or Kruydt-boeck*, 1670. Incidentally, Nylandt does include a small number of exotic herbs that in his view are indispensable.

37 'Lang verdroogt, verschimmelt en verrot', Ockenburgh: J. Westerbaen, *Gedichten, Verdeylt in Vijf Boecken*, 1657, part IV, p. 137; ''tghene wij ons seluen soo uijt onse eighen droogisterije ingeuen, sal ons min walghen, dan 'tghene van buijten werdt gebracht', Huygens, *Dagh-werck* [1658] (1973), p. 357. The

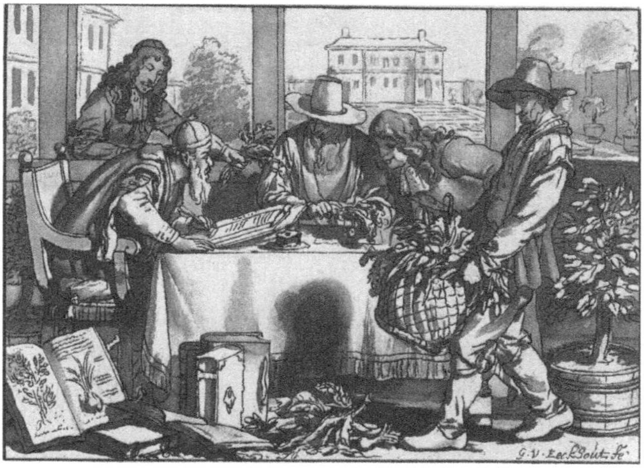

Fig. 4.3: Cornelis Ploos van Amstel after Gerbrand van den Eeckhout, *Botanicus*, c. 1780–1787. Ink and brush. Illustration on title page of Petrus Nylandt, *De Nederlandtse Herbarius of Kruydt-boeck*. (© Rijksmuseum, Amsterdam).

this ecologically oriented discourse, which places green herbs above dried drugs, also influenced Six's poetics. At the same time, I will mention texts by doctors and botanists that are relevant here.

'Necessity is enough'

One would expect this capitalist, this self-confident burgher who is wealthy thanks to international trade, to reject ideas that undermine the very basis of his existence, but surprisingly, there are actually poems in *Poësy* that support Van Beverwijck's views.

One poem directly related to Van Beverwijck's argument is 'Nooddruft is genoegh' ('Necessity is enough') (J133). As the title suggests, the theme of the text is the opposition between the 'nooddruft', *i.e.* 'necessitie of nature, as victuals; meate, drinke, and cloathing', and what is superfluous, *i.e.* luxury goods from foreign

rhyming pair 'doogen' – 'droogen' ('function – drugs') is important in this context. It is also found in *Lof der Geldsucht* by Jeremias de Decker: 'Sijn kruyderen en droogen / Soo droog somtijds en dor, dat sij niet veel en doogen, / En maaken niet alleen een openingh in 't lyf, / Maer in de geldbors oock, al slootse noch soo stijf' ('His spices and drugs [in the city apothecary] so dry sometimes and arid, that they do not function much, and make not only an opening in the body, but in the money purse too, even though it is closed so firmly') (p. 40). *Cf.* the same opposition between the natural pleasures of the garden and the unhealthy perfumes of the city in English literature, Holly Dugan, *The Ephemeral History of Perfume. Scent and Sense in Early Modern England*, 2011, pp. 154–181.

lands.[38] 'Wie leeven kan te huis, in vree, / Wat jaaght hy naa de ryke zee?' ('He who can live at home, in peace, what drives him to the rich sea?' (l. 5–6), Six asks rhetorically at the beginning of the text. He then gives a picture of those who are satisfied with what the local environment has to offer (l. 19–34):

Luksaaligh is hy, die genoegen,
In land, schept, als geleent te ploegen:
Wat schraaler dan Ismenias,
Wat vetter dan 't by Kodrus was.
Een simple borger leeft veel blyder,
Nooit schroomich voor den bitsen nyder.
De nachtmeer van 't ontslaaprigh geld
Doet, hem vermoeit, vergeefs geweld.
De suchtvloek van de goude scherven
Verdoemt hem niet: gedenk te sterven,
O gierge dwaas, in deesen nacht.
Wat baat hem rykdom dan, en pracht?
Syn ziel gaat moedernaakt versinken,
Om 't vuur oneindelyk te drinken.
Hy die gepurpert swolgh den wyn,
Smeekt, om een druppel, uit den Rhyn.

Blissful is he who is satisfied
To plough the land that is entrusted to him:
A little poorer than Ismenias,
A little richer than Codrus,
A simple citizen lives more happily,
Never afraid of the backbiting, jealous ones.
The nightmare of money that startles him awake
Harasses him in vain when he is tired.
The accursed desire for gold coins
Does not condemn him: remember death,
O greedy fool, in this night.
What good does wealth or splendour do him, then?
His soul will sink, stark naked,
And drink forever from the flames.
He who, dressed in purple, drank up the wine,
Now begs for a drop of the Rhine.

38 'Nootruft' in Hexham 1658, unpaginated.

Ismenias of Thebes, a character from Plato's *Meno*, was renowned for his riches, while Kodros was a Greek prince who dressed like a beggar.[39] The ideal Six proposes is to be neither rich nor poor, but to live as 'een simple borger' ('a simple citizen'). The rich man has nightmares about money. When his wealth sends him to hell, he begs for a drop of water from the Rhine. In the next line, the punishment for harbouring a desire for goods is described with a play of words: 'O goed, niet goed, dat uw besitter / Betaalt, met zulken heilich bitter' ('O goods, not good, that pay your owner with such a holy bitter') (l. 35). 'Bitter heilig' could be interpreted in a figurative sense as 'bitter fate'. But given Six's playful style of writing, the word can also be understood literally: 'bitterheilig' (*herea picra*) was an ill-tasting purgative.[40] Thus the introduction of the rich man to a fiery hell is immediately experienced as bitter and dirty. At the same time, the metaphor is reminiscent of the products of the early modern apothecary. The 'bitterheilig' compound consisted of various exotic ingredients in which the early modern druggist traded, including aloe and cinnamon. The criticism in this poem has to do, then, with Six himself. He himself is a trader in hellish substances. This quotation also echoes the humoral-climatic theories: the rich man, dressed in purple and drinking wine, is swallowed up in a pool of fire, where he begs for a drop of the opposite humoral component: water.[41] But it is not just any water that will quench his thirst, but a drop of water from the Rhine, a river in his own country.

Six's image of the 'simple borger' in his pastoral landscape corresponds to Van Beverwijck's autarkic ideal: the Batavian happily ploughing a field in his own country. He succeeds in curbing his excessive desires and rejects exotic luxury.[42] And these are the words of a wealthy merchant! But one may also wonder how significant the self-critical element in the text is. If we put the poem next to Horace's famous *Beatus ille* (Epode II), it becomes clear that the text is partly an *imitatio*.[43] Should 'Nooddruft is genoegh' thus be read as a literary exercise – a half-hearted penance from someone who also knows that commercial interests always take precedence? I will consider this possibility in more detail below in my discussion of Six's medical history.

39 Jacobs, 1991 II, p. 247.

40 See the meaning in *WNT*.

41 The image is derived from the Bible – see Luke 16:19. *Cf.*, too, the explanation given about this biblical site in Wittewrongel, 1661 II, p. 1115.

42 The ideal of necessity is frequently discussed in Coornhert's ethics. See Johan Koppenol, *Leids heelal. Het Loterijspel (1596) van Jan van Hout*, 1998, pp. 350–351.

43 Six also bases himself on other sources, including Horace's Ode II, 16, and, as we have seen, on texts by other poets. See Jacobs, 1991 II, pp. 247–248.

Visits to botanical gardens

The rejection of exotic luxury is reflected in several texts in *Poësy*. A good example is 'Wild tuilken, aan Raimond Smeth' ('Wild Bouquet, to Raimond Smeth') (J109), which Six dedicates to an old merchant and distant cousin, who has replaced the uncertain life of a trader with a quiet life on his estate by the river Vecht.[44] The original way in which Six presents himself in this poem is interesting: it is not Six, but a bouquet of wild flowers that is speaking (l. 25–36):

Merk myn verscheiden reuk, en kleur
Meer dan met tachtich eige naamen,
Die meenigh bloementuin beschaamen,
Verciert met weingerleije keur,
In Holland al te kostelyk geplant,
Ontbooden uit geen naageleegen land.
Van sulk aanloklik veldgewas
Weet Koridon een krans te vlechten,
En die syn lief, om 't hoofd, te hechten,
Wyl sy de schaapjes hoed, in 't gras:
Dat bly cieraad behaaght de harderin,
Voor sorglik goud, op Medens Kooningin.

Notice my different smells and colours,
More than eighty plant names,
Which put to shame many flower gardens
Decorated with a less extensive selection
Of plants imported from foreign countries,
Planted at excessive cost in Holland.
From such appealing field plants,
Coridon braided a wreath,
Which he attached to the head of his beloved,
While she herded the sheep in the grass.

44 For the relationship between Six and Raimond de Smeth, see Appendix II. On the many risks associated with trading in the early modern era, see Kooijmans 1995, pp. 65–92. Bankruptcy in particular had major social consequences, including the withholding of the Lord's Supper. See R.B. Evenhuis, *Ook dat was Amsterdam. De kerk der hervorming in de gouden eeuw*, II, 1967, pp. 150–154. Some trading partners of Six's also went bankrupt, including Manuel Spranger in 1658 (whereupon he fled to France), and Isaak de Bra, the merchant who gave Six a bezoar stone (J476), in 1665 – see http://research.frick.org/montias/browserecord.php?-action=browse&-recid=2351 and http://research.frick.org/montias/browserecord.php?-action=browse&-recid=2535 (consulted 17 May 2019).

That happy jewellery pleases the shepherdess,
More than worry-making gold
On the head of the Queen of Meden.

We read that the wildflowers 'embarrass' many Dutch gardens, which are decorated with precious plants imported from abroad. The pastoral motif in the quotation is accompanied by elements from peasant scenes from ancient literature. For example, among classical writers, Corydon is the usual name for shepherds.[45] The wildflowers then give their verdict on precious plants from foreign climes: they are as reprehensible as 'worry-making gold on the head of the Queen of Meden' – Vasthi's famous golden crown (see Esther 1:10–19). The position of the poem in *Poësy*, in the Spa series, reveals more about the function of these flowers. In this series of texts, Six portrays himself not only as a patient but also as a medical adviser. Besides drinking the mineral Spa water, he also emphasises the importance of physical exercise out in the open air, among the invigorating 'bloemen, die daar schoon in 't wilde tieren' ('flowers, which grow beautifully in the wild there') (J101, l. 339). The scent of wildflowers in the Ardennes is therefore part of Six's Spa treatment. They have a therapeutic effect.

Poësy also contains a series of poems dedicated to botanical gardens. In these texts, too, the debate about local green plants and exotic dry drugs has a central place. During his business trips through the Southern Spanish Netherlands, the Calvinist grocer was not afraid of having contact with Catholics (although his many outbursts against Catholicism in other texts give a different impression. I will come back to this below). He visited the city of Ninove (near Aalst) on two occasions, and befriended the Norbertine Amandus Fabius, a monk and the supervisor of the local monastery garden (Fig. 4.4). Fabius is a Latinisation of the actual surname of the priest: Boon, Boonen, or Boonaert. Six's maternal grandfather came from Ninove. It could be that Six also went there to visit family. The encounter will likely have had something *gentlemanly* about it, because Fabius was a scholar and the author of neo-Latin works, in addition to being an herbalist who had even garnered some fame abroad.[46] I will discuss here the two poems that came out of Six's second visit to Ninove in 1654, when he was on his way to visit England for the first time. The first poem is a lyrical poem of praise for the monastery garden. In 'Erkentenisse, aan Amandus Fabius, priester in St. Kornelis Klooster, en opsiender des hofs daar aan geleegen, te Nineve' ('Recognition to Amandus Fabius, Priest in St. Cornelis Monastery, and Supervisor of the Garden There, in Ninove') (J368). Whereas in the text to Raimond de Smeth, Six creates an identity in direct opposition to his work as a druggist, he once again bases himself on

45 The name is known from Ecloga VII by Virgil, for example (Jacobs, 1991 II, p. 202).
46 Jacobs, 1991 II, p. 735; for details on Amandus Fabius, see Robrecht Lievens, 'Dichterlof voor de Ninoofse kloostertuin', *Land Aalst*, 1999, pp. 148–159.

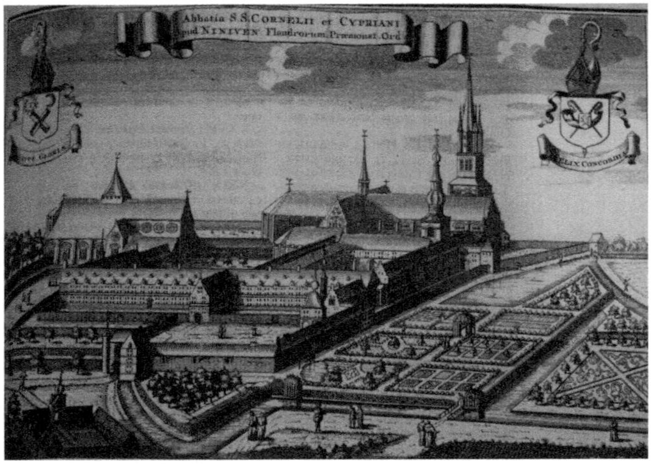

Fig. 4.4: *Ninove Abbey*, illustration from Antonius Sanderus, *Flandria Illustrata*, 1735. (© University Library of Oslo).

a poetics of *dryness* in this poem: he presents himself as a 'dry' rhymester who needs just a 'dropjen geestgen inkt' ('a small drop of spiritual ink') (l. 10) to be able to write a poem to the monk. Six praises the garden, the 'earthly paradise' (l. 14) where the plants are the monk's 'miracles' (l. 19). 'Wat rost, en reist men Oost, en West? / Hier siet men, t' huis is allerbest' ('Why travel and rush off to the East and the West? Here one sees that staying at home is best') (l. 25–26). In 'Op het Latynsche Dankdicht, Van Amandus Fabius, Norbertyn te Nineve, Voor het geschenk van syne Hoogheid Leopold Wilhelm, Aertshertoch van Oostenryk, steedehouder der Spaansche Nederlanden' ('On the Latin Poem of Thanks by Amandus Fabius, Norbertine in Ninove, for the Gift from his Highness Leopold Wilhelm, Archduke of Austria, Stadtholder of the Spanish Netherlands') (J428), Six again plays on the meaning of the surname Fabius, which once again has a deeper significance (l. 1–5):

Damaskus vruchtbre daadelstam
Geeft malse daadels, naa veel jaaren,
Maar van u, goede boonaard, quam
Al vroegh de vrucht der baakelaaren,
Die God Apol zyn toegewydt.

The fertile date plants of Damascus
Give tender dates after many years,
But from you, good bean-earth, there already came
Early the fruit of the laurels,
Which are dedicated to the God Apollo.

Six portrays Fabius as 'bean-earth' – soil that produces beans that are as healthy and evergreen as the leaves of the 'baakelaaren' – the laurel, the tree of Apollo, god of poetry. Six thus metaphorically describes the neo-Latin poem that Fabius presented to Stadtholder Leopold Wilhelm as one of Fabius's 'healthy beans'. But Six also insinuates himself into the quotation: in contrast to fresh and fast-growing beans, the tender dates from the Damascus 'date plants' were an article that could be found in drugstores in the early modern period. After picking, dates are 'hung to dry in the sun / so that they can be sent away more skilfully and kept well for longer', Dodonaeus tells us. Taking as a starting point the contrast between dried and exotic plants on the one hand, and fresh, native ones on the other, Six offers a double portrait of himself and his friend, in which the uprooted druggist-rhymester considers himself to be inferior and, moreover, deficient when compared to the native botanist-poet.[47]

The contempt for foreign plants is expressed even more clearly in a poem of praise for the first prefect of Amsterdam's first *Hortus Medicus*: 'Steetuinkroon aan Joannes Snippendal' ('Crown of the City Garden, to Johannes Snippendaal') (J146).[48] Six compares the botanist Johannes Snippendaal (1617–1670) and his botanical garden to the famous Carolus Clusius and his extensive *hortus* in Leiden. Six emphasises that the work Snippendaal does promotes the health of the city's population. Thanks to Snippendaal's continual search for new medicinal plants, and to his catalogue of the many plant species present in the *hortus*, the sick no longer have to resort to 'wydgehaalde droogen / Die dikwils schaars zyn, of niet doogen' ('drugs fetched from afar that are often scarce or do not work well') (l. 10–12): 'Gebruik, maar fris, en deughdsaam kruid' ('Use only fresh, wholesome herbs') (l. 13), Six advises his readers. Snippendaal thus follows Van Beverwijck's ideal: laying the foundations for an urban *hortus* will make trade with remote parts of the world superfluous. In the Amsterdam *hortus* one could also find herbs from foreign regions, as we read later in the poem. Six explains that this is thanks to modern techniques: growing in greenhouses or, indeed, in artificial shade, makes it possible to grow, in the Netherlands, herbs of a 'verkouwende aard' ('cold origin'), from Arctic areas (those areas that are, we read, under the constellations of the Great Bear or the Small Bear), l. 23–28:

47 'In de Sonne te droogen gehangen / op dat sy bequamer wegh gesonden ende langher goedt bewaert moghen worden', Dodonaeus 1644, p. 1283; Jacobs, 1991 II, p. 735. It could be that Six sold dates to the monastery of Amandus Fabius. Lievens (1999, p. 158) assumes that Six visited Ninove for commercial reasons, in addition to a possible visit to family in the area.

48 For more on Johannes Snippendaal and the first Amsterdam *hortus*, see Ferry Bouman, Bob Baljet & Erik Zevenhuizen (eds.), *Kruidenier aan de Amstel. De Amsterdamse Hortus volgens Johannes Snippendaal (1646)*, 2007.

Het Oost, noch West, noch Suiden queekt
Zoo fraaijen bloem, die hier ontbreekt.
Al heeft ons Noorde korter hetten,
Met kachels weet hy son te setten.
De kruiden uit verkouwende aard,
Ontrent den Noordschen beer vergaart,
Of met, of sonder schaaduw wassen,
In schraaler sand of vettere aschen.

Neither the East nor the West, nor yet the South cultivates
So beautiful a flower, which is missing here.
Although the North, where we live, has less prolonged heat,
With stoves [in greenhouses] he succeeds in prolonging the sun.
Herbs from freezing soil,
By the Northern bear [Ursa Major or Minor],
Thrive with or without shadow,
In poorer sandy, or richer soil.

The text confirms important innovations that took place under the leadership of the manager of the *hortus,* Johannes Snippendaal: the number of plants increased from 300 to 800 around 1646, and the Amsterdam *hortus* was probably the first to have a greenhouse installed. But Six's argument apparently contains deviations from Johan van Beverwijck's autarkic ideal. There is no flower that grows so beautifully in the East, the West or the South that there is no example of it in Snippendaal's garden, the poet argues. Exotic drugs may therefore be used by the Dutch as long as they thrive in Dutch soil. This thought was not unusual in the Republic. A few decades after *Inleydinge tot de Hollandtsche Genees-middelen*, a medical treatise was published that once again called into question the issue of exotic versus indigenous medicines: *Dissertatio de re herbaria* (1683), written by pharmacist Lambert Bidloo. The treatise was bound up with, and functioned as an introduction to, the first extensive native flora of the Netherlands: *Catalogus plantarum indigenarum Hollandiae*, by the above-mentioned Jan Commelin. Bidloo repeats many of Van Beverwijck's arguments. As far as the effects of foreign drugs on society are concerned, he even uses stronger words than his older colleague: 'Due to the wares of foreigners, weakness, luxury, and gluttony are now stealing our people, as happened to the Romans in their day [...]'.[49] But at the same time he blurs the contrast between exotic and native plants by accepting foreign plants in Dutch gardens as long as they are able to acclimate to their new environment.

49 Bidloo, 1683, p. 34. I have taken the quotation from Cooper, 2007, p. 47.

This apothecary reports that he knows at least 600 plant species that have become accustomed to the Dutch climate. However, Bidloo does not give the whole list: he mentions only two examples of exotic plants that have become acclimated, such as potatoes and tobacco, which are grown on a large scale by Dutch farmers. That Bidloo earlier in the treatise had warned against tobacco now seems to have been forgotten.[50]

Were such ideas already in vogue when Six wrote his praise poem to Snippendaal? For him, this does not mean any legitimisation of his trade in exotic drugs. Bidloo's criticism of drugs does not necessarily concern tropical plants as such. But he is sceptical about the treatment process that foreign drugs usually undergo: the preservation of fresh herbs to make them suitable for long-distance transport, which diminishes their medical potency and obscures their geographical origin. For Snippendaal, on the other hand, there is no need to engage intermediaries: for him, fresh medicines can be had directly from the *hortus,* regardless of whether they are of Dutch or foreign origin.

Could it be that, in addition to his professional interest in botany, his search for remedies for the ailment in his spleen was another reason for his visit? A year before Six travelled to Spa for his medical treatment, in 1655, he wrote a poem praising the marriage of his friend and travel companion Abraham Grenier: 'Trouwdagh, van Abraham Grenier, rechtsgeleerden' ('Wedding day of Abraham Grenier, jurist') (J410). In a tribute to the wealth of colours and smells of the Dutch spring, Six mentions an herb from which he personally benefits (l. 29–32):

Tamme hoppe, dat kostelik kruid,
Voor verstoppingh der miltepynen,
Eert myn taafel, met spruitjen, op spruit,
Als salaadjes in porcelynen.

Domesticated hop, that precious herb
For constipation in those with an ailment of the spleen,
Graces my table with sprout upon sprout,
Like salad in a porcelain bowl.

In *Inleydinge tot de Hollandtsche Genees-middelen,* Van Beverwijck recommends this plant, which grows wild in the Netherlands, as an indigenous medicine against 'verstoptheyt' ('blockage') and 'gele-sucht ('jaundice').[51] One could regard Six's

50 See Cooper, 2007, pp. 46–49.

51 Van Beverwijck, *Inleydinge tot de Hollandtsche Genees-middelen*, p. 20. And *cf.* Dodonaeus on hops, the leaves and stem of this herb 'openen de verstoptheydt van de lever, milte ende nieren, ende reynighen

therapeutic suggestion as a pronouncement in its own right, but even in the texts addressed to the Greniers family, the merchant makes moral statements about global trade. In a text addressed to his friend's father, Six writes, 'Blyde begroetinge, aan Abraham Grenier den ouden, oover de weederwelvaarentheit van synen soone' ('Cheerful Greetings to Abraham Grenier, on His Son's Return to Health') (J314, l. 47–48). 'Men zou hier [in Nederland] raad voor sieken graaven, / En niet na verre ryken draaven' ('Here [in the Netherlands] one should unearth remedies for patients and not rush off to faraway realms'). It could be that Six received hops from Johannes Snippendaal's botanical garden.

Ambergris

Many texts in *Poësy* have the history of Six's ailment as their theme. I will discuss the texts that can shed some light on the relationship between this ailment and his trading in drugs. I will focus on three druggists' wares: ambergris, gold and the horns of exotic animals. In this section, too, I will suggest that the debate about foreign drugs versus fresh, homegrown herbs also plays a role in Six's self-portrayal as a patient seeking a remedy.

We will look first at ambergris. This substance is discussed in 'Dankdicht aan Simon Dilman' ('Poem of Thanks for Simon Dilman') (J142), which is addressed to Six's regular doctor. Before I start the analysis, we should dwell for a moment on the addressee of the poem: ''s Amsterdammers winter' ('Winter in Amsterdam') (J96), the longest poem in *Poësy*, is dedicated to him. This indicates the importance of the place that Dilman occupied in Six's life. Six seems to have built up a close friendship with him. Their families were also bound together by marriage: Simon Dilman was a cousin by marriage, since he was married to the cousin of the poet, Janneke Hartgers.[52] In those poems of Six's in which Dilman features, the contact between them is not really like what we would find in a relationship between a patient and a doctor, but is all about encounters between a learned poet-druggist and a humanistically trained physician.[53] Six even dedicates poems to other members of

dat bloedt van alle onsuyverheydt [...]' ('open the blockage of the liver, spleen and kidneys, and clean the blood of all impurity [...]'). I have taken this quotation from Jacobs, 1991 II, p. 712.

52 See Appendix II.

53 It seems that Dilman's circle of friends included several poets. See Jan Vos, 'Toen den E. Heer Dylman, Geneesmeester t'Amsterdam, op zyn vertrek stondt, om te Wormer, op zyn Hofsteê, te gaan woonen' ('When the Noble Mr. Dylman, Physician in Amsterdam, was about to go and live in Wormer, on his estate'), *Alle de gedichten,* part 1, 1662, pp. 253–254; and the assignment from Oliver van den Tempel in his *Torquato Tassoos: Vierde Gezangh van Ierusalems Verlossinge*, 1644, which is dedicated to the *'medicus ordinarius* Symon Dylman' (pp. III–V).

Dilman's family. One gets the impression that he was more or less a poet in residence to the Dilman family. One of Dilman's sons even served as an apprentice in Six's drugstore.[54] But despite the nice tone in the druggist's poems to his doctor, some texts show that this was not a friendship without disagreements. As we shall see, Six was not pleased with Dilman's medical treatment methods.

As the title suggests, the poem was written as an expression of thanks for a piece of advice Dilman had given to Six. What that advice entailed is not said, but it seems that moderation and austerity in one's diet were at the heart of it. Six emphatically states that he has understood the dietary lessons well: 'Ik haat de wys der slempren, en, de reên / Der brassende Apiciaanen' ('I hate the song of the gourmands and the talk of the guzzling Apicians') (l. 11–12): Apicians are imitators of the Roman gourmet Apicius, whose cookbook has come down to us. Six continues: 'Een graage maagh brenght self het soetst banket. / De saus werd van den honger opgeset' ('A hungry stomach itself ensures that the banquet tastes well. The sauce is served by your own hunger') (l. 13–14). As we have seen, sauce was a synonym for the use of rich spices. Writing as though he were present at one of Plato's symposia, Six acknowledges that a 'schootel wyse spreuken' ('dish of wise sayings') (l. 28) that Dilman served is more valuable than any culinary delicacies.[55]

In the following passage, Six shows that he knows the pathological consequences of excessive eating: if 'men veel de keel begiet, en smeert, / De volle maagh, / met neevelen, verteert, / in 't vadsich hoofd' ('you fill and stuff your throat, the full stomach, while digesting, produces dimming vapours that rise to the head') (l. 29–31). Nutrition causes constipation not only in the stomach, but – given the major role that Galenic physiology assigns to digestion – also in central bodily

54 For example, Six wrote poems about the birthday of Dilman's wife, about the birth of a child, and about the couple's daughter: 'Geboortuur, aan Johanna Dilman, myn nichte' ('Birthday, to Johanna Dilman, My Cousin') (J194), 'Geboortlaurier aan Joanna Dilman' ('Birth Laurel to Johanna Dilman') (J344), 'Op het geestigh dochtertjen, van Simon Dilman, geneesheer' ('On the Wise Daughter of Simon Dilman, Physician') (J328). A son, Jacob Dilman, appears to have been apprenticed to the Six family business – see ''s Amsterdammers winter' (J96), l. 820–852 and 'Aan Simon Dilman geneesheer' (J281). One can even track the highlights of the life story of the physician's older son, Joannes Dilman, through the occasional poems Six wrote to him, from the beginning of his medical training through his academic disputation to his wedding: 'Lauwerier, aan Joannes Dilman, beweert hebbende de inleidinge der geneeskonste' ('Laurel, to Joannes Dilman, Having Completed the Introduction of Medicine' (J295), 'Welkomst, aan Joannes Dilman, van Leiden, naa hy geneesheer was gemaakt, alvooren hebbende beweert, wat raasernye was' ('Welcome to Johannes Dilman, from Leiden, after He Was Made Physician, Having Shown What Frenzy Was') (J381), and 'Trouw van Joannes Dilman geneesheer, met Elisabeth de Vry' ('Wedding of Joannes Dilman, Physician, to Elisabeth de Vry') (J403). And not to forget: even if it is not clear at first glance, the longest text in *Poësy*, ''s Amsterdammers winter' (J96), is actually an invitation to Simon Dilman to come to dinner.

55 *Cf.* the meaning of 'sauce' in ''t Huisblyvens beede, aan Jan Druivestein, te Venecie' ('Plea to Stay Home, to Jan Duivestein, in Venice') (J287), l. 30.

processes. This causes undigested spirits to come back up, thus creating a haze in the brain – a scenario often portrayed clinically in early modern medicine. This results in various disorders, such as confusion and weakened judgment, and that in turn means that one succumbs to other passions. Six closes out the text with a testament to the satiating effect of Dilman's advice. The taste of that advice is better than that of delicious food (l. 33–40):

> Ghy saaght met wat een smaaklikheit ik at,
> En dronk, ook hoe leerhongrigh dat ik sat,
> Om uit uw praat van artsenye wat
> Besonders op te leggen.
> Dat smaakt myn geest langhwyliger dan spys
> Van Ambar of een kostelyker prys [...]
>
> You saw with what appetite I ate
> And drank, and how eager to learn I was,
> In order to gather some details
> Of your lessons on medicine.
> That is a taste with with a longer-lasting effect
> Than food made of Ambergris or [an ingredient] of a higher price [...]

In ancient times it was thought that ambergris (the fragrance from the sperm whale's intestinal canal) and amber (fossilised tree resin) were the same thing. Early modern naturalists and doctors, for example, distinguished between grey amber – *ambergris* is the old French word for 'grey amber' – and yellow amber. The 'Ambar' in this poem probably refers to grey amber, which is found floating in the sea or washed up on the beach.[56] There was still a great deal of mystery surrounding this substance in the seventeenth century: Van Beverwijck wrote, 'no one yet knows what grey amber is'.[57] But in *Schat der gesontheyt,* the physician offers possible explanations for the origin of the precious substance – almost as many as there are conditions against which the drug would work. I will mention a few of them here. The first is not far from the truth, but is not considered to be the most credible: 'Some believe that it is the Seed of Whales, others, a droppings of some Sea monster, some foam of the Sea. But more credible is the saying of those who claim it to be a Glue, which is cast out of the sea upon the beach'.[58] In other

56 *Cf.* 'amber' and 'barnsteen' in the WNT.

57 'Het is noch niemant bekent wat Ambergrijs is'.

58 'Eenige meenen, dat het Zaet is van Walvisschen, andere, een uytworpsel van eenich Zeemonster, sommige schuym van de Zee. Maer geloofflijcker is het seggen van de ghene, die het stellen te zijn een Lijm, die onder uyt de Zee op strandt gheworpen werdt', p. 39.

words: a typical item in an early modern drugstore. Incidentally, Six links the confusion caused by voraciousness to the consumption of ambergris. Elsewhere in his medical reference work, Van Beverwijck writes, in reference to the Italian doctor Pietro Andrea Mattioli, 'that ambergris put into wine makes one drunk'.[59] Six occupies a humble position with respect to Dilman. He relates to him as a grateful patient.

So this time, it is not about non-native substances in relation to Six's role as an importer, but about exotics in relation to his sick body. As a druggist, Six had ready access to exotic drugs, either as a stimulant or as a remedy for his ailment. The mere exposure of his body to *exotica* in the course of his daily professional activities would have been a risk to his health. Six had to use his senses actively in testing and controlling his merchandise mainly through the physical observation of substances. As I mentioned above, Pamela H. Smith emphasises the great role that the artisan played in the seventeenth century in acquiring knowledge. A good illustration of this can be found in Sijbrand Feitama's 'Op de vyf Zinnen' ('On the Five Senses'). Without these, there is no 'volleerd Drogist' ('fully trained druggist'), Feitama declares in the first strophe. In strophe five, on taste, he elaborates on what he means by this: 'Die twyffelagtig zyn in d'een of d'and're zaak, / Die neemen ten behulp de proeve van de Smaak' ('those who are doubtful in one or the other matter carry out a taste test as an aid') (Fig. 4.5).[60]

'Dankdicht aan Simon Dilman' shows that Six's medical history is important for a good understanding of his experience of exotic substances in *Poësy*. Other poems, such as 'Op de reedenstryd, oover de kooninghlyke siekte, te Leiden gehouden, door Geeraard Worst, voor syn geneesheerschap' ('On the Disputation on the King's Evil, Held at Leiden by Geeraard Worst, for His Doctorate in Medicine') (J423), show that Six followed developments in medical science closely.[61] One of the reasons for writing such poems to academically trained doctors was probably that Six was keen to portray himself as an erudite druggist. But even though he does not explicitly mention his ailment in the text, it is worth asking whether its theme can also be linked to his ailment. The seventeenth century was characterised, after all, by medical experiments and uncertainty, and ailments of the spleen and drugs are malleable concepts in Six's writing.[62] In 'Op de reedenstryd, oover de

59 'Dat Amber in Wijn geleyt droncken maeckt', Johan van Beverwijck, *Schat der gesontheyt*, 1656, p. 89. I will come back to early modern views on drunkenness in Chapters 7 and 8.

60 Feitama, 1684, p. 260. See also my discussion of *cachou* in Chapter 8. *Cf.* also the emphasis on sensory experience in the widely read *Merchant's Map of Commerce* (1634), see Holly Dugan, 2011, p. 129.

61 In his poem, Six mentions most of the arguments that come up in Worst's thesis, *cf.* Geeraard Worst, *Disputatio medica inaugaralis de Morbo regio*, 1655.

62 Van Beverwijck reports, for example, that there are various theories about the function of the spleen (*Schat der ongesontheyt*, 1656, pp. 149–150), *cf.* note 72. See also the discussion on the removal of the

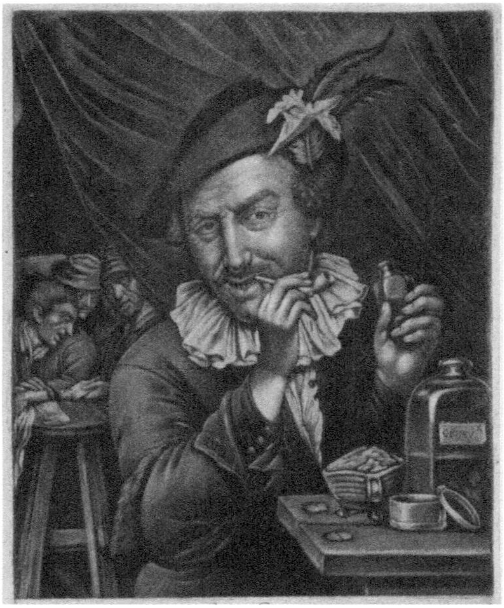

Fig. 4.5: Anonymous, *The Taste*, c. 1683–1684. Etching. (© Rijksmuseum, Amsterdam).

kooninghlyke siekte', we find several phrases that evoke associations with Six's own medical history. Six is himself, after all, a trader in 'royal substances' – *cf.* 'Rariteiten te koop'. Gluttony is highlighted in the text as one of the potential causes of the ailment dealt with in this text – jaundice – including the so-called 'King's Evil', an illness I will come back to in Chapter 9. After all, greed was something that Six as a merchant had to watch out for. In a text on his illness, Six also mentions 'jaundice' as one of the symptoms.[63] The perspective our spice merchant has on his ailment colours how he judges his merchandise: the decisive factor for him is whether it is pathogenic or medicinal. I will discuss this in more detail below.

spleen from the human body in 'Raad om naa 't Spa te koomen, aan alle miltsuchtigen' ('Advice to Come to Spa, to all People with a Spleen Illness') (J114). Such a removal of the spleen did not occur in humans in Six's time, but it turned out not to be impossible. The function of this organ was already the subject of much debate in ancient times. The anatomist Erasistratos of ancient Alexandria calls it a body part without use, while Aristotle saw it as a 'twin sister' of the liver. Vesalius observed that an animal could continue to live for a few days after its spleen had been removed. Dissectors made the same observation in Six's day: Baumann 1949, p. 98; Luuc Kooijmans, *Gevaarlijke kennis. Inzicht en angst in de dagen van Jan Swammerdam*, 2007, p. 79.

63 See 'Aan Rafäel – – –' ('To Raphael – – – ') (J271). Van Beverwijck mentions, among other things, an ailment of the spleen as a cause of jaundice (*Schat der ongesontheyt*, 1656, p. 159).

The merchant's body

According to Six's text to Dilman, early modern medicine devoted a great deal of attention to the moral life of the patient: whoever wanted to cleanse their body first had to cleanse their mind. Such a purging of unhealthy lusts and cravings takes place in 'Dankdicht aan Simon Dilman'. The poem 'Vraage, om aaderlaatinge, aan Simon Dilman, Geneesheer' ('Request for Bloodletting, to Simon Dilman, Physician') (J159), which once again demonstrates the close contact between the sick druggist and his regular doctor, takes us to the next step in medical treatment: the purging of the sick body.

Purging, it was believed, served to remove excess and contaminated bodily fluids. There were three treatment methods: administering an enema, giving vomiting agents, and finally bloodletting, a treatment that was applied for a great many diseases and disorders. The poem deals with the question of how and where Six would undergo this last, harsh treatment. He wants a bloodletting at a time that, according to Galenic medicine, is not suitable: during the hot dog days.[64] He had already swallowed emetics and had had an enema administered. The text concentrates on the effect of this on his body. It does not seem particularly pleasant. First, Six describes the dizziness caused by a high dose of purgative, Mexican *jalap* and Arabic *scammone* (l. 18–19). Six could have got these medicines from his own shop. Van Beverwijck describes the *scammone* as an herb 'that grows in Syria and Antioch', and says that it 'draws the gall-like and aqueous Humidities by great force, and fierce dismay out of the whole body'. Lemery says that *jalap* is a root from a plant growing in the West Indies, which 'expels very strongly all the fluids through the bowel movements'.[65] Everything was spinning around (l. 31–36):

't Gesicht besweek van duisterheit.
De keuken, in tiras geleit,
Ia 't huis, dat vast, op kooten, staat,
Dat tuimelde om, en om, op straat.
Den Heemel, en het aardryk viel
Te naauw, voor myn benaauwde ziel.[66]

64 For suitable times for bloodletting, see Van Beverwijck, *Schat der ongesontheyt*, 1656, p. 10.

65 'Groeyende in *Siryen*, en *Antiochyen*', '[t]reckt de galachtige en waterachtige Vochtigheden met groot gewelt, en felle ontstellinge uyt het gansche lichaem', *Schat der ongesontheyt*, 1656, p. 26. 'Hy dryft alle vochten door de afgang zeer sterk af', Lemery, 1743, p. 353.

66 *Cf.* Van Beverwijck's description of the effect of drunkenness: 'door het draeyen van de Herssenen, meenden [de dronkenen], dat de kamer beweeghde, ende gedraeyt werde' ('by the turning of the brains, the drunken thought that the room moved and was being turned around') (*Schat der ongesontheyt*, 1656, p. 89).

Everything went black before my eyes,
The kitchen laid in tuff blocks,
In fact, the whole house, which stands on bricks,
Tumbled round and about on the street.
Heaven and earth seemed
Too close to each other for my anxious mind.

This is followed by bowel movements and vomiting. Six rushes to the toilet to 'het stinkend vet, van 't ingewand, / Te lossen', 'anders had / Ik my, van achtren, seer bekladt' ('dissolve the smelly grease of the intestine', because 'otherwise I would bedaub myself awfully behind') (l. 41–44): in this text, Schenkeveld-van der Dussen praises the realistic descriptions and the ingenious allusions, combined with the playfulness with literary differences in style.[67] It is also worth asking why someone would make such intimate details public by publishing them in a collection of poems. As in the case of 'Dankdicht aan Simon Dilman', my own view is that this text is a medical self-profile meant for Six's regular doctor. In the early modern period, illness was seen as a matter of behaviour and morality. As we have seen, Six was the target of rumours. By publishing this literary 'health record', Six shows that he takes his doctor's medical advice seriously and is prepared to undergo painful treatment in order to become a better person.

The body is also at the heart of another text that focuses on therapeutic cleansing: 'Dankoffer, aan gesondheit' ('Poem of Gratitude, to health') (J184). Just as in the previous text, this poem contains an account of the course of a treatment, even as it is distinguished by an allegorical narrative form. The text is a tribute to Hygieia, the goddess of health (Fig. 4.6).[68] The poem describes how Six is abandoned by Hygieia and how he experiences the absence of the goddess: as wandering in the dark. The poet confesses that it is only after experiencing this darkness that he learns to appreciate the light of Hygieia. The text thus refers to Six's personal medical history: health is possible only if one shows respect for light and life. This allegorical story is accompanied by a description of the harsh therapy Six had to endure in order to welcome back the light of Hygieia (l. 23–38): once again it is purging, followed by bloodletting, which gave the poet hallucinations.

Two aspects of the text deserve extra attention. The first concerns the allegorical language. The struggle between disease and health is described as a struggle between the elements fire and water. As soon as Six has lost Hygieia's favour, he feels he is descending into the first of these two elements (l. 19–22):

67 Schenkeveld-van der Dussen, 2007, pp. 119–122.

68 The text is partly an *imitatio* of 'Van de Gesontheydt, en hare weerdigheydt' ('On Health and its worthiness') by Jacob Cats (included in Van Beverwijck's *Schat der gesontheyt*, 1656, pp. 13 and 14). Cats's poem is in turn an adaptation of an ode to Hygieia, translated from the Greek by Julius Scaliger (Jacobs, 1991 II, p. 333).

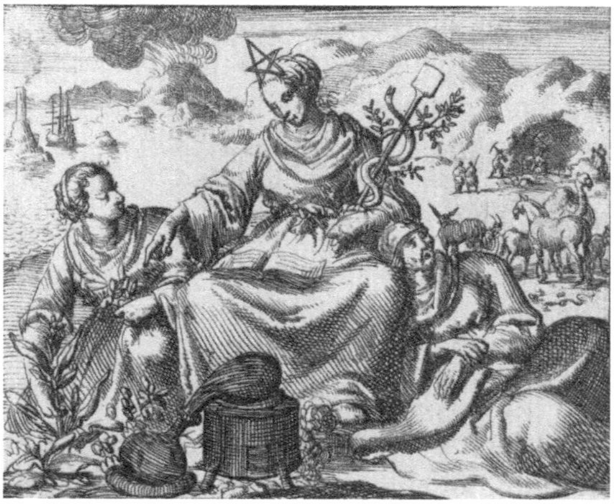

Fig. 4.6: Jan Luyken, *Health*, c. 1688. Etching.
(© Rijksmuseum, Amsterdam).

Myn val was, in een vuur,
Dat, als een schrik, dee trillen myn natuur.
Die korts daar aan, van sulken binnevlam,
Verteerde, als nooit, uit eenen vuurbergh, quam.

I fell into a fire,
That made my inner being tremble with terror,
Which shortly thereafter consumed a fire deep inside,
Such as never came from a volcano.

Six then describes how doctors come to give him medical treatment. They supply his body with the opposite element, water, which apparently serves as an antidote to the poisonous fire. But in this case, the collision between the elements meant an immediate deterioration in Six's condition. He experiences his body as a battlefield between the life-giving water and the deadly fire, where the fire has the supremacy. He feels that death floats above his bed, and that he himself is about to leave his body and be united with death. But then, at the moment that the evil fire is driven out by the bloodletting, the life-giving element gets control of the body again (l. 24–39):

My wierd van uw naaneeven toegebracht,
Al wat men kon van vocht, met kroes, op kroes.
Al 't leschen docht my gift, en doodlik moes.
In 's rechters erm daar kreegh het lichaam tocht,

Daar sprongh het nat uit bloedigh, in de locht.
Toen drongh een damp, door duisend sluisjes uit.
Toen dreef het lyf, gelyk een waaterschuit.
De gierge dood vloogh somwyl oover 't bed:
Ik schrikte en docht, daar, daar mee vliegh ik med.
Wat veete dat het waater heeft met vuur,
Onsoenelyk, ervoer ik binnens muur,
In lanke en pense, aan scheut, aan steek, aan snee,
In 't stryden van die werselende twee.
Eerst eeven sterk, doch 't minder vuur lee nood,
Zoo dat het jongst, met stank, de poort uitvloodt.

Your nephews [the physicians] brought me
All that could be brought of liquid, mug after mug.
All the softening medicine seemed as poison to me, and deadly mush.
In my right arm, there my body was given a gap,
There the liquid burst out, bloody, into the air.
Then a vapour forced its way through a thousand pores.
Then my body drifted, as a water boat.
Voracious death hovered for some time over the bed.
I gave a start and thought, there, there, I am flying too.
All discord that the water has with the fire,
Irreconcilable, I experienced within my body,
Inside and belly, with [each] sprout, sting and cut,
In the struggle of these two [water and fire] that oppose each other.
First equally strong, but the fire, which was in the minority, loses,
So that, in the end, it flows out of the gateway.

It is striking to note all the words related to physical boundaries, such as 'myn sieke muuren' ('my sick walls') (l. 14), 'a thousand pores' (l. 29) and 'gateway' (l. 38). These physical 'passages' play an essential role in driving healthy and unhealthy into and outside of his body, and in restoring the balance of humours. As we saw, the excessive fire was extinguished by adding the opposite element: water.

With this humoral dualism we have come to the second remarkable aspect of the poem. The two conflicting elements of nature connect to a moral choice between two life paths that are described in the poem. Once again, we are dealing with the early modern link between illness and morality. Hygieia prefers to live a simple life 'in een arme boereschuur, / Dan in den arm van een Vorstins natuur, / Die, in een hof, vol gouds, van krankheits sucht' ('in a poor farmer's shed than in the arms of a woman of Princely birth, who sighs in a court full of gold and disease') (l. 3–5).[69] We read that only when one adheres to a sober, Spartan lifestyle does one share in the grace of Hygieia. The description of the medical treatment is followed by a warning about various forms of opulence: chic houses, luxury merchandise and furniture, copious meals and licentious music (l. 39–52). Six reports in the text on his fight against dangerous vices such as lust (*luxuria*) and greed (*gula*). In the advice that Hygieia gives at the end of the poem about a sober diet, we hear echoes of Van Beverwijck's opposition between, on the one hand, the indigenous and good health and, on the other, the exogenous and illness. Hygieia offers Six 'roggenbrood en water' ('rye bread and water') (l. 57) instead of the 'taafel van Lukul, vol lekkre spys' (the 'table of Lucullus, full of tasty food') (l. 49) – the opulence of a Roman table – and a 'deuntjen, op de fluit' (a 'tune on the flute') (l. 59) instead of an exotic 'Musentoon' ('tone fit for the Muses') (l. 52). In this context, 'dieet' should be read in the original sense of 'way of life'. For not only culinary opulence that enters the mouth, but also musical pleasure that enters the ears, is an exotic element that Six has to guard against if he wants to stay healthy.[70] 'Dankoffer, aan gesondheit' pathologises the consumption of opulence. The excess of fire in Six's body was, in other words, caused by his temptation to consume luxury goods.

Poësy contains several literary self-portraits that focus on the sick body of the poet. The recurring motif in this group of texts is that Six is riddled with cancer inside, even though he looks fine from the outside. Things are so serious that he fears that he will soon die. See, for example, 'Verdorventheit der Natuure' ('Corruption of [Human] Nature') (J340) (l. 37–44):

> Wanneer ik nu my, laas, besie,
> 'k Ben sieker, dan ik pleegh te weesen:
> De kanker voormaals, in een knie,
> Sloegh voorts, door aaders, en door peesen.
> De kanker die heur wortlen schoot,
> Zoo diep, tot in myn swarte lenden,
> Is 't teiken van een wisse dood,
> Die niemands handwerk af kan wenden.

> When I, now, unfortunately, look at myself
> I am more certain than I used to be:
> The cancer that I had earlier brought to its knees,

69 *Cf.* Johan van Beverwijck's definition of 'hygiene': 'een Konste om ghesondt te leven' ('an Art of healthy living'), *Schat der gesontheyt*, 1656, p. 19.
70 See my discussion of moral warnings against 'the pleasures of the ear' in Chapter 6, pp. 218–219.

Developed further, through veins and tendons.
The cancer, which shoots its roots,
So deeply into my black loins,
Is the sign of my certain death,
No one's skills can avert that.

Six not only mentions his spleen as the core of his illness – he also links it concretely to sin and guilt. That is how the text reads in 'Schyn bedrieght' ('Appearances are Deceptive') (J420): 'Maar in den milt steekt, onder 't hart / Die oude slangh' ('But in the spleen, beneath the heart, the old snake stings/sticks') (l. 17–18).[71] Six points to the underlying reason for the weakness for vices: original sin. But this emphasis on the spleen can be also explained in the light of the content of 'Dankoffer, aan gesondheit'. In the early modern period, the stomach and its spleen were regarded as the most important organs for digestion: the spleen served as a purification system for contaminated matter from the stomach.[72] Once again, health is a matter of ethics. It is about self-knowledge and self-discipline: about control over bodily borders. The poem therefore not only tells us that things have improved after medical treatment. The trader in luxury goods also indicates which elements are dangerous to his health and which ones he must be careful about in the future. He tells us that he is constantly struggling against the non-Dutch toxins related to his profession as a druggist.

71 *Cf.* 'Aandacht op myn dertighjaarigen ouderdom en quellycke miltsucht' ('Attention to My Thirties and Agonising Spleen Disease') (J56), 'Myns leevens sukkelinge. Op de wyse van Mariaas Lofsangh' ('The Suffering of My Life. In the Manner of the Song of Maria') (J222), 'Op kostelyke kleeren' ('On Costly Clothes') (J309), 'Aan Venus' ('To Venus') (J388). I will come back presently to 'Schyn bedrieght'.

72 See Van Beverwijck's explanation of the function of the spleen in *Schat der gesontheyt*, 1656, p. 17, and *Schat der ongesontheyt*, 1656, pp. 149–150. As noted above, the spleen was considered to be a sort of purification system for contaminated matter from the stomach; it 'strekt voor een tweede Lever' ('serves as a second liver'), which 'het grofste van de Gijl [de 'spijsbrei'], eer dat aen de Lever komt, nae haer trekt, en tot bloet maeckt, op dat de Lever het overige van Gijl in suyverder soude konnen veranderen' ('attracts the coarsest of the chyle [the thick liquid, that, according to Galen, food is transformed into when it reaches the stomach], before it reaches the liver, and turns it into blood, so that the liver could turn the rest of the chyle into purer blood'). If the spleen is prevented from performing this task, 'de Aderen van de Lever door dit grof bloet [...] verstoppen, waer door het bloet-maken niet alleen soude belet gheweest hebben, maer oock veroorsaeckt hebben Geel-sucht, Water, Koortsen en dierghelijcke Sieckten' ('the veins of the liver would have been blocked by this coarse blood, which would not only have prevented the making of blood, but would also have caused jaundice, water, fevers and similar diseases') (p. 150). And *cf.* 'Raad om naa 't Spa te koomen, aan alle miltsuchtigen' ('Advice to Come to Spa, to All People with a Spleen Illness') (J114), where Six describes the spleen as 'vuilnis maagh, die boose milt' ('stomach for refuse, that evil spleen') (l. 9). The iatrochemist Franciscus de le Boë Sylvius held that a ferment – a 'tincture' – was produced in the spleen that stimulated the transformation of the 'chyle' and made the blood 'more perfect', see Baumann 1949, p. 98.

To whom is 'Dankoffer, aan gesondheit' written? One possible addressee is Simon Dilman, a doctor who, after all, belongs to 'Podaliers geslacht' ('Podalirius's family') (Podalirius was the son of Asclepius and a renowned physician in classical mythology), and is one of Hygieia's 'naaneeven' ('nephews') (l. 23–24) – the epithet used for doctors in this text. In view of the considerable weight the poet accords to moral responsibility, it is striking that, in addition to the many references to classical mythology and history, the text does not contain any references to Christianity. This shows once again that, in the seventeenth century, being ethically engaged was a matter not only for pastors, but also for humanistically trained doctors. But negative descriptions of the actions of physicians also reveal an ambivalent view of them. According to the quotation in 'Dankoffer, aan gesondheit', Six refers to medicines as 'deadly mush'. I will come back to this presently.

Gold as a medicine

Amber was mentioned in 'Dankdicht aan Simon Dilman'. The allegorical 'Dankoffer, aan gesondheit' is not about specific drugs, but rather evokes the decadent atmosphere in which luxury goods play a role. The next pharmaceutical product I will discuss in this chapter is gold, which Six discusses in detail in several of his poems.

Johan van Beverwijck also discusses gold in his reference works. In *Inleydinge tot de Hollandtsche Genees-middelen*, the physician points to the adverse effect that this metal is having on the Dutch economy. Dutch merchants export indigenous, 'necessary food' in exchange for gold and silver. The doctor warns that gold arouses a desire for more gold, and that it seduces earthy Dutchmen to take to risky journeys to unknown climes. He advocates instead a local barter trade based on homegrown products.[73] Van Beverwijck talks here about gold as a means of payment. But other properties were also ascribed to gold. For example, it was also known as a medicine.[74] This characteristic of gold is also discussed in Six's *Poësy*. The poem 'Goudsucht' ('Desire for Gold') (J279) deserves special attention in this context.

'Hoe komt het dat de mensch, van goud, zoo is beseeten, / Als loutre toovery?' ('Why is it that people are so obsessed with gold as pure magic?') (l. 1–2), the merchant-poet asks himself at the beginning of the text. Because there is nothing special about this metal in itself, he argues on the basis of Van Beverwijck's reasoning, what appears to us to be exotic is quite quotidian for the inhabitants of Cuzco

73 'Nooddruftigen voeden', Van Beverwijck, *Inleydinge tot de Hollandtsche Genees-middelen* 1642, p. 2.

74 This use is not discussed in Van Beverwijck's apology. However, *Schat der ongesontheyt* does contain several discussions of gold as a medicine.

in Peru, the area where most gold came from in Six's day.[75] And in countries where one has never even heard of gold, one does not need it, '[w]ant in Karibis land / Een land, als Adams eeuw, daar leeft men niet, op brokken / Van goud, maar wat men plant' (l. 18–20) ('For in the Caribbean, a land with the same blissful conditions as in the time of Adam, there people live, not off lumps of gold, but off what they plant'): Six sees their 'time of Adam', a utopian, innocent life, as an ideal for the early modern Dutch – a notion that is in line with Van Beverwijck's idea of an autarkic society.[76] In addition to demonstrable qualities such as beauty and scarcity, Six wonders whether its reputed ability to bring about miracle cures may also determine the attraction gold exerts (l. 14–17): 'Altoos het heeft geen kracht, / Al swetst geneesery, om 't leeven aan te fokken' ('Regardless of how it may be, it has no power, even though the doctors boast that it has the power to bring things to life'). Gold was indeed taken as a medicine in the seventeenth century. Van Beverwijck presents it as follows in *Schat der ongesontheyt:* 'Gold is the most respectable and the most temperate of all Metals'; it strengthens 'the Heart, cheers up the Mind, and is therefore suitable for Melancholy, Palpitation, Dizziness, and other like diseases'.[77] The idea of gold as a royal substance prevailed especially within alchemy. Many chemists in Six's time were still preoccupied with the original purpose of alchemy – making gold by means of 'transmutation' through the use of the 'philosopher's stone'. Gold was also included in official seventeenth-century pharmacopoeias. Two well-known drugs that contained gold were *aurum potabile,* a potable gold tincture, and gold-plated pills (a thin layer of gold leaf was applied to pills to promote the effect and to take away the unpleasant taste). Six discussed both.[78]

Our druggist believed that gold had hidden powers, but that these had a negative character. This medicine is a poison and gold fever is a disease, he argues in an allegory (l. 21–28):

Goudsiekte ontsoogen, van de borst der helsche borsten,
Gelykt een zee van sucht:
Die hoese meerder drinkt, hoe dat se meer blyft dorsten,
Hartnekkigh teegen tucht.
De bloedgraage ecchel suight sich wel, aan 't lichaam dronken,
En slindt een hoopen bloed,

75 See l. 9–11, and Pomet, 1737, p. 306.

76 See Schmidt, 2006.

77 'Gout is het treffelijckste, en gematighste van alle de Metallen'; it strengthens 'het Herte, verheugt het Gemoet, en is daerom seer bequaem voor de Swaermoedighheyt, Hertkloppinge, Qualickheyt, en dergelijcke', Van Beverwijck, *Schat der ongesontheyt*, 1656, p. 47.

78 Snelders, 1993, pp. 11–36; Lemery, 1743, pp. 81–86; H.A. Bosma-Jelgersma, *Poeders, Pillen en Patiënten*, 1983, p. 18; Gregory J. Higby, 'Gold in Medicine: A review of its use in the West before 1900', *Gold Bulletin*, 1982, pp. 130–140.

Geswollen vol, en rond, maar met se was beschonken,
Zoo was de lust geboet.

Gold disease, sucked out of the breast of hellish breasts,
Like a sea of desire:
The more she drinks, the thirstier she gets,
Obstinately against all standards.
The bloodthirsty leech sucks himself drunken to the body,
And swallows a large amount of blood,
Swollen, full and round, but at the moment she was intoxicated,
The lust was satisfied.

The personification of greed in this quotation illustrates the real effect of gold in Six's eyes. The gold fever works just like a bloodsucker: 'The more she drinks, the thirstier she gets' (l. 23). The attraction of gold is addictive, as if it were a modern drug.[79] In this passage, we recognise the main character from 'Gierigheits woninge en gestaltenisse', Madam Miserly. Six speaks directly to her in l. 29–36:

Ghy vrekke tooveres, en hoopt, en schraapt de kassen,
En kisten vol van schat,
En mest uw gierigheit, nooit, als de Maan, volwassen,
Maar als een seevigh vat.
De roest, en schimmel slaan haar tanden, in de schyven,
De mot, en schieter kluift,
Aan 't onbescheenen doek, de rotte knaaght de lyven,
Van keutlen swart bestruift.

You stingy sorceress, who stacks and scrapes the boxes
And chests full of treasures,
And fertilises your greed, never full as the Moon,
But as a barrel leaking like a sieve.
The rust and mould put their teeth on the coins,
The moth and silverfish gnaw
On fabrics stored in the dark, the rat gnaws these bodies,
Dirtied with black pellets.

79 Van Beverwijck takes the nature of a spider as a point of departure and presents a similar insatiable thirst as a symptom of avarice: 'hoe vele dat hy heeft, hy en is evenwel nimmermeer te vreden, noyt versadight, vol nijts, als hy siet dat een ander wat meer heeft: ende hoe hy selve meeder krijght, hoe hy altijdt meer hebben wil' ('For no matter how much he has, he is never content; never satisfied and full of envy when he sees that another person has something more; and when he himself gets more, he always wants to have more') (*Schat der gesontheyt*, 1656, p. 51).

Even international politics cannot escape the addictive effect of this gold fever. Three European trading powers are fighting for the wealth of the weakened Spanish Empire. Besides his own country, Six presumably means England and France. The toxic effect of the mineral is indeed puzzling, and that is, in the end, the refrain of the text: 'Is dit geen toovery, / Dat die het goud besat, van goud, zoo wierd beseeten? / Dat die het goud nooit at, van goud nu werd gevreeten?' ('Is this not witchcraft, that the one who possessed the gold will become obsessed by gold? That the one who never ate gold now becomes eaten by gold?') (l. 48–50). The toxin is deadly; it eats away at people from the inside out. Spain has already suffered this fate. Now the same fate awaits England, France and the Netherlands.[80]

Six is present in this poem at several levels of meaning. First of all, we hear the voice of Six the merchant. After all, in the early modern period gold was primarily a means of payment. We then recognise the other roles that Six assumes in the text, based on the medicinal use that gold is put to. The dealer in medicines once again expresses his aversion to a typical pharmaceutical product: gold radiates exclusivity like no other product in the range of items available in the early modern drugstore. At the end of the text, he refers to the harmful effect that gold has on the disposition of great European powers, but here we also recognise Six as the patient: his own body is at stake. Several texts in *Poësy* focus on his own consumption of gold as a medicine. A chronological medical history can be reconstructed from his *oeuvre*, which ultimately leads to a rejection of exotic and expensive medicines in favour of Spa water, which costs nothing. Gold is specifically mentioned in this process. We do not know when 'Goudsucht' was written, but it may have been after a medical cure that Six had undergone and that entailed the use of gold. Space does not allow detailed interpretations of these poems, but I will discuss those passages that go into Six's relationship to gold as a medicine.

In 'Klachte oover ingenoomen artsenye, aan Simon Dilman, geneesheer' ('Complaint about Medicine Taken, to Simon Dilman, Physician') (J231), Six distances himself from gold as a medicine. This text also reports on the progress of his healing process – or the lack of it. Six expresses his displeasure at the medication his regular doctor has prescribed him – namely, 'vier bedriegers goude wikken' ('four deceitful vetches of gold') (l. 3): 'Die pillen werkten niet te deegh, / Al seid ghe die vry sterk te weesen' ('Those pills were not reliable, even though you said they were rather strong') (l. 6–7). He accuses the pharmacist, from whom he bought the medicine, of having taken it out of a box of old, useless medicines. ''k Ondank my zulken pillegift' (l. 14) ('I do complain about a poison/gift such as this'), concludes the disappointed patient. Six is playing here, of course, on the double meaning of 'gift' in Dutch, which translates to both 'gift' and 'poison'. The dissatisfaction that creeps

80 Jacobs, 1991 II, p. 293.

into Six's relationship with Simon Dilman is more evident in the poems he wrote during his stay in Spa (Fig. 4.7). In 'Aan Simon Dilman Geneesheer t'Amsterdam' ('To Simon Dilman, Physician in Amsterdam') (J116), Six announces that he no longer relies on his friend's academic-medical methods of treatment. This is how he addresses Dilman: 'Neef, zoo geleerd, en zoo ervaaren [...] waarom hielpt ghy / My, die zoo langh gingh krochen, steenen, / Van pyn der miltesy, / Vergeefs, met kunst van God gegeeven' ('Cousin, so learned, so experienced, why did you help me in vain with the skills that God gave you, me that so long did groan and complain because of the pain in my spleen') (l. 1–9). These lines testify to a turning point in the medical history of the druggist-poet. The Spa water seems to have had a good effect on Six's spleen ailment, in contrast to the medications he got from doctors and pharmacists. This is evidenced by the parallels Six draws between the Spa water and foreign drugs: the healing power of the water is '[b]equaamer dan een balsemboom' ('more suitable than a balm tree') (l. 26), Six writes in 'Raad om naa 't Spa te koomen, aan alle miltsuchtigen' ('Advice to Come to Spa, to All People with a Spleen Ailment') (J114), referring to a group of drugs in which druggists trade: oriental gum resins. And in 'Om geneesinge myner miltsiekte, aan de Spafonteinen' ('To Cure my Spleen disease, to the Spa Springs') (J102), we read that the Spa water 'verlenght het leeven' ('extends life') in a more purifying way than 'het drinklik goud' ('potable gold') (l. 55). Six is referring to gold tincture. The Spa water, which costs nothing, has managed to do what a distinguished physician tried in vain to do with the help of reputable science.[81]

The last poem that has gold as its theme, and which I will briefly discuss here, is 'De vreese des Heeren, het begin der wysheit' ('Fear of the Lord, the Beginning of Wisdom') (J451). The aversion to gold is set here within a theological framework. The poem elaborates on the well-known biblical imagery of the narrow versus the wide path. Surprisingly, this does not result in a general reflection on the dangers life holds for us, but in a very specific consideration of two different types of therapies. The broad path – that of foolishness – stands for the use of gold as a medicine, while the narrow path suggests a different kind of medical treatment (l. 31–42):

> Myn kinders, spreekt de wyse man:
> Schuuw smetten, die u hangen an,
> Als smeer, en teer, die leelik stinken:
> Schuuw pillen, die van gulsel blinken,
> Maar opgeswolgen in den maagh,

81 A disagreement between Dilman and the Six family appears also from a notarial deed, but this time it concerns Six's mother. In February 1661 Dilman approaches Sara Juliaens for outstanding debts concerning doctor's visits in the period 1651–1654. See Appendix II.

Aan al het lichaam zyn een plaagh.
Gaa met de balsemdoosen om,
En winkeliers van geurge gom,
Die soeten aadem van sich geeven:
Al wat u liefliks aan zal kleeven,
Smaakt meede, aan uws gelyk, na wensch,
Vermaakt den goeden God, en mensch.

My children, the wise man says,
Shun stains that hang on you,
Like grease and tar, which stink awfully:
Shun pills that shine of gilding,
But that, swollen up in your stomach,
Become a bother to you.
Deal with boxes of balm,
And tradesmen of fragrant gum,
Who give off sweet breath:
Everything that sticks lovingly to you
Also tastes the same to your fellow human beings,
And brings joy to the good God, and to people.

In early modern pharmacopoeias, gold had a purgative effect, but in Six's opinion it causes constipation and physical pain. 'The wise man' in the text – a kind of prophetic figure – advises the sick to reject such seductive but foul medicines and instead to seek medical help from 'tradesmen of fragrant gum' who give a 'sweet breath'. At first glance, this advice could be seen as an inconsistency on Six's part. 'Fragrant gum' – Eastern resin gum – was, after all, referred to as a fake medicine in the Spa poems we have just been discussing. However, we should not take 'tradesmen of fragrant gum' literally. Rather, we should read it as a metaphor for ministers of the Dutch Reformed Church . 'Fragrant gum' and 'sweet breath' thus refer to their sweet, edifying words.[82] Six's metaphor is in line with a *topos,* used in the early modern period, of Jesus as an apothecary, and with the exegetic interpretation of the numerous references to fragrances and perfumes in the Bible (Fig. 4.8). In an annotation on Song of Songs 3:6, myrrh, incense and 'allerley poeder' ('powders of all kinds'), in which (according to the translators of the Bible) 'kruydeniers' and 'droguisten' trade, are allegorically interpreted as the benefits of Jesus Christ, 'which are a fragrant scent for God

82 Jacobs, 1991 II, p. 762.

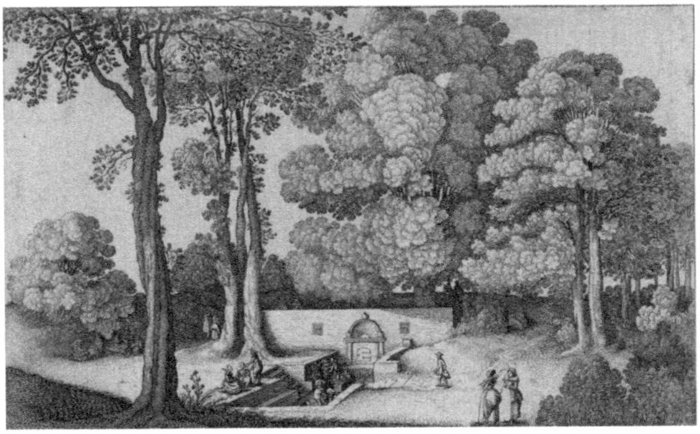

Fig. 4.7: Wenceslaus Hollar, *Mineral Spring in Spa*, c. 1625–1677. Etching. (© Rijksmuseum, Amsterdam).

the Father'.[83] Preachers are the *good* 'druggists': they trade, not in treacherous drugs, but in healing words.[84]

'De vreese des Heeren, het begin der wysheit' posits, not indigenous herbs (as was the case in the poems discussed above) but the salutary words of the Bible as an alternative to foreign drugs. 'Stinking' gold brings forth vices; the 'fragrant' words of pastors, virtue. Sickness and health are created by a God of both punishment and forgiveness.[85] The choice between the narrow and the broad path of exotic medicines is also the theme of the next medicine I will discuss here.

A miracle horn from Spain

The last medicine discussed in this chapter is of animal origin and forms a separate category in the range of products that early modern drugstores carried: the horns of exotic species. This is the subject of 'Uitroep om hoornafsetters' ('Buyers of Horn Wanted') (J244). The product in question is a very attractive and unique specimen within this group of commodities.

'Uitroep om hoornafsetters' opens with a list of ethical rules that a traveller must observe in foreign countries – whether he is 'leergierigh' (a humanistic scholar) or a trader who is just out for 'profyt' (l. 1–2): 'die oeffent sich, in deuchd, in taalen, en in seeden, / Of wint licht syn wingraagen tyd ('he practises in virtue,

83 'Die Godt den Vader eene welrieckende reucke zijn', *Statenbijbel*, 1657: dbnl.org/tekst/_sta001stat02_01/ (consulted 17 May 2019).

84 For fragrances as symbol of the 'fragrant words of God', see Chapter 7, pp. 231–232.

85 *Cf.* 'Blyde begroetinge, aan Abraham Grenier den ouden, oover de weederwelvaarentheit van synen soone' ('Cheerful Greetings to Abraham Grenier, on His Son's Return to Health') (J314), l. 41–44).

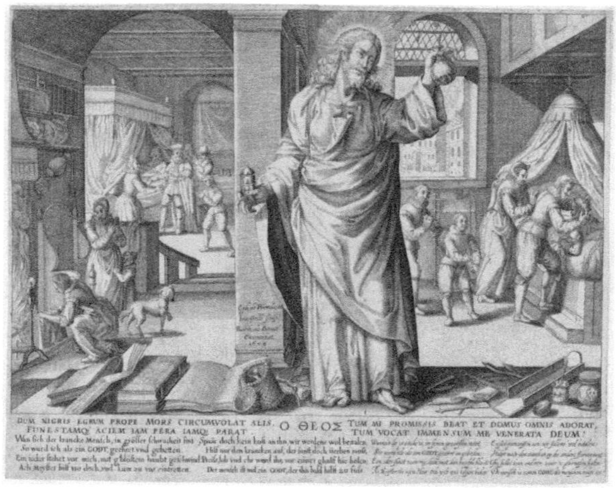

Fig. 4.8: Johann Gelle, *Christ as Apothecary*, 1609. Engraving. (© Rijksmuseum, Amsterdam).

in languages and in morals, or spends [in case he is a merchant] the time he wants to make a profit, undoubtedly good') (l. 3–4). This is one of the advices to the foreign merchant traveller that Caspar Barlaeus expresses in his *Mercator sapiens*.[86] But Six recognises that, as a traveller, he himself has paid more attention to the pursuit of profit ('handelingh') than to learned virtues: 'Ik blyf selven meest een swaare boete schuldigh, / Om achtloosheit, op 't eerste, en 't best: / Maar op myn handelingh beken ik sorrighvuldigh / Geweest te zyn, in elk gewest' ('I owe myself most of all a heavy penance, for being careless with the former, but in relation to my business, I confess to have been meticulous, in every region') (l. 5–8): Irony is coming through already in these lines. The poet is ashamed not only of preferring profit to learning, but also of the kind of business he has been engaging in. Six is on a commercial trip to Madrid. Here – in 'dat ontyge vuilnisgat' ('that dirty rubbish hole') (l. 14), the capital of the Dutch Republic's traditional enemy – he has made an unfair deal, for which he is apparently feeling some remorse. He says that he met a Spanish merchant who offered him a very special commodity (l. 17–25):

Hier quam een koppelaar, of maaklaar, tot my loopen,
  Wie arrigh denkt, vaar argh, in 't hart,
Opveilende vast goed, om niet met al, te koopen,
  Ja bood noch penningen te bard.

86 Barlaeus, 2019, pp. 108–109, and *cf.* Christine Skeeles Schloss, *Travel, Trade, and Temptation: The Dutch Italianate Harbor Scene (1640–1680)*, 1982, p. 71.

Ik vraaghde, vriend, wat is 't? syn antwoord was, 't syn hoorens,
Madrils uitsteekenste cieraad:
Want op haar kerken staan, gelyk men siet, geen toorens,
Om dat de man getoorent gaat.
Het quelt hem langer een doorboorden hoed te toonen.

Here, a middleman, or broker, came walking towards me,
– He who suspects the worst, gets his worst suspicions confirmed in his heart –
he offered fixed goods for sale, which I could get for nothing,
Yes, he even offered to pay money for it.
I asked, friend, what is it? His answer was, it is horns,
The most outstanding jewel of Madrid,
Because on the churches of the city, as one sees, there are no steeples,
Because the men wear steeples [on their heads].
It torments him more than showing a pierced hat.

The subject here is the trade in an exclusive type of horn. The Spaniard not only offers Six a free horn, but even wants to offer money. In view of the nature of the situation, it is clear that 'a middleman, or broker' means a 'pimp'.[87] However, this poem is not about a prostitute, as one might expect, but about the materialisation of the shame caused by cheating, the 'horn' of the 'hornbearer'. The seller himself is a cuckold, because he is 'horned' by this product: it 'doorboort' ('pierces') and torments his body (Fig. 4.9). Despite the clearly immoral nature of this merchandise, Six does not shy away, but is tempted by the urge to make the purchase.

However, there is one problem: these 'fixed goods' (l. 19) – a play on 'onroerend goed' ('immovable property'); it is, after all, safer to invest in real estate than in movable property – are attached to the Spaniard's body. If Six has some advice to fix this problem, his profit will be all the greater, promises the man: 'Hebt ghy tot deese raad, en sin? / Men zal, voor elken tak, u hondert goude kroonen / Betaalen, als een vast gewin' ('Do you have advice and a plan for us? We will pay you a hundred golden crowns for each horn, as a fixed reward') (l. 26–28). The Spaniard addresses Six in his capacity as an importer. Not only does he wear a horn at his side, but this 'horn ailment' has spread throughout Madrid. Those who manage to help the horn-bearers get rid of their horns can earn a fortune by bringing the 'Spanish horns' to the Dutch market as a new miracle cure.

In the last part of the text, Six turns to practitioners of various medical professions in Amsterdam. He promises that he will share the profit with whoever can pull

87 For the orginal meaning of 'makelaar', see the comments on 'Rariteiten te koop' in the Appendix I. See also Jacobs, 1991 II, p. 439.

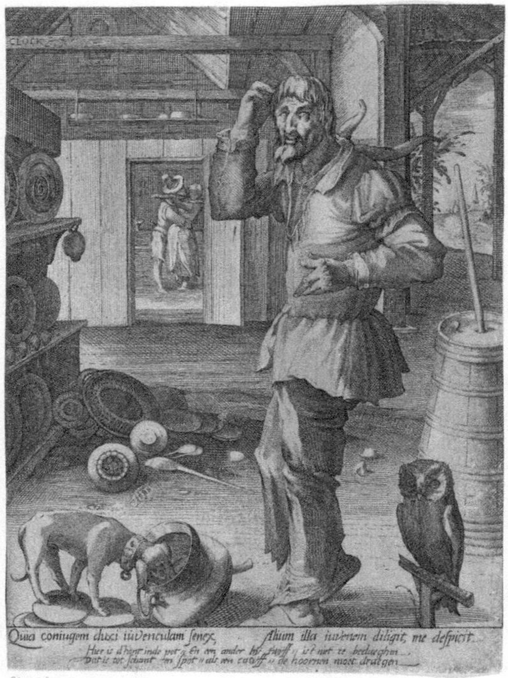
Quia coniugem duxi iuvenculam ſenex, Alium illa iuvenem diligit, me deſpicit.

Fig. 4.9: Nicolaes Jansz. Clock, *A Cuckold*, c. 1586–1602. Engraving. (© Rijksmuseum, Amsterdam).

off this master stroke. The ironic tone of the first part of the poem becomes clear at the end, when Six shows moral indignation towards the bearers of such horns, 'those monsters' in Madrid (l. 41–54):

Maar om die monsters, van dat ooverwight, t' ontlaaden,
  Heb ik geen oeffningh, noch verstand:
Dies soek ik iemand, die my konstigh weet te raaden,
  En hulp te bieden met syn hand.
Hoor, Amsterdammers, hoor, hoor weetende doktooren,
  Hoor meesters in de sirurgy,
Komt u iets, uit Pare, of uit Galeen te vooren,
  Gedienstigh tot die artseny:
Hoor, quakkesalvers, hoor, hebt ghy een sprookje onthouwen,
  Of daar, of elders van een bes,
Die 't by de spinrok vondt, probatum, by de vrouwen,
  Ai oopenbaar die goude les.
Wie 't beste pleistren kan, om hoornen af te heelen,
Zal al 't profijt, met my, van al de hoornen deelen.

But as for how to release these monsters from that nuisance,
I have neither the skill nor the knowledge:
Therefore, I call for anybody with the expertise to counsel me,
And give me a helping hand.
Hear, Amsterdammers, hear, hear, learned doctors,
Hear, masters of surgery,
Will you come up with something from [Ambroise] Paré or Galen,
As a solution for this medical operation?
Hear, quacks, hear, reveal your fakery,
Either there or elsewhere from a crone,
Who heard it at the spinning wheel – a *probatum,* according to the women,
Oh, reveal that golden lesson.
Whoever knows the best way to apply plaster, in order to remove the horns,
Will share the profit of all these horns with me.

Six states that he has no experience with 'horns' – thus implying that he has no experience with infidelity or visits to prostitutes. His conscience is clear. And since trade is not in fact what this is all about, but rather the actual removal of a stain, Six passes on the offer to quacks and empirics – unauthorised people on the periphery of medicine, with their miracle cures for all kinds of shameful venereal diseases – and to the gentlemen doctors in Amsterdam: the distinguished physicians, the surgeons and the practitioners of the 'golden lesson' – alchemy.[88]

It is clear that Six's encounter with the 'horned' Spaniard did not actually take place. It is an invented story about a fictional wonder drug. But the satire addresses phenomena that were real in the early modern period: moral dangers to which people who travelled to distant climes were actually exposed. But that is not the whole story. The text also introduces the horn as a desirable commodity on the medical market. So the horn has all kinds of symbolic meanings. 'Uitroep om hoornafsetters' is full of typical Sixian ambiguity: Six discusses the different contexts in which he and the versatile horn play a role. We recognise Six as a travelling bachelor, patient and merchant-druggist, while the horn is presented as a medicine, an exhibition object, a showpiece, an aphrodisiac and ultimately as a social stigma. I will explore these different facets in more detail below.

The introspective character of the poem becomes clear when we consider that Spain belonged to the area in which our travelling apothecary traded. Six stages a test by means of a danger to which he was exposed in Southern Europe – countries

88 After all, one of the Dutch words for 'chemistry' is 'scheikunde', a way of separating one substance from another: *cf.* the lemma 'stofscheikunst' in the WNT.

that in the eyes of the Dutch Protestants were full of sinful temptations.[89] Other poems in *Poësy*, such as 'Dank voor gesonde geneesmiddelen, aan Abraham Grenier Rechtsgeleerden te Middelburgh' ('Thanks for Healthy Medicines, to Abraham Grenier, Jurist, in Middelburg') (J367), which is about one of Six's trips to Italy, give us some clues about this. How did this travelling bachelor get his illness? From Italian courtesans, of course, Six hears his suspicious compatriots say (l. 33–46):

Maar booven al dit lyden,
Zoo dunkt hem een rapier, door 't ingewand, te snyden,
Wan hy onnoosel hoort, uit een vileine keel,
't Zyn ooverblyfsels van een Veneciaansch bordeel.
Indien hy dan, heel veiligh,
Het teegendeel besweert, zoo noemt men hem een heiligh,
Die, oover gloenden turf, gegaan heeft ongeschendt,
Hoe wel men huidendaaghs geen heiligen meer kent.
O! tyd, o! boose seeden,
Voortteelende 't gevolgh schier vast van zulke reeden,
Wat baat hem goeden raad, te weesen bly gemoedt,
Daar siekte, en zulk verwyt, swaarmoedigheit self voedt?
Maar weer heeft hy beslooten,
Sich, wyl hy suiver is, aan laster, niet te stooten:

But worse than all this suffering,
It is like a sword that cuts through his intestines
When he unsuspectingly hears from a villainous mouth
That it [Six's illness] is the consequence of having been at a Venetian brothel.
If he should – with great certainty –
Claim the opposite, then he should be called a saint,
Who, unscathed, managed to walk on glowing peat,
Even though there are no longer any saints.
Oh, what times! Oh, what evil customs!
Which such words are the result of, which will make them spread,
How can good advice help him to be happier,
While illness, and such reproach, just cause melancholy?
But once again he has decided,
Since he is pure, not to let himself be affected by slander.

89 See Schloss, 1982, pp. 70–73; Kooijmans, 1995, pp. 65–92, especially pp. 83–86; and Maurits Ebben, 'Lodewijck Huygens' *Spanish Journal*, 1660–1661: Perceptions of Spain and Confirmation of the Identity of the Dutch Republic', *Dutch Crossing*, 2018, pp. 118–134. See also the next chapter, pp. 182–185.

Worse than his painful illness is this backbiting, which he says he feels cut through his intestines like a sword. According to the slanderers, no one is strong enough to resist the temptations of Venetian prostitutes, and Six would have to be a saint to accomplish something like that. But Six knows that this is not how things are, and he promises to suppress these rumours.[90]

At the same time – and no less important – as a druggist, Six was, of course, interested in wondrous horns. If we read the text again, we notice how much attention Six pays to horns as a commodity. He confesses that the horn of the Spanish horn-bearer is of particular interest to him as a druggist. Six is, after all, looking out for new, unknown medicines, and the horn would fit well with the other horns he has collected and which adorn his shelves (l. 29–40):

Ik wingraagh seide, ik daar aandachtigh op zou letten,
Als zynde koopwaar, die my past,
Om onse winkelton geleeght weer voor te setten,
Die juist op myn versorgen vast:
't Zy 't blanke hoornen zyn, als van de Rusche harten,
Of van een Libische Olifant,
Die 't vinnighste fenyn, als teegenstrydigh tarten:
't Zy datse rauw zyn, of gebrandt.
't Zy swarte hoorenen, als van Rhinocerooten,
Ook kostlik om hun teegengift.
't Zy van een eenhoorn, die zoo fraai verguldt komt stooten,
Voor uit, om hoogh, aan ons gestift.

In my desire for profit, I said that I would pay close attention to it,
As merchandise that it would suit me to
Set in front of our empty shop barrel,
Which is 'fasting' now while I am gathering 'food' for it:
Whether it be white horns, as from the Russian deer [reindeer],
Or from a Libyan Elephant,
Which defy the sharpest venom,
Whether they are raw or burned.
Whether they are black horns, as from a Rhinoceros,
Also expensive because of their antidote,
Whether it be from a unicorn, which, so beautifully gilded, stands out
High in front of our store.

90 *Cf.*, too, 'Weeromslach aan W.B. oover syn laster teegen my, neeven dry andren' ('Rejection to W.B. about His Slander against Me, besides Three Other Persons') (J134) and 'Misleide onnooselheit' ('Misguided Innocence') (J170).

They are all rarities with miraculous healing powers; substances that thus 'defy the sharpest venom' and are 'expensive because of their antidote'.[91] Among these one will also find the most beautiful of all horns, 'which, so beautifully gilded, stands out / high in front of our store'. This is, of course, the horn of the unicorn, the sign on the gable of Six's shop. Horns constitute a category of pharmaceutical products that touch on the world of fables and myths, and are therefore a good example of the fantastic as a hallmark of the early modern druggist.

The quote also mentions another quality of this fictional, yet tangible, preciousness. 'The most outstanding jewel of Madrid' – as the horn was called in the passage cited above (l. 22) – ensures not only commercial gain for the owner, but also greater social standing. As a collector's item, it is suitable to 'set in front of our empty shop barrel'. Six also presents the horn as a *curiosum*.[92] The name Six gives to the 'horned' Spaniards in his text is striking in this respect: he calls them 'monsters' (l. 41) – see the quotation above. As we know, Sijbrand Feitama used the same term in his poem to Jan Norel, in which the attraction of the 'monsters' in his collection of *naturalia* was discussed.[93] The reason for this terminology is clear if we compare the 'monsters' from 'Uitroep om hoornafsetters' with those in 'Gierigheits wooninge en gestaltenisse'. Once again, the fascination and the desire for the strange and the frightening in the early modern curiosity cabinets are mocked. But in the early modern period, horns were also used for other purposes. Many exotic spices were considered aphrodisiacs, as we saw above. The same goes for the phallic horns. A transfer of the Spaniard's horn to Six means an exchange of sexual identity (in terms of both vitality and shame).[94]

91 Horns were grated and used in powder form or as a decoction. For other horns, such as elephant ivory, see Lemery, 1743, p. 262. 'Rauw' probably refers to the assertion that the Moors ate elephant ivory both raw and 'burned' (ibid.). Although Van Beverwijck is sceptical about the existence of unicorns, he still tells us that their horns had medicinal qualities, especially the alleged anti-toxic effect of the miracle cure. See *Schat der ongesontheyt*, 1656, p. 47. For discussions in the early modern Republic about the existence or otherwise of unicorns, see Jorink, 2010, pp. 299–300. For the anti-toxic effect of unicorn horn, see also 'Wensch des Eenhoorns' ('Wish of the Unicorn') (J182), which, like this poem, is about Six's social prestige as a merchant-druggist.

92 Horns were popular in curiosity cabinets. A good example of this is the *exoticotamia* of the aforementioned druggist Joan Breyne. The auction catalogue of his collection includes rhinoceros horns, horns of the bezoar ibex, antlers, and a drawer filled with hundreds of small horns. Also mentioned are walrus teeth and carved elephant's tusks (p. 4). We recall Knorr von Rosenroth, who looked at a walrus tusk in 'Den Eenhoorn in Kalverstraat' (Chapter 3, p. 94). Although they are not horns, they belong to the same category as the horns in Six's poem: they were considered to be aphrodisiacs.

93 *Cf.* 'monster' in Daston & Park, 1998, pp. 173–214.

94 For the apparently stimulating power of horns, especially rhino and unicorn horns, see Humphry Humphreys, 'The Horn of the Unicorn', *Annals of the Royal College of Surgeons of England*, 1951, pp. 377–383; and Francisco Vaz Da Silva, 'Sexual Horns: The Anatomy and Metaphysics of Cuckoldry in European Folklore', *Comparative Studies in Society and History*, 2006, pp. 396–418. The Dutch exported rhinoceros

We saw earlier how Six, in 'Dank, aan Manuel Spranger. Voor kaaviaar' (J135), took pains to emphasise his lack of experience with caviar as an aphrodisiac. This has to do with his status as a young, travelling bachelor. We see a similar act of self-exoneration in 'Uitroep om hoornafsetters'. The Spanish pimp is in many ways a mirror image of Six: the pain that torments his side is reminiscent of the splenetic ailment Six suffers from. But Six tells us emphatically that he has 'neither the skill nor the knowledge' of hot horns. However, this does not alter the fact that Six did in fact own copies of rare animal horns, in his capacity as a trader. It is possible that the Russian caviar and smoked salmon discussed earlier also included reindeer antlers (horns of 'Rusche harten') – goods that Six received from Russian contacts and exported to Southern Europe. The other animals in the quotation, 'a Libyan elephant' and 'Rhinoceroses', come from countries to the south of Spain. Ivory and rhinoceros horns were pharmaceutical products that Dutch merchants probably acquired through Spanish 'brokers' – in the sense, not of 'pimps', but of 'middlemen'.

Foreign drugs were therefore regarded as both socially and physically harmful. 'Uitroep om hoornafsetters' is a good illustration of this. You are what you eat: if you eat lust-inducing horns, then an unbreakable horn grows out of your side, like a venereal disease. There will be intolerable physical pain coupled with a social stigma: an indelible stain on your reputation. But 'Uitroep om hoornafsetters' is not only about a possible consumer of hot horns, but also about a middleman dealing in such products. He is not only a trader in physically harmful substances, but also a dealer in dangerous desires or, in the words of Six's favourite author, Horace, 'a trader in shame'.[95]

Conclusion

We know that the premises of 'De Vergulde Eenhoorn' was sold in 1675. However, Six continued his activities as a merchant after that. The family firm was still registered in the ledger of the Wisselbank until Six's death, although the volume of trade changed significantly from one year to the next. We also know that, in the last decades of his life, Six spent a lot of time at 'Ceulen', the estate in the Diemermeerpolder, which he had inherited from his grandmother Catharina Jeheu

horns to Japan. See Wim Wennekes, *Gouden handel: De eerste Nederlanders overzee, en wat zij daar haalden*, 1996, p. 232. See also the painting 'An Interior with a Seller of Curiosities' by Cornelis de Man (1621–1706), on which horns of different foreign animals can be seen among the erotic *exotica* of the trader in curiosities: Bergvelt & Kistemaker, 1992, II, pp. 123–124.

95 See the description of a 'Spanish trader in shame' in Horace's Ode III, 6, l. pp. 29–32: Was Six influenced by Horace as he wrote 'Uitroep om hoornafsetters'?

in 1669.[96] In 1674, almost twenty years after the publication of *Poësy*, a new book by Six finally appeared, *Davids Psalmen*, a versed translation of the psalms of David. For the study and conversion of David's sacred words, Six isolated himself in 'Ceulen', where, according to the introduction to the collection of translations, he 'was pregnant for twenty years, and about ten years in heavy labour'. For these biblical contemplations, he sometimes stayed in the solitude of 'the harsh, unpleasant winter' in the Diemermeerpolder, as though this were some penance by a repentant sinner.[97] This shows that *Davids Psalmen* should be seen, not as an isolated work, but in relation to Six's work as a poet of 'earthly' verses and as a trader in luxury goods. An analysis of the texts introducing the collection of poems confirms this impression. In addition to Six's own introduction, there is also a series of laudatory comments by theologians. In the text by Professor of Theology Frans Burman (Franciscus Burmannus), we find a reference to the former life of the author: Six's translations should 'give many merchants lust and love for this commerce in truth, which is more precious and far superior to all commerce in gold or silver, and of all treasures'.[98]

In the last years of his life, the merchant himself led a *pastoral* existence. In 'Ceulen', he emerges as a 'pastor' in the original sense of the word: a shepherd. This can be interpreted in two ways: first, in terms of his location in a Christian *Arcadia* – the reference being to his work as a 'spiritual shepherd', following the example of the biblical David; and second, as a botanical-scientific *shepherd*. According to Six's will, the poet had a gardener who inherited an amount of money. Six thus created a garden with homegrown herbs near his estate in the Diemermeerpolder.[99] In this way he himself realised the ideal of the poems I have discussed here: the botanist in the monastery garden in Ninove and in the botanical *hortus* in Amsterdam, and the livelihood that Raimond de Smeth earned as a gardener in the Dutch countryside – thus taking his distance from the uncertain livelihood of the merchant.

96 According to the ledger of the Wisselbank, see Appendix II. Six's grandmother, Catharina Jeheu, died in 1652; his mother, in 1666 (Peters, 2012, p. 77). Three years later, Six became the sole owner of 'Ceulen'. But apparently he had been responsible for the estate long before that – for, after the breach of the dyke in Diemen in 1651, when the estate suffered serious damage, repairs were carried out 'on behalf of Jan Six van Chandelier'. Thus he had already stayed on the estate before 1669. See Jacobs, 1991 II, pp. XXXVII–XL.

97 'Oover de twintig jaaren swanger, en ontrent de tien jaaren in swaaren arbeid', 'de guuren naaren winter', Six 1674, p. VI.

98 'Veele kooplieden geven lust ende liefde tot desen koophandel der waarheid, die kostelikker is, en verre te stellen boven allenhandel van goud of silver, ende van allen schatten', Six 1674, pp. XI–XII.

99 In the will of Joannes Six van Chandelier, the gardener Cornelis de Haan and his wife, Maria Heijmans, are mentioned – see Appendix II. *Cf.* also 'Wanhoop om vruchtverlies, aan de sonne' ('Despair at the Loss of Fruit, to the Sun') (J346) and 'Mooi weer, aan Simon Dilman Geneesheer' ('Nice Weather, to Simon Dilman, Physician') (J148), which probably refer to Six's garden.

The self that Six creates in the texts discussed in this chapter is paradoxical, to put it mildly. The wholesaler of luxury goods portrays himself as an ascetic on a strict diet of 'hop sprouts', and as a guilty patient who undergoes severe bloodletting treatments to cleanse his body and his mind of 'fiery' elements. We have seen how Six locates his texts at the heart of a debate between indigenous herbs and foreign spices. He does this not only theoretically – in 'Nooddruft is genoegh' – but also medically and clinically, in his poems on therapeutic treatments. The connections between his blocked spleen and 'slimme apteekery' ('malignant pharmaceutics'), as Six calls his profession in one poem, and between illness and sin, are central to my textual analyses.[100] The meaning of many poems, especially the Spa series, is the same as that of *Inleydinge tot de Hollandtsche Genees-middelen*: what is native, natural and inexpensive is associated with health; what is exotic, artificial and precious, with disease. Six developed, as it were, an ecological poetics for the seventeenth century. Although it is not explicitly stated, it is difficult not to read his poems as a way of coming to terms with the global trade in plants and spices. But Six's poetics remains ambiguous: as we saw in the first chapter, he continued to present himself, even in his later years, as a merchant, even if this was more or less in an ironic tone.

In this chapter we have once again seen the poetics of the *sober* druggist, whereby Six renounces a whole series of drugs that he considers dangerous both to himself and his society. In addition, this chapter has simultaneously introduced us to a new meaning of 'droog': in his poems to Amandus Fabius, Six presents himself as a 'droog' – in the sense of 'flawed' – druggist-poet: whereas he portrays himself as the producer of 'tender dates', he presents his friend Fabius as a wholesome 'bean-earth' who produces 'evergreen' poems. We can of course locate Six's humble tone within the *topos* of modesty that is found in Renaissance poetry, but this play of words also reflects Van Beverwijck's botanical contrast again: herbs from Fabius's southern Dutch monastery garden are superior to foreign drugs. I should emphasise here that Six's rejection of foreign spices and plants is not consistent. The Spa poems also praise various exotic foodstuffs. We also saw how Six even used Mexican jalap as a purgative in 'Request for Bloodletting'. But his condemnation of gold, ambergris and balm, medicines that he refers to as 'deadly mush', cannot be missed. This is also the case with other early modern moralists. Christine R. Johnson, whom I mentioned in the introduction, shows in her study how the German Reformation polemicist Ulrich von Hutten encouraged the use of some New World imports, while at the same time condemning Old World drugs.[101]

100 In 'Aan Venus' ('To Venus') (J388), l. 56.
101 Johnson, 2008, p. 123.

Six's identification with the Spanish 'broker' in 'Uitroep om hoornafsetters' is more earnest. His argument here is also based on humoral-climatic concepts. 'Wellust' (*luxuria*) is referred to in 'Uitroep om hoornafsetters' as a local pathological characteristic of Madrid – as a disease of that city, so to speak. The introduction and spread of Spanish horns in the Netherlands would have unhealthy consequences. As we saw, the Spanish pimp can be interpreted as a mirror image of Six: not only is he a trader in *curiosa* and miracle cures – he is also a representative of an illness that resembles Six own ailment. At first glance, Six finds himself drawn to the Spanish merchant, but he quickly realises that his merchandise is a trap: it is not a medicine, but an epidemic disease. This interpretation is in line with Christine R. Johnson's research: the spice merchant was, in the eyes of the critics of Germany's overseas involvement, a carrier of disease. According to early modern moralists, importers of exotic medicines should be aware of their crucial role: they are partly responsible for the health of their country. This is the ultimate theme of 'Uitroep om hoornafsetters'. Six uses the dangers of an internationally transmissible toxin to sketch out what we could call a divine trial. According to early modern theology, God has allowed the devil to test his chosen ones. But Six emphatically lets us know that he has 'neither the skill nor the knowledge' of sinful horns. In this way he tells us that the Batavian constitution he was born with has remained unchanged, despite his illness and his risky profession. The link between exotic spices and sexuality was a commonplace in early modern culture, and it is also a theme in the next chapter, which discusses spices as cosmetics.

5. Drugs as material and linguistic cosmetics

Abstract
In many of his poems, Joannes Six van Chandelier discusses the use of cosmetics as both material and literary ornaments. He writes about the use of make-up by Spanish women, and about incense and colours in Renaissance love poetry. In this chapter, I show how, in these texts, he perceives cosmetic drugs as substances that have a transformative effect and that are thus threats to the human body, in both the medical and the religious sense. Through a development of a 'flawed poetics', Six demonstrates a distance to the un-Dutch, aristocratic values of expensive dyestuffs. Nevertheless, this does not prevent him – by means of the rhetorical device of *praeteritio* – from writing colourful poems on the occasion of a wedding and on the landscape of Oostkapelle.

Keywords: Cosmetics, literary ornaments, love poems, civet, incense, *praeteritio*

> And if the outward splendour of the clothing worn by Kings and the greatest Princes of the World is a stain and a sin, how much more dreadful would that splendour be if our Merchants and Shopkeepers, and their Wives and Children were to go about all decked out like so much Royalty, as if they themselves were Kings and Queens?
> – Petrus Wittewrongel[1]

Roosters without combs

In the literary self-presentation of our merchant-poet, colours do not seem to occupy a significant place. In one of the opening poems of *Poësy*, 'Afscheid aan myn rymen' ('Farewell to My Rhymes') (J120), which I discussed in Chapter 2, Six

1 'Ende indien de uyterlicke pracht in de kleedinge, in de Koningen, ende de grootste Princen van de Wereldt, eene schantvlecke ende sonde is; hoe grouwelick moet dan sulcken pracht zijn; wanneer onse Koop-lieden, ende Winckeliers, hare Vrouwen, ende Kinderen, met een Princelik, ende Konincklik cieraet, te voorschijn komen; ende soo gekleet gaen / als of sy Koningen, ende Koninginnen waren?', *Oeconomia Christiana ofte Christelicke huys-houdinghe* (1661 II), p. 1149.

Spaans, R., *Dangerous Drugs: The Self-Presentation of the Merchant-Poet Joannes Six van Chandelier (1620–1695)*. Taylor & Francis Group, 2020
DOI 10.5117/9789462983543_CH05

describes his poems in this way: 'Wat haanen zyn dit sonder kammen' ('What kinds of roosters are these, without combs'). He presents his verses as misshapen, drab creatures that will generate negative criticism. This identification with drab species of birds also occurs in other places in *Poësy,* often in comparisons with the texts of the great Poets in the Dutch Republic, whom Six depicts, by contrast, as noble, colourful birds. A good example of this is 'Huldekroon, aan den heer Geerard Bikker, Drost te Muiden, Baljuw van Gooiland, en Weesperkarspel' ('Crown of Praise to Gerard Bicker, Bailiff of Muiden, Gooiland, and Weesperkarspel') (J173), in which Six presents himself as a contrast to the colourful splendour and the beautiful singing voice of the prince of the poets, Joost van den Vondel (l. 1–4):

> Een gaggelende gans zal singen, by een swaan:
> Een swarte blinde staart der Kalekoetsche haan
> Zal pronken, by een paauw, vol glans, en siende veeren,
> Nu ik den Muider Drost, als Vondel, gaa vereeren.

> A giggling goose will sing, next to a swan:
> A black, blind tail of a Turkey cock
> Will show off next to a peacock, full of lustre and feathers that see,
> Now that I am going, like Vondel did, to honour the Bailiff of Muiden.

Six is a simple black rooster compared to Vondel, the bright peacock of Dutch poetry. Behind this apology for his lack of linguistic colourfulness, however, lies some pride. Six's drabness is not a handicap, but a testament to his roots in Dutch culture. This lack of colour must be interpreted, then, in the light of his distinctly down-to-earth poetics and the iconography of the Batavians. Drabness symbolises humility and austerity, while colourfulness is in keeping with a non-Dutch, counter-Reformation poetics.

Having said that, if we study the form and content of the poem in more detail, we see that, although Six presents himself with self-hatred as a 'basterdkeel' ('bastard throat') (l. 5), the text sounds downright Vondelian in tone. At the end of the text, the 'black rooster' turns out to be 'the colourful bird', the type of bird that Six initially opposed. Six writes that spring, in which season this poem is set, is full of colourful plants. Just as the Queen of Sheba lavished gold and spices on King Solomon, 'Kooninginne Maai' ('Queen of May') (l. 33) approaches Bicker and showers him with 'diere bloemen' ('precious flowers') and 'varsch ontlooken groen' ('fresh-budded green [plants]'). And where else in this allegory does Six place himself but in her procession, where the druggist-poet gives his 'crown of praise' (*cf.* the title of the text) to Bicker (l. 39–42):

Lyk d'Arabierster, met veel gouds, en speceryen,
Uit Scheba quam, om aan den Kooningh bly te wyen,
Naa sy syn wysheit sach. Dies ik, in haaren stoet,
Reik, met een saalge wensch, dees kroon, met oopen hoed.

Just as the Arabian woman, with much gold, and spices,
Came from Sheba, happily, to dedicate them to the king,
After seeing the evidence of his wisdom. Therefore, in her [the queen of May's] cortege,
I present [Gerard Bicker] with this crown, with best wishes and hat in hand.

Why this inconsistency? Perhaps we will find the answer when we look at who the recipient of this text is. The poem was written in praise of the appointment of Gerard Bicker, a young descendant of the renowned Amsterdam patrician family, as Bailiff of Muiden on 5 May 1649 – a post that had opened up after the death of P.C. Hooft. The inauguration ceremony took the form of a Joyous Entry, a ritual usually reserved for royalty. The performance of the ceremony with triumphal chariots fits in well with Six's poem. The druggist-poet takes a place, as it were, in one of these chariots. Around the middle of the seventeenth century, the taste of the well-to-do bourgeoisie was no longer marked by Spartan austerity.[2]

'Huldekroon, aan den heer Geerard Bikker' once again shows up the ambivalent character of Six's writing. The theme of many poems in *Poësy* is a critique of showiness among Six's contemporaries. Both the literary excess of the Golden Age – the pompous writing style of his contemporaries – and the sumptuous Dutch interiors and clothing styles make them ready targets for Six's satirical mockery.[3] The subject of this chapter is the use of drugs as cosmetics. By 'cosmetics' I mean both make-up and aromatic products. We saw from my survey of the historical meaning of 'drogerij' in Chapter 2 that the early modern druggist traded in dyes and fragrances. Humoral, transformative properties were ascribed to fragrances and perfumes, as they were to medicines: their supposed degree of coldness, heat, and so on, were held to influence the human constitution.[4] The transformative

2 The aristocratisation of the merchant class in this period can readily be seen if we compare Bartholomew van der Helst's portrait of the father (Andries Bicker) with his portrait of the son (the young bailiff of Muiden). See Kees Zandvliet, *De 250 Rijksten van de Gouden Eeuw. Kapitaal, macht, familie en levensstijl*, 2006, pp. 73–75; Roberts, 2012, p. 60–62. For details on the inauguration ceremony of the new bailiff of Muiden, see D.P. Snoep, *Praal en Propaganda. Triumfalia in de Noorderlijke Nederlanden in de 16de en 17de eeuw*, 1975, p. 82. It could be that Six's poem was recited in the Amsterdam theatre to celebrate this event. See Chapter 7 for more on Royal Entries.

3 See for example 'Kraampracht' ('[The use of] Decoration during Childbirth') (J221) and 'Op kostelyke kleeren' ('On Costly Clothes') (J309).

4 Dugan, 2011, pp. 102–113.

power of pigments and dyes was also explained through chemical theories. Art and alchemy were deeply related to each other, writes Sven Dupré; one of the ancient roots of alchemy lay in the 'art of dyeing'. A change in colour appeared to constitute a transformation of substances, even if only the surface of an object was affected.[5] The relationship between fragrances and medicine is also evident at the linguistic level. For instance, Carolus Clusius rendered the original title of Portuguese Garcia da Orta's *Coloquios dos simples e drogas da India*, as 'Aromatum et simplicium [simples]' when he translated the work into Latin. And it is worth mentioning here that the verb 'medicare' has two meanings: to 'medicate' and to 'dye'.[6] The correlation between these two activities is also evident in Six's poetry, as we shall see.

This chapter takes the same approach as the preceding one, in that it asks what literary strategies Six makes use of in his self-presentation as a *level-headed* druggist-poet. Early modern Dutch art contains warnings to be cautious when approaching dyes. In Job Adriaensz. Berckheyde's 'The Merchant of Colour', the merchant holds a scale in his hand that illustrates his careful use of colours (Plate 7). This merchant could have been Six. I would like to show here that *aromatics* also formed a large but problematic part of Six's professional identity, and that Six likewise took a balanced disposition to dyes and perfumes in his poems. But first I will discuss poems in which cosmetics – both material dyes and artistic ornaments – are presented. Six is not at a safe distance from the subjects of his mockery. As a druggist, he himself was associated with bright and alluring colours.

The colours of love poetry

A natural starting point for a study of the aromatics in Renaissance literature is love poetry. In Six's collection of poems, we find two types of love poetry: on the one hand, there are Petrarchan love poems to a girl whom Six calls Roselle, and on the other, a series of *epithalamia*: wedding poems that Six wrote to family members and fellow merchants. In one of the verses in the first group of texts, 'Kontrefeytsel van Roselle' ('Portrait of Roselle') (J138), he makes use of a well-known Renaissance *topos*: the poem as a painting. Six commissions a painter to make a portrait of his beloved, but the artist does not have to see her for that. The poet instructs him personally how to paint Roselle by describing her in words. I will quote a few lines here. This is how her face is to be (l. 39–50):

5 Sven Dupré, 'Art and Alchemy: An Introduction', in: Sven Dupré, Dedo von Kerssenbrock-Krosigk & Beat Wismer (eds.), *Art and Alchemy. The Mystery of Transformation*, 2014, pp. 11–17, esp. p. 13.

6 Harold J. Cook and Timothy D. Walker, 'Circulation of Medicine in the Early Modern Atlantic World', *Social History of Medicine*, 2013, p. 339.

Vergeet geen roo koraalen,
Heur lipjes aan te maalen,
Die meer dan amberklippen,
Verlekkren myne lippen.
Haal sachtjes, naa beneeden,
Heur gladde kin deursneeden,
Lyk 't aardigh abrikokje,
d'Een syde plooit van 't rokje.
Heur blonde krullge draadjes,
Als pluksel van kaffaatjes,
Bestrooi met Cipers poeder,
Vol geurs der minnemoeder.

Do not forget to colour
Her lips with red coral,
Which sweetens my lips
More than do pieces of ambergris.
Brush gently
Downwards, across her smooth skin,
Just as the nice apricot,
[That] on one side of the peel shows a fold
Sprinkle her curly blonde hair
With Cyprus powder,
Full scent of the mother of love [Venus],
As with threads of caffa [a rich silk cloth with a printed or woven design].

Six follows the Neoplatonist and Petrarchan traditions in this portrayal: red coral, 'pieces of ambergris' and 'apricot' give the reader a good impression of the youthful freshness and charm of Six's young beloved. But not only that: Roselle's outward beauty also reflects her inner virtues. And at the same time, we must remember how exclusive and costly such substances were in early modern Northern Europe.[7] 'Cipers poeder' refers to the 'Cypriot' Venus, goddess of love and beauty – the nickname is related to the great fertility cult in Cyprus – but also to existing early modern cosmetics. The make-up of these *composita* goes back to the Roman recipe for 'Venus powder', a fragrance of dried pine moss mixed with fragrant substances such as musk, rose water, civet and sandalwood. It is described as a coveted, luxurious fragrance.[8] In this poem, Six seems to have no objections to adorning his beloved with expensive cosmetics.

7 Ambergris scent – see Chapter 4, pp. 140–141. For red or blood coral, see Appendix I.

8 *Cf.* a Dutch description of the fragrance, in which oak is replaced by pine: 'Van Lernica, de Laadplaats van 't Eiland Cyprus, krygt men, behalve veel Wasch, Ladanum en andere welriekende Drogeryen, het

But this poem has a moderate tone compared to the sonnet 'Op de schoonicheit van Roselle, aan de selve' ('On the Beauty of Roselle, to the Same Person') (J27), the most baroque text in the group of poems on Roselle. Not only is a whole range of cosmetics covered in the text, but Six makes Roselle the object of a religious cult. The pharmacist-poet depicts the body of his beloved as a temple that is adorned with precious decorations, and in which solemn religious ceremonies take place. Her cheeks are coloured with purple, her eyes are like turquoise chandeliers, and so on (l. 1–7). According to the text, this house of worship even surpasses in its splendour the temple of Artemis in Ephesus (l. 8), which was the largest temple in antiquity and one of the seven wonders of the ancient world. The poet himself enters this building as a high priest, to honour his beloved with devotional songs. As the temple is an embodiment of his Roselle, this entry takes shape as an approach to her mouth and teeth, an ivory choir. The fairly crass symbolism we see here borders on the parodic (l. 9–14):[9]

Tweedeurich klein poortaal, vol roosende festoenen,
Dat oopengaande toont een elpenbeene koor,
Ter plaats der galmen, die God looven, en versoenen:
Rosel myn Afgoddin, ik recht een needrigh spoor,
Naa uw verheeventheit, met uitgetrokke schoenen,
Verleen den lofsangh van uw schoonte een gunstigh oor.

A small portal with two doors, festooned with rosy garlands,
Which opens onto an ivory choir
Where resounding songs praise God and ask for His mercy.
Roselle, my idol, with timid steps, shoes discarded,
I approach you in your sublimeness,
Lend a favourable ear to the song in praise of your beauty.

The pharmaceutical background of the druggist-poet can also be seen in Six's wedding poems; Six wrote a series of poems in this genre. This is evident from the first poem I will discuss, 'Bruiloftnacht van Kaspar van Keulen, en Katarina Opmeer' ('Wedding Night of Kaspar van Keulen and Katarina Opmeer') (J131), a text that illustrates the Latin term for the genre, *epithalamium,* which means 'in

Poeder van Cyprus, zynde niet anders dan verwormd Pyn-boomen-Hout, met Water tot een Deeg gemaakt, welke te Venetie parfumeert, en dan zeer gezogt wordt' ('From Larnaca, the port on the isle of Cyprus, you get, except from wax, labdanum, and other fragrant drugs, powder of Cyprus, which is nothing but heated pinewood made into a dough with water and then perfumed in Venice. It is highly sought after'), Anonymous, *Hedendaagsche Historie, of Tegenwoordige Staat van Frankrijk*, 1757, second part, first section, p. 468.

9 *Cf.*, also 'Aan Roselle oover een stuk meloen' ('To Roselle, about a Piece of Melon') (J200).

the bridal chamber'. In this text, Six literally locates himself next to the bed of the wedding couple. The bride's arms are (l. 35–40):

Bestrooit met roosen, mirt, en kruid,
Die, door heur geur, den min verwarmen.
Het bedde, een outaar van 't juweel
Van Katarine, is nu een Heemel,
Haar oogjes 't licht, en al 't gespeel
Des bruilofts, Engelen geweemel.

Strewn with roses, myrtle and spice,
Which, with their scent, heat up the love.
The bed, an altar of Katarine's jewel,
Is now a Heaven,
Her eyes are the sun, and all those
At the wedding are a host of angels.

Adorning the bride with myrtle and roses is a common *topos* in the wedding poem. These adornments are presented as the holy plants of Venus, the goddess of love. But at least as interesting, for our grasp of this text, is the fact that myrtle and roses were physically present in the seventeenth-century drugstore. Although the evergreen myrtle was considered 'cold' in the Galenic system, it had, according to Van Beverwijck, a warming, healing effect.[10] The sensual fragrance of the plants Six refers to in the quotation was supposed to have been understood more literally than it would be today. In 'Bruyloftbed Van Joos de Smeth den jongen, en Maria Fassin' ('Wedding Bed of Joos de Smeth the Younger and Maria Fassin') (J348), where Six talks about 'heavenly medicines' and 'Venusian spices', he is very specific when it comes to their effects: the love herb 'verquikt en bly geneest' ('invigorates and brings healing through happiness') (l. 14–16). Venusian herbs are multifunctional products with both decorative and medicinal qualities. In 'Trouwdagh, van Abraham Grenier, rechtsgeleerden' ('Wedding Day of Abraham Grenier, Jurist') (J410), the poet also shows himself to be a flamboyant dealer in herbs and spices. With the spring season in mind – it is March – Six places the bridal couple in a Golden Age (l. 26) in the 'Garden of Eden' (l. 60), the utopian state of well-being, where Venus ploughs the fields with love (l. 65) and makes plants grow.[11] At the end of the text, as a final wedding gift, Six encourages the cupids – Venus's helpers – to 'konfyten' the couple with spring flowers (l. 77–80):

10 See Johan van Beverwijck, *Schat der ongesontheyt*, 1656, p. 33.

11 In the Chapter 7, I will discuss in more detail the notion of the 'Golden Age' in the culture of the early modern Netherlands.

Kupidootjes, mindienende schaar,
Gaat alvooren Bruids bedtapyten,
Mooi bepalmen, met psalmen, en snaar,
En met bloempjes van lent konfyten.

Cupids, a host of servants of love,
Adorn the bed curtains, before the wedding,
With palms, to strains of psalms and strings,
And with edulcorated spring flowers.

'Konfyten' is a direct reference to the profession of the apothecary. It refers to the technique of putting substances into sugar (such as jam) – a storage method that is described in early modern pharmacopoeias.[12] It is well known that sugar acts both as a sweetener and as a conserving agent. Jam therefore turns out to be an excellent metaphor for the desired qualities of marriage. On the one hand, it provides the necessary sweet decoration and, on the other, symbolises the durability of the marriage contract: till death do us part.

A final example clarifies the context in which Six's *epithalamia* should be read: 'Bruids inhaal. Aan Francois de Koster, en Anna van Baseroode' ('Welcoming the Bride: to François de Coster and Anna van Baseroode') (J145). The rhyming dealer in herbs and spices is also right there on the spot: as soon as he hears music and discerns candles 'met loovergoud, en rosmaryn, en palm' ('with sequins of gold, rosemary and palm leaves') (l. 2), 'Poësys natuurelyke boeken / Ontstaaken vuur, tot dichten' ('books of poetry appropriate to the situation, inspired me to write poems') (l. 7–9). This time it is François de Coster (1626–1653) and Anna van Baseroode (1626–1669) who are getting married.[13] The social pattern repeats itself: marriage was advantageous for the bridegroom's social career. The bride's father was a wealthy owner of a 'Suyker-bakerij', a sugar refinery.[14] Like the texts discussed

12 See 'konfijten' in the WNT and in *Pharmacopaea Amstelredamensis*, 1686, pp. 89–91.

13 Coster plays a role in the life of Rembrandt van Rijn a short time before his early death: Rembrandt hired him as a lawyer to demand payment from his debtors. See Paul Crenshaw, *Rembrandt's Bankruptcy: The Artist, His Patrons, and the Art World in Seventeenth-Century Netherlands*, 2006, p. 56, where Coster's wife is also mentioned. Jacobs presumes on the basis of l. 54 ('Voor Vrankryks kust kuss' hy nu Annes wangh' ('On the coast of France he kisses Anne's cheeks')) that Coster was a trader in France. Coster, then, worked as a lawyer in addition to earning his livelihood as a merchant. But the reference to France could also be to where Coster trained. Like another friend of Six's, Abraham Grenier, he would have obtained his law degree at a French university. See 'Aan Abraham Grenier den jongen, rechtsgeleerden van Middelburgh, tegenwoordigh te Angiers' ('To Abraham Grenier the Younger, Jurist of Middelburgh, These Days at Angiers') (J53).

14 Crenshaw, 2006, p. 56. See the lemma 'suikerbakkerij' in the WNT. In the seventeenth century, Amsterdam was the most important centre in Western Europe for the production of refined sugar. On the

earlier, the poem is full of complimentary allusions to the classical world of the gods. Not only is the bride compared to figures such as Cleopatra (l. 12) and 'Pafos Kooningin' (l. 18), the queen of the Greek city of Paphos, on the island of Cyprus. She is also adorned by a goddess, Minerva (l. 25–28):

> Al praalt de paauw veelverwigh van natuuren,
>   Natuur pronkt hier, met fraaije konst, verselt,
> Daar silver, goud, en parlen sich borduuren,
>   Op syde, van Minerves hand, bestelt.

> Even though the peacock, which nature made colourful, struts about,
> Nature shows off here, accompanied by beautiful art,
> Now when gold and pearls are embroidered
> On silk ordered by Minerva.

Six goes on to say that Anna van Baseroode, 'besaait, met silver, en groen kruid' ('sprinkled with silver and green herb) (l. 38–39), is like the beautiful Paeonic woman with whom Darius fell in love (Herodotus V, 12). Six does not describe reality, but creates a new reality. Using the beautifying herbs of Renaissance cosmetics, Six turns the bourgeois confectioner's daughter into a Greek queen.

The addressees of Six's wedding poems reveal the language and style of the texts discussed: they are the poet's rich business friends and relations. The bridegrooms in the first two poems, Caspar van Ceulen (1620–1680) and Joost de Smeth (1626–1704), were both wealthy merchants who, just like Six, traded with Mediterranean countries. De Smeth is described as 'a very distinguished merchant in England, Spain, Italy and the Levant – a wholesaler of silk and a banker'.[15] Van Ceulen was of Southern Dutch descent, and came from one of the Protestant families who had fled the Alva regime. The same applied to the De Smeth family, who were also relatives of Six.[16] The names of the brides also tell us a lot about the social aspirations of these young businessmen. However sweet and lovely the poems may be, these marriages were partly opportunistic: they were a way for the grooms to realise their ambitions to acquire official positions. For instance, Katarina Opmeer (1627–1712) came from an Amsterdam family of officials and regents. We already know the groom, Six's good friend Abraham Grenier, from the wedding poem we have just seen. As the title makes clear, he

Dutch sugar industry, see A.H. Poelwijk, *'In dienste vant suyckerenbacken'. De Amsterdamse suikernijverheid en haar ondernemers, 1580–1630*, 2003. See also Chapter 10.

15 J.E. Elias, *De vroedschap van Amsterdam*, 1903–1905, Part II, p. 797.

16 Jacobs, 1991 II, pp. 124, 617. See Appendix II.

was not a trader but a legal scholar. For him, the wedding also brought with it a rise in social status: he married Anna Arentse Westdorp, the daughter of the burgomaster of Middelburg.[17]

The social background of those who are portrayed also says a lot both about Six himself and his poetry. He places himself in higher social circles, in the midst of the well-to-do bourgeoisie, which prefers classical metaphors and *topoi*.[18] And Six, as a Renaissance poet trained in the literary repertoire of ancient writers, is well able to supply these. Allusions to classical gods and heroes place the wedding couples in idyllic landscapes. But Six's profession also resonates throughout these poems: with his particular, materialistic approach to metaphors, from the *colores rhetorici*, he not only shows his pharmaceutical expertise as a druggist-poet, but also pays tribute to the bridal couples. He acts, so to speak, as a donor of paradisiacal 'love herbs': heavenly substances that guarantee the sweetness and longevity of their marriages. Presumably the poems also serve as advertisements for the products in his selection. One possibility is that Six sold dyes to Joost de Smeth's silk company. Six had cultural, social and commercial ties with wealthy citizens. Wedding poems full of decorative drugs make for excellent commercial contracts.[19] The bridal couples portrayed in these poems in no way stand for the Batavian values of humility and austerity. However, it is Six himself who undergoes a metamorphosis here: the druggist-poet reveals himself to be a creative poet with the capacity to improve the world.

This social reality also relates to the Roselle who appears in Six's own love poems. No one has been able to find out who Roselle actually was. It would seem from 'Afbeeldinge en wydinge van Roselle, en haare bestraffinge. I-VI' ('Depiction and Consecration of Roselle, and Her Punishment') (J59–64) that her name was actually Mary (Maria in Dutch). I will return to this group of poems presently. Her beauty, whose praises Six sang in his verses, was certainly not the only reason he

17 For sources, see Jacobs, 1991 II, pp. 47, 243, 617, 707.

18 Frijhoff & Spies, 2004, pp. 448–458. These were also rich merchants who decorated their houses with expansive paintings. The aforementioned physician Johannes Dilman also dealt in paintings. For instance, in 1662 he sold a 'baars', a bass, painted by Rembrandt. See Appendix II.

19 We know that Joost's son, Pieter de Smeth, was a cloth dyer. See Elias, 1903–1905 II, p. 797. *Cf.*, too, wedding poems by Six van Chandelier's druggist colleague, Sijbrand Feitama, which look more like an advertisement for the selection of products in a druggist's shop than a wedding poem, referring as they do to more than a hundred exotic perfumes and dyes: 'Ter bruilofte van monsr. Jan de Wys, en juffr. Katharina van Os, vereenigd in den huuwelijken staat op den 5 van Louwmaand 1683. binnen Amsterdam' and 'Ter bruilofte van monsr. Jan Kaspar Lemp en juffr. Geertrui Hoofd. Vereenigd in den Huwelijken Staat, op den 14. van Sprokkelmaand, 1683. binnen Amsterdam' ('At the wedding of Mr Jan de Wys, and Miss Katharina van Os, on the 5th of January 1683, in Amsterdam') and ('At the Wedding of Mr Jan Kaspar Lemp and Miss Geertrui Hoofd, on the 14th of February, 1683, in Amsterdam'), Feitama, 1684, pp. 192–204.

was in love. Like Maria Fassin and Katarina Opmeer, she probably came from the Dutch social elite.[20]

Outer versus inner beauty

I will now turn my attention to another type of text in *Poësy*, which problematises more strongly the colours and smells of the early modern pharmacy. In this connection, those poems in which Six has it that a beauty brought about by make-up is incompatible with inner virtues are striking. In 'Roosekrans, aan Roselle' ('Wreath of Roses, to Roselle') (J176), we recognise many arguments from the preceding chapter. In this text, Six discusses which items might make the more suitable gifts to his beloved Roselle: flowers that grow naturally in the Netherlands or luxury goods from the Far East. The classical gods know what to choose, Six tells us: Jupiter prefers 'den schoonsten bloem' ('the most beautiful flower') – the rose (l. 5) – to exotic fragrances and gems. 'Het [de roos] aasemt niet dan liefde, en min' ('it [the rose] breathes nothing but love') (l. 21). Six tells us that, because the rose has no artificial smell or colour, it stands, not for false flattery, but for real feelings: it is 'des aardryks seedigste gelaat' ('the most decent face on earth') (l. 15), and its 'bloosend licht' ('blushing light') (l.17) outshines that of the other flowers of a garden. In 'Roosekrans', the 'blushing' of the rose thus emerges as a true manifestation of love. This is in contrast to the artificial blush on a made-up face, since make-up makes it hard to tell whether blushing is fake or real. Real, innocent love thrives among austere, simple people, not in the world of luxury and decadence. Many of the beauty products mentioned in the poem are recognisable: gold, diamond, sapphire (l. 3–4), amber, civet (l. 22) and ruby (l. 25). Earlier, we discussed grey and yellow amber. Civet is a substance with a strong musky odour and is obtained from the civet cat, which is found in the wild in Southeast Asia (Fig. 5.1). Amsterdam druggists bred civet cats themselves in their shops, according to Pierre Pomet. Drugs made from animal products were among the most valuable commodities in the early modern period.[21]

The clearest example of a contrast between inner and outer beauty is 'Blaame van gemaakte schoonheit' ('Rejection of Artificial Beauty') (J195), in which Six criticises women who go about dressed up too fancily. Six calls them members of 'het pauw geslachte' ('the peackock's family') (l. 19) – thus the same 'family' he

20 Monique A.F. Peters proposes a candidate: Maria de Kempenaer (born 1628), daughter of Dankert de Kempenaer, who was a druggist in the Kalverstraat, just like Six. See Peters, 2012, p. 29. But it is also possible that her surname was 'Kasteel' and that she lived in Zeeland. See 'Proef van liefde aan Roselle' ('Proof of Love, to Roselle') (J10), and Jacob's comments on the poem (Jacobs, 1991 II, pp. 9–10). For the social ambitions of merchant families and their marriages, see Kooijmans, 1995, pp. 65–92.

21 Pomet, 1737, pp. 241–242; Freedman, 2008, p. 14.

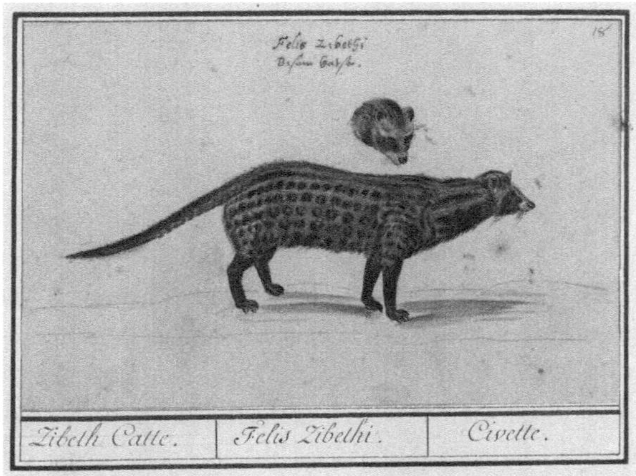

Fig. 5.1: Anselmus Boëtius de Boodt, *Civet cat,* c. 1596–1610. Brush. (© Rijksmuseum, Amsterdam).

considers Vondel to belong to. In his discourse against cosmetics, he discusses various pharmaceutical substances (l. 1–12):

Laat andren zyn geneegen,
Tot Juffers, fraai bereegen,
Om 't hoofd, met fyne parlen,
En diamente karlen,
Langs haair bestrooit, met poeder,
Van Ciprus minnemoeder.
Laat andren, met vermaaken,
Vry vryen, aan de kaaken,
Met rood, en wit bestreeken,
Tot deksel van gebreeken:
Of om wat mooi te schynen,
Wie weet, met wat fenynen?

Let others be inclined
To call themselves damsels, decorated with cords
Around their heads, with fine pearls,
And diamonds pebbles
Sprinkled over the hair with powder
Of the Cypriot mother of love.
Let others, with joy,
Feel free to make love, with cheeks
Painted red and white,

To cover up flaws:
Or to seem beautiful,
Who knows with what poisons?

The woman he loves is not a 'Juffer' – originally a noble title ('jonkvrouw'), which became popular among women from the lower social classes in Six's time – but a morally upstanding, honest woman who does not resort to artificial make-up to pretend to be more noble.[22] Interestingly, this social argument is supported by a medical argument: a woman who does not do herself up is not at risk of being poisoned by the 'poisons' (l. 12), from which, he says, perfume and cosmetics are made (l. 21–30):

Ik min een simple vryster,
Onkundigh van valsch plyster,
En lieflik stinkende aschen,
Tot treurasch best te passen.
Ik acht noch eel gesteente,
Noch parlende gebeente,
Noch waarde van borduuren,
Noch andre dartle kuuren.

I love a simple girl,
Who knows nothing of false make-up,
And lovely stinking ashes,
Which work better as mourning ashes.
I value neither noble gems,
Nor ivory pearls,
Nor costly embroidery,
Nor other lascivious artefacts.

The various cosmetics Six refers to in these two citations are substances with which he was undoubtedly familiar as a druggist. 'The Cypriot mother of love' is the 'Cyprus powder' we discussed above. Cheeks 'painted red and white' may well be a reference to powders containing white lead and vermilion, two chemicals that were popular in early modern times as medicines and as colouring agents in both painting and cosmetics. Although the high toxicity of both pigments was less well known at the time than it is today, Six seems to know what he is talking about when, as we have just seen, he labels them 'poisons'.[23]

22 See 'Juffer' in the WNT. *Cf.* also Jongman, 1951, p. 33.
23 For vermilion, see also note 32.

More pharmaceutical substances are discussed in 'Blaame van gemaakte schoonheit'. 'Noble gems' refers to gems that were used as earrings, among other things. Pearls – the quote has 'ivory pearls' (or literally: 'pearly bones'), possibly referring to ivory decorated with pearls – were among the most important commercial products the Dutch East India Company traded in.[24] These *animalia* (since pearls come from shells) were used not only as ornaments, but also for medicinal purposes.[25] The last cosmetic mentioned in the text, 'lovely stinking ashes', refers to the use of ashes as cosmetics. Ash is in fact one of the oldest beauty products we know of. As an ingredient in mascara, it has been used since ancient times to darken eyelids.[26] We can recognise the argumentation Six uses in this poem from verses we have discussed above. By referring to dead and inanimate ingredients in cosmetics – 'bones' and 'ashes' – Six underscores the contrast between women who wear make-up and those who do not. The latter stand not only for naturalness, but also for vitality and vigour; the former, for filth and lifelessness. Ash is also a substance that should prompt the user to feel remorse and to repent, Six argues, referring to the biblical habit of sprinkling oneself with ashes in times of mourning (see Joshua 7:6 and Isaiah 58:5). Although Six does not refer to himself by name in the text, my view is that the satire is just as much about the satirist himself as it is about what it is taking aim at. The detailed list of all cosmetic products serves as an indication of this.

While criticism of make-up is the theme, Christian ethics must also be taken into account. As my research into the reception of Six's writings has shown, the poet had an affinity with the Calvinistic ministers of the Further Reformation. Petrus Wittewrongel, whom we mentioned earlier, is referred to at several points in *Poësy* (Fig. 5.2).[27] 'Blaame van gemaakte schoonheit' would likely have been welcomed by this circle. The use of cosmetics was considered by Calvinistic pastors to be a great sin. Wittewrongel devotes a separate chapter to this in his monumental *Oeconomia Christiana ofte Christelicke huys-houdinghe*.[28] In his discourse, we find the usual theological arguments against beautification, but just as interesting for us is the strong emphasis on medical arguments in the battle against cosmetics.

24 Jacobs, 1991 II, p. 346. *Cf.* the information on pearls in 'Voorwind, naa nieuw Batavie, aan 't Schip de Paarle […]' ('Tailwind, to the new Batavia, for the ship De Paarle […]') (J374), l. 63–66.

25 Van Beverwijck, *Schat der ongesontheyt*, 1656, pp. 46–48.

26 Richard Corson, *Fashions in Makeup: From Ancient to Modern Times*, 1972, p. 50.

27 'Troost aan Sirikzee, oover 't verlies van Pieter Wittewrongel, Kerkenleeraar, hier beroepen' ('Comfort to Zierikzee over the Loss of Petrus Wittewrongel, Doctor of the Church, Who Has Received a Call to Come Here [Amsterdam]') (J123). Six praises the clergyman for his criticism of Amsterdam theatre in 'Op blaamrym' ('On a Rejection in Rhyme') (J391).

28 Wittewrongel, 1660 II, pp. 1140–1166.

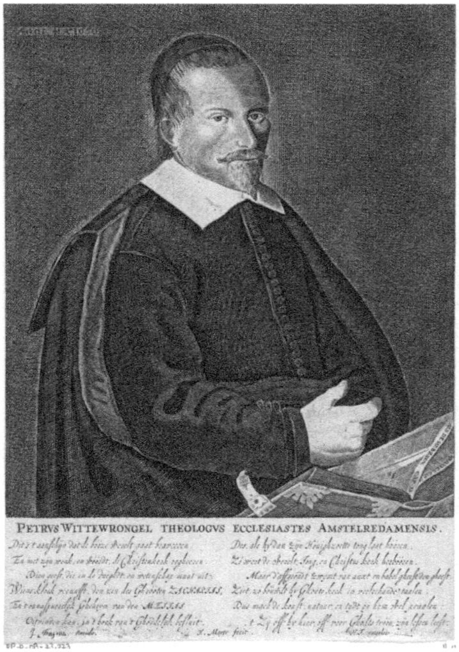

Fig. 5.2: Harmen de Mayer, *Portrait of Petrus Wittewrongel*, 1650. Engraving. (© Rijksmuseum, Amsterdam).

Wittewrongel, for example, describes the effect of an insatiable desire for new, strange cosmetics on the bodies of Dutch people:

> For, just as we make ourselves spiritually miserable in this life with splendour and adornment, if we are constantly, and with all five senses, busy and concerned with studying it till we are exhausted, with finding something new to do ourselves up with, we will never get peace of mind. And so it is that we overwhelm our bodies with many mishaps and heavy plagues.[29]

We recognise Johan van Beverwijck's argument in the quotation: foreign drugs are dangerous for European bodies. The pastor appears as a doctor concerned about the pathological state of his compatriots. In the early modern debate on the use of make-up and perfumes, medical issues are therefore indistinguishable from ethical ones. I will discuss this phenomenon in more detail below.

29 'Want gelijck wy met onse pracht ende prael / ons selven in desen leven, na de ziele gantsch ellendigh maecken; wanneer wy geduerigh met alle onse vijf sinnen besigh zijn / ende daer op studeren tot vermoeyens toe / om steets wat nieuws tot onser versieringe uyt te vinden; sulcs dat wy nergens ruste des gemoets en kommen hebben. En so ist / dat wy ook na den lichame ons selve vele onheylen, ende sware plagen over-dringen', p. 1160.

Skin whitener

When it comes to dyes, we cannot overlook the series of sonnets 'Op het blanketten van 't vrouwvolk in Spanje' ('On the Skin Whiteners Used by the Women in Spain') (J41–50). As far as the cosmetic use of early modern drugs is concerned, these are the most important texts in *Poësy*. 'Blanketten' means 'brightening the skin by means of skin whitener', but the word also has a second, figurative meaning: 'something that serves to hide or disguise a defect'.[30] The series, which consists of ten sonnets, is the largest part of *Poësy's* first book, the section entitled 'Klinkdichten' ('Sonnets'). It is remarkable that Six devotes a whole series of sonnets to the use of make-up by Spanish women, in Dutch – not in their own language. Is this again about the poet himself, as a trader in dyes travelling in Southern Europe?

The first poem introduces the theme of the series to the reader (l. 1–4):

Zoo, naa men segt, de Spaansche vrouwekaaken,
Met afgangh van Hegdissen, grys fenyn,
En rooserood van floers geschildert zyn,
Zoo dar ik dat er schoone zyn versaaken.

If, as they say, the cheeks of Spanish women
Are painted with lizard excrement,
Grey poison, and concealing pinkish-red pigment,
Then I daresay there are no beautiful Spanish women.

Although Six apparently wants to give the impression, with these opening lines, that he is ignorant when it comes to make-up, the contents of the poem give him away.

First, I will discuss the make-up mentioned in the quotation. 'Pinkish-red pigment' does not refer to a specific dye. Perhaps Six is referring to the vermilion we discussed earlier, which was used to give a red tint to the cheeks and lips. The fact that lizards served as cosmetics is evident from the pharmaceutical reference work by Ambrosius Paré. According to his recipe, one of the ingredients of skin whitener is 'droppings of small lizards'. Naming the foul, horrible origin of many of the cosmetics and ornamental pieces used in early modern times is, as we have seen, a *topos* in Six's work.[31] Six rejects lizard droppings as 'grey poison'. Its dangerous effect is elaborated on at the end of the sonnet (l. 11–14):

30 See the definition of the word in the WNT. See also Six's epigram on skin whitener: 'Blanketsel' (J537).

31 'Dreck der kleyne aketissen', Ambrosius Paré, *De chirurgie, ende alle de opera, ofte wercken*, 1636, p. 877. *Cf.* also Epode XII by Horace, which denounces the showiness of Roman women. One of the cosmetic powders and creams discussed in the poem is rouge made from the excrement of another reptile, the crocodile ('tercore fucatus crocodili', l. 10–11).

Zoo schudt een bes alle uur wat oudheits uit.
O poppery ontvonkt in aarde leeden,
Prometheus schort er maar met Heemelbuit,
Voor schooner steen, van Fidias gesneeden.

In that way, a crone gets rid of old age.
O idolatry that catches fire in earthy limbs,
All that is missing is Prometheus with his heavenly fire,
So he could make a statue more beautiful than that sculpted by Phidias.

According to the quotation, make-up is a transformative power that allows it to manipulate the human body, in this case by erasing the effects of old age (Fig. 5.3). Six condemns the use of such a secret power as 'idolatry', similar to the actions of Prometheus in all his hubris. This mythological figure stole fire from the gods and wanted to breathe life into a man kneaded out of clay – a creature that would be more beautiful than the work of the famous Greek sculptor Phidias. In other words, cosmetics have a physical influence on bodily functions and fluids. These are not only ointments that are smeared on the skin – that is, externally – but also mysterious drugs with transformative effects on the interior of the human being. It is possible that Six is referring here to the chemical nature of vermilion. In the seventeenth century, Amsterdam was the leading manufacturer of artificial vermilion, and as mentioned earlier, the production of chemical colours was intertwined with alchemical ideas. The alchemical laboratory and the pursuit of transformation of base metals into precious ones – the so-called transmutation – were associated with the fire of Prometheus.[32] Six bases himself on medical aspects as well as on the technical aspects of colouration throughout the entire series of sonnets, as we shall see. He also derives arguments from theology.

At the heard of his argument is *fire*. We have seen how 'hotness', in the theory of humours, was seen as a symptom of uncontrollable passions. The reader sees this in the main part of the sonnet series (IV–VII), in which the moral dangers of applying 'verwery' ('pigments') are discussed. 'Vurigheid' ('fieriness') arouses

32 'Vermilion (or Cinnabar)' is 'a mineral Matter, solid, hard, weighty, bright, crystalline, of a very Red Colour, distinguished with streaks, shining and sparkling like Silver, compos'd of a Sulphur, and Quicksilver, and a little Earth [...] Cinnabar is an Indian word, meaning Dragon and Elephant Blood': Pierre Pomet, *A Compleat History of Drugs*, with additional comments from Nicolas Lemery, 1737, p. 328. By the fifteenth century, artificial vermilion, synthesized by combining mercury and sulfur, dominated the market, see Elisabeth Berry Drago, *Printed Alchemists: Early Modern Artistry and Experiment in the Work of Thomas Wijck*, 2019, p. 226–238. For transmutation, see Sven Dupré, Dedo von Kerssenbrock-Krosigk, Beat Wismer (eds.), *Art and Alchemy. The Mystery of Transformation*, 2014, p. 56. For alchemy and Prometheus, see William R. Newman, *Promethean Ambitions: Alchemy and the Quest to Perfect Nature*, 2004.

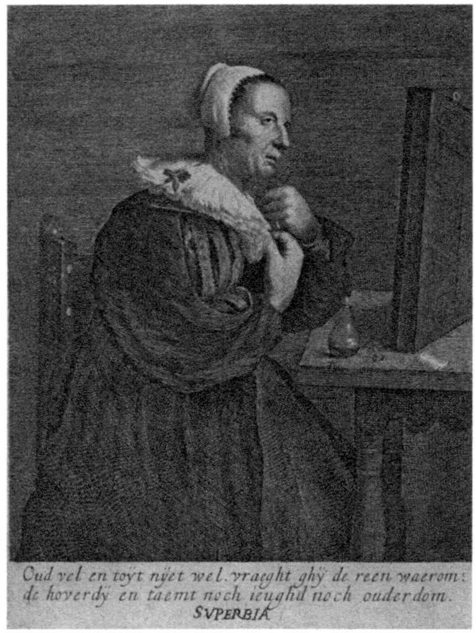
Oud vel en toÿt nÿet wel. vraeght ghÿ de reen waerom:
de hoverdÿ en taemt noch ieughd noch ouderdom.
SVPERBIA

Fig. 5.3: Lucas Vorsterman (I), after Adriaen Brouwer, *Superbia*. An old woman is putting on make-up, c. 1619–1675. Engraving. (© Rijksmuseum, Amsterdam).

dangerous passions: lust and jealousy, which cause unfaithfulness, divorce and revenge. Men who are 'aangelokt door 't kruydige geryf' ('allured by the spicy delight') (IV, J44, l. 6) – thus, seduced by women who are made up with 'cosmetic spices' – commit atrocious acts. Thanks to make-up, the number of *crimes of passion* in Spain has increased: 'Leon, o Leeuw, Kastilie o Kasteel, / Wat kryt al bloeds, om wraak, naa 's Heemels daaken' ('Leon, O Lion, Castile, O Castle, / How the blood already shouts to heaven for revenge') (VII, J47, l. 9–10). We recognise this fiery temperament, which was attributed to the Spaniards, from my discussion of 'Uitroep om hoornafsetters'.[33]

Elsewhere in the series, the idea of artificiality versus naturalness is discussed in more detail. Cosmetic powders disrupt genuine, natural, God-given beauty, according to the second sonnet (J42, l. 1–4):

33 *Cf.* Lodewijck Huygens' comment on *crimes of passion* in Spain, Maurits Ebben, *Lodewijck Huygens' Spaans Journaal. Reis naar het hof van de koning van Spanje, 1660–1661*, 2005, p. 229. Unfortunately, space does not allow a full treat of the entire series of sonnets here. I will thus concentrate on the significance of the poems in relation to Six as a druggist and poet. His view of women is not only negative, although the reader might be forgiven for thinking it is at first glance. Men who take the initiative to divorce or murder women are the primary targets of Six's ridicule. He also emphasises who the real losers of cheating are: the children – see sonnet IV (J46), for instance. In this sense, the series feels rather modern; but that is also in keeping with the attention lavished on children in the Republic – see Schama, 2004, pp. 481–561.

De schoonheit van de reedelyke dieren
Schuilt in geen konst van verwen fyn, of grof,
Schuilt in geen nooit vergankelyke stof,
Of die vergaan men weer weet op te cieren.

The beauty of the reasonable animals [that is, human beings]
Does not lie in any art of painting, whether fine or coarse,
Or in any eternally imperishable substance,
Or in the fact that the substance can be restored if it perishes.

The last three sonnets (VIII–X) return to this motif. When Six finds a woman who spoils her God-given beauty with artificial make-up, he prefers to kiss one of her dirty garments rather than her mouth, VIII (J48), l. 7–14:

Ik kusse liefst uw ooverrokte knie,
Of hemde, van u seevenmaal beslaapen.
Waarom zoud ghy 't goede eevenbeeld van God,
Als Adams, wiens gebeente u tot een deure
Ten leeven wierd, daar naa met vleisch in slot
Geslooten, met quaksalvery koleuren?
Zoo dryft sy met Gods welgeval den spot,
Die 't fraai panneel, om fraayer gaat besmeuren.

I would rather kiss your knee covered with a skirt,
Or a shirt you have slept seven times in.
Why should you colour yourself with quackery?
You who are the true image of God,
And of Adam, whose bones became a door to life
For you, which thereafter were closed off with flesh.
In that way, she mocks God's creation,
She who besmirches the beautiful panel
In order to make it more beautiful.

According to the poem, make-up is tantamount to blasphemy. Adam, the first man, was created in God's image. The 'beautiful panel' of the great Artist – God's work of creation – is sacred and inviolable, in accordance with the Renaissance commonplaces of the argument put forward by Farah Karim-Cooper, who is mentioned in the introduction: the notions of the Creator as an artist, of the human body as God's sacred work of art, and vice versa – the artist as a creator of perfect divine worlds.[34] The make-up artist thus appears as a 'creator' who 'improves' God's work. In the following sonnet, Six writes that an artist does not allow others to paint over their paintings. Six subscribes to the notion of the artist as creator, as a god. Honesty and authenticity are more important than perfection, he writes (IX, l. 5–8):[35]

Een schilder heb mismaakte schilderyen
Uithangen, om te veilen, voor syn poort,
Sulks wie se siet mispryst, en laakt se voort,
Hy wil nochtans 't penceel van andre my'en.

A painter hangs paintings that did not turn out right
In front of his gate to sell them,
So that those who see them can comment on and disapprove of them.
He will nevertheless avoid the paintbrush of another painter.

The last sonnet also discusses the medical risks associated with using cosmetic creams and powders. Six addresses this issue in the light of a fundamental debate about the function and role of medicine, and eventually warns against too much faith in science. He opens his argument with two rhetorical questions, X (J50, l. 1–6):

Hoort niemand dan gebreeken te geneesen?
Want smetten in 't gelaat zyn een gebrek.
Wat baaten ons geneeskonst, en 't gerek
Des artsenys, zoo Goddelyk gepreesen?
Dat heilsaam licht geensins vergeefs gereesen,
Heeft eevenwel syn lynen van bestek [...]

Is nobody then allowed to cure defects?
For blemishes on the face are defects.
What advantage do medicine and the convenience
Of physicians then offer us, so divinely praised though they are?

34 See Karim-Cooper, 2006. Also *cf.* Simpha Brinkkemper and Ine Soepnel, *Apollo and Christ: Klassieke en christelijke denkbeelden in de Nederlandse renaissance-literatuur*, 1989, pp. 174–175; Boudewijn Bakker, 'Een goddelijk schilderij: Vondel over landschap en schilderkunst in zijn *Bespiegelingen* van 1662', *Neerlandistiek*, 2005, pp. 1–36.; Frances E. Dolan, 'Taking the Pencil out of God's Hand: Art, Nature, and the Face-Painting Debate in Early Modern England', *PMLA*, 1993, pp. 224–239.

35 See also Cyprian, a Church Father, who said, as Wittewrongel put it: 'Soude (seght hy) wel een konstigh Schilder dat verdragen / dat een anders handt / eenige nieuwe verwe soude op sijn werck leggen? in het minste niet' ('Would (he says) a painter tolerate that another man's hand would put any new colours on his work? Not at all') (1660 II, p. 1152).

That beneficial light, certainly created not for nothing,
Nevertheless has its boundary lines [...]

Six stresses that there are ethical boundaries that science should not cross, and that the use of cosmetics is permitted only by those who are disfigured, and when it has God's blessing: 'Ten waar de kunst een wangebooren kind, / Of ouder van wat leeliks kon verschoonen, / Sy sie dan, of sy 's Heemels seegen vindt' ('the only exception is if the medicine could help a disfigured human being – a child or an adult – and then in the hopes of getting a heavenly blessing') (l. 9–11). In all other cases, transgressing the limits set by God should, he says, be regarded as a rebellious act. The cycle ends as it began, with a reference to a myth about hubris. Attempts to defy nature with artificial make-up ensure that 'de slangh syn vleijige appels [komt] toonen' ('the snake comes to show its tempting apples') (l. 14). Women who want to use make-up to transform their appearance are guilty of 'hoovaardy' ('hubris') (l. 12), the most serious of the seven deadly sins. Such *curiositas* – the urge to gain hidden knowledge about creative forces – will be met with divine vengeance, just as, in the Bible, Adam and Eve were expelled from paradise and, in Greek mythology, Prometheus was condemned to unending torment.[36]

And that is what the series of sonnets on make-up has to say about make-up. What at first glance seems to be a moral appeal addressed to Spanish women turns out to be a philosophical discussion about the functions and limitations of medicine. And what is equally remarkable is that the series was written, not by a theologian or a doctor, but by a trader in dyes. Six emerges as a humanistically learned merchant in accordance with the ideal of Barlaeus and Coornhert: he draws his arguments in equal measure from the writings of the ancient world and from theological authorities. But why is so much attention paid to Spanish women's make-up? Is Six once again distancing himself from his own merchandise here? If we compare his objections to cosmetics with his criticism, which we looked at in the Introduction, we see many parallels. In both cases, it is a matter of aversion to decadence, artificiality and obfuscation – vices that the moralists attributed to foreign drugs. Skin whitener provokes 'vlammen die de jonckheyt met vleeschelicke lusten ontsteken' ('flames that ignite youth with fleshy lusts') warns Wittewrongel, quoting Hieronymus, a Church Father.[37] It is in this light that we should read 'Op

36 *Cf.* Karim-Cooper, 2006, pp. 57–58.

37 Wittewrongel, 1660 II, p. 1152. Other pastors, whom Six probably knew of, also gave this theme some attention. One example is Michiel Spranger's in *De geblanckette Izebel; Dat is: Een Waerschouwinghe tegens alle Blancketselen, ende wat daer mede gemeynschap heeft* (1654). Spranger was a relative of the aforementioned Manuel Spranger. See nikhef.nl/~louk/SPRANG/generation3.html, and http://research.frick.org/montias/browserecord.php?-action=browse&-recid=2351 (consulted 17 May 2019).

het blanketten van 't vrouwvolk in Spanje'. In addition, two things are important for a good understanding of the poem. Both came up earlier in my interpretation of 'Uitroep om hoornafsetters': the fact that Six travelled through Southern Europe as a young bachelor and the fact that he was the carrier of a disease that his contemporaries attributed to visits to brothels.

The elegant nature of Southern European women, a *topos* in Dutch travel descriptions, is also discussed when Six, in his poetry, talks about prostitutes and other women. No one can resist the temptations of Venetian prostitutes, the slanderers claim in 'Dank voor gesonde geneesmiddelen'. And Six himself acknowledges that the beauty of Spanish women has not left him unmoved. 'Aanvechtinge geleeden te S. Lukas' ('Assailment by Sanlucar de Barrameda') (J55) is testament to a tempestuous love for a girl from 'Andalusy, dat Paradys' (l. 3). The girl, as beautiful as the Greek Helena, ignites such a roaring fire in his body – ''k voel de lieve min het ingewand strax quellen' ('I feel the sweet love immediately tormenting my guts') (l. 4) – that the 'aanvechtinge' ('assaults') on this fiery passion degenerate into a struggle to preserve his reason and his health. It is mainly the intensity of her eyes that Six finds somatically disruptive (l. 5–8):

> Maar wend ik myn gesicht dan naa uw oogeschellen,
> Waar uit dat paar zoo glanst van diamente steen,
> In 't bloosend blanke veld, met syn volkoomentheên,
> Zoo voel 'k de heete min myn leever meer ontstellen.
>
> But I turn my face towards your eyelids,
> From under which your two eyes glow like diamonds,
> In your blushing white face, with its perfect qualities,
> In that way, I feel the hot love stir my liver even more.

Her perfect beauty is expressed in the shine of her eyes, in the middle of her 'blushing white face'. Does Six mean a white face with red cheeks? If so, her face possesses the artificial, enchanting beauty that Six warns against in his series of sonnets.[38]

According to early modern moralists, Eastern powders and ointments had a devastating, debilitating effect: they were sources of infection that had to be avoided if they were not to corrupt society.[39] The transformative power of dyes and

38 On the enchanting power of eyes and the concepts of 'fascinatie'/'fascie', see Thijs Weststeijn, '"Painting's Enchanting Poison": Artistic Efficacy and the Transfer of Spirits', in: C. Göttler and W. Neuber (eds.), *Spirits Unseen: The Representation of Subtle Bodies in Early Modern European Culture*, 2008, pp. 141–178.

39 See Mark Breitenberg, *Anxious Masculinity in Early Modern England*, 1996; Dolan, 1993, pp. 224–239. See also various satirical poems on make-up in classical literature, such as satire II, 'Weakness of Men', by Juvenal, *Juvenal and Persius*, 2004, pp. 147–165.

pigments would have been perceived by Six as threatening his physical and mental personhood, including his gender identity. Six was, after all, a young bachelor when he travelled through Southern Europe. In my view, the criticism he levelled against the many homosexuals in Florence – for example, in 'Op de sodomiterye' (J68), which contains a warning to Dutch parents to keep their sons at home, should also be read in this context. It is more about his self-presentation to the recipients of the poems – reformed ministers – than it is about the actual conditions in Florence. According to the poem, there is no cure for this sinful disease, except the rain of fire with which God 'gaf te drinken' ('gave Sodom to drink') (l. 12–14). Male prostitutes in Italy also used cosmetics.[40] In another poem, 'Aan Florencen' (J69), Six talks about the freedom that the Florentines enjoy in their city. He urges the city dwellers to keep their freedom under control, so that they do not fall into depravity (l. 9–11): 'Sy [vrijheid] dartelt op uw grond, en lydt noch toom, noch wet, / Gelyk ten tyde van aaloude Tiberynen, / Van 't weelich Asien, in vrye vree, besmet' ('Freedom waltzes on your ground, and obeys neither bridle nor law, just as in the times of the Romans, who, when living in Peace with the East, were infected by lascivious Asia'). Six viewed the contagious wealth of Asia as the source of the decadence and the cause of the Roman Empire's collapse.[41]

We should thus read 'Op het blanketten van 't vrouwvolk in Spanje' in light of Six's profession. The series of sonnets is aimed at those among the Dutch who were suspicious of the druggist-poet travelling through Southern Europe, not only because of the pathogenic temptations he would potentially be exposed to, but also because of the nature of his commercial interests in Spain and Italy. We are already familiar with Six's own affinity for Southern Europe. 'Schetse van Venecie' ('Sketch of Venice') (J97), one of the longest poems of *Poësy*, reveals a fascination for Italian life and culture – although the message of the poem is that Amsterdam has taken over Venice's role as the leading European centre for spices.[42] Was Six himself involved in the trade in skin whitener and other cosmetics? In a humanist discussion of 'Op het blanketten', he shows that he knows the limitations of science and that he is aware of the boundary between the use and the misuse of medicines. Misuse includes the cosmetic use of early modern drugs. He does not want to be associated with this. After all, skin whitener is defined, in this series of sonnets, not as a druggist's commodity, but as a product of 'quaksalvery' ('quackery') (VIII, J48, l. 12).

40 N.S. Davidson, 'Sodomy in Early Modern Venice', in: Tom Betteridge, *Sodomy in Early Modern Europe*, 2002, p. 67.

41 *Cf.*, too, Six's verdict on a Dutch libertine travelling in Italy (probably the poet Matthijs van de Merwede van Clootwijck): 'Dwaasen roem' ('Foolish Fame') (J91). See also Hooft, 2001, pp. 24–27; Koopmans, 1915, pp. 25–49.

42 See Buyens, 2005.

Taking a distance from poetry as decoration

In 'Op het blanketten van 't vrouwvolk in Spanje', Six makes his drugstore colourless, as it were, by means of a theoretical discussion of vices that he links to the use of 'blanketsel'. The same systematic approach to fragrances and colours, but this time in relation to his writing desk, can be found in two poems that I would like to discuss here: 'Bruiloftsangh, aan Joannes Abeels getrouwt met Anna de Bra' ('Wedding Song, to Joannes Abeels, Married to Anna de Bra') (J171) and 'Oostkappele, aan Abraham Grenier den jongen' ('Oostkapelle, to Abraham Grenier the Younger') (J172). We saw in the Introduction that, in classical rhetoric, instructions on literary production include references to dyes: an orator should decorate his texts with 'rhetorical colours' in order to make his work engaging to the audience. We have seen how George Puttenham compared the production of poems with the use of make-up: the 'coulours in our arte of Poesie', he wrote, must not be 'well-tempered' or 'well-layd'. The classical vision of rhetorical imagery as alluring art is reflected in the literary theory of the Renaissance.[43] For Six, however, the ideal turns out not to be a balanced distribution of oriental colours from poetry, but a categorical rejection of these. This iconoclastic approach to poetry is expressed in the two poems I will discuss here. In 'Bruiloftsangh, aan Joannes Abeels getrouwt met Anna de Bra', the self-critical poet carries out a systematic investigation of the classical tropes of the *epithalamium*, and proceeds to reject each of them in turn.[44] For example, the part in which the decoration of the bride is mentioned reads (l. 19–24):

O neen. Ik swygh ook van uw schoone bruid,
Als een Goddinne, muntende uit,
In reijen ooverschoone maaghden:
Gelyk de son, wanneer hy klom,
Verdoofde al wat er scheen, en glom,
Aan 't bruin gewelf, waar mee het daaghde.

No, I am silent about your beautiful bride,
As a Goddess, standing out
In rows of extraordinarily beautiful virgins:

43 George Puttenham, *Arte of English Poesie*, 1589, p. 115.

44 Joannes/Jan Abeels was the son of Jonas Abeels, a trader in peppers, silk and yarn who did business in Venice. The bride was the sister of Isaac de Bra, the merchant who gifted Six with a bezoar (J467) – see Jacobs, 1991 II, p. 309; and see: http://research.frick.org/montias/browserecord.php?-action=browse&-recid=2535 (consulted 10 May 2019). Members of the well-to-do bourgeoisie had an affinity for glorifying classical art and poetry.
Frijhoff & Spies, 2004, pp. 448–458.

Just as the sun, as it rose,
Outdid all that shone and gleamed,
On the dark vault [the firmament] that it dawned on.

Lavishing attributes of a pagan goddess on the bride was hardly appropriate for a Christian. The tone is clearly different from that of the wedding poems discussed at the beginning of this chapter. The rejection is explained later on in the text: the linguistic cosmetics of poetry obscure the truth. It is vain flattery that the poet uses only as self-promotion (l. 37–40):

Wegh ydelheit van fleeuwery, vol wind,
Waar deur een dichter sich bemint,
Gemeinlik tracht by elk te maaken:
Want prysen kost hem kleinen prys.

Away with the vanity of flattery, full of wind,
Through which a poet tries
To be loved by everyone,
Because praising [others] costs him little.

'Ik eindige op een andre wijs, / En wil myn laffe rymen staaken' ('I finish in another way, and want to stop my pallid rhymes'), Six concludes (l. 41–42). He stops playing his pagan lyre, and instead asks the Christian God, the creator of the sacred institution of marriage, to bless the bridal couple.

Six applies the same deconstructive approach to another subject of the praise poem: the *laus urbis* or praise for a town. We see this in the poem that follows 'Bruiloftsangh': 'Oostkappele, aan Abraham Grenier den jongen'. At the beginning of the text, the poet turns to his subject, the village of Oostkapelle in Zeeland, and tells how beautifully he would paint this landscape in verse if he were Horace, l. 12–20:

Mocht ik een dagh maar zyn Horaats,
Wat deftigh werk zou ik bedryven?
Hoe schilderachtigh zou ik looven
U, die geheel niet anders zyt,
Dan een prieel, of mooi tapyt
Van akkers, duinen, daalen, hooven?
Ik liet my dan, op wielen, sleepen,
Met een penceeltjen, in myn hand,
Van Walchrens hoofdstad, langs uw land,
En haalde weer te voet die streepen.

If only I could be Horace for one day,
What stately work would I carry out?
How picturesquely would I praise
You, who are no different
From a garden or a beautiful tapestry
Of fields, dunes, valleys and courts?
I let myself, then, be taken on wheels
With a small brush in my hand,
From the capital of Walcheren [Middelburg], through your land,
And repeated these strokes on [metrical] feet.

If he had the colours of the Horatian palette at his disposal, he tells us, the result would be astonishing: a literary landscape so perfect that birds would rise up out of it (l. 25–36):

Ik wed, als die verscheide verven,
Zoo glommen afgeset, in 't oogh
Der beestjes, langhs den sonneboogh,
Se streeken alle die er swerven.
De geelvink beesigh, om in 't kooren,
De leeuwerk om, in 't bloeijend hooi,
De musjes om, hun elsenkooi,
Langs slooten, aassiek op te spooren.
Lyk Zeuxis, met syn konstge druiven,
De voogels, van den Heemel, trok,
Die hongrigh, voor een lekkren brok,
Bemaalde doeken wouden kluiven.

I bet – as these different colours
Jumping out brilliantly to the eye
Of the beasts along the sun's arc [*i.e.*, in the air],
– That all flying animals would alight [on this poem].
The yellow finch, busy in the wheat,
The lark, in the flowering grass,
The sparrows, with their nests in the alder grove,
Along the ditches, greedy for food.
Like Zeuxis, who with his artificial grapes,
Allured the birds of the Sky,
Which, greedy for a tasty crumb,
Would pick on painted canvases.

In this text, too, we can spot a number of commonplaces from Renaissance art. Perhaps the most famous of these is the reference to the story of the competition between the Greek painters Parrhasius and Zeuxis – a story that was popular in Dutch Renaissance art. According to the quotation, Zeuxis was able to paint a bunch of grapes so realistically that birds (and thus also spectators) were tempted to believe that it was not a work of art, but the real thing. Six's reference to the story, however, is not so much a plea for truthful art as a warning against the bewitching properties of colours. This warning is reinforced by the imagery Six uses elsewhere in the poem. If he were Horace, he tells us, he would use his music to bewitch plants and animals, as Orpheus did, or make stones move and build a city, as Amphion made the city Thebes rise by playing the lyre; or enchant a dolphin so that it brought him to France, just as the mythical poet Arion attracted a dolphin with the music of his lyre so that it saved him from drowning (l. 40–52). The whole discourse rests on another magical-religious concept: the realisation of such a transformation requires faith in Pythagoras's doctrine of the transport of the soul (l. 9–10).[45] But Six does not believe in that.

This passage is followed by the anticlimax. Six emphasises that he cannot make such exalted poetry – that his poetic 'brush' lacks the magical colours of Horace (l. 53–56):

Maar om den Venusyn te lyken,
En met een puik penceel te gaan,
Waar zoo een stuk van dient gedaan,
Zoo mis ik verw, om net te stryken.

But to resemble the Venusian [poet – *i.e.,* Horace],
And to handle a fine brush,
Which is necessary to make such a masterpiece,
To that end, I lack the pigments to paint with fine strokes.

To understand this turning point, we need to see who the recipient of the text is. In addition to Abraham Grenier, who is mentioned in the title, the text is addressed to Peter Duivelaer, a preacher and Grenier's brother-in-law, who was a minister in Oostkapelle in 1649 and then, in 1654, in Middelburg.[46] Six addresses him directly in lines 62–64, and apologises for his negligence when it comes to singing the praises of the beautiful village of Duivelaer. What follows proceeds along the same lines as with the wedding poem to Joannes Abeels and Anna de Bra: he prefers to quietly praise Oostkapelle in his

45 See Vossius, 2010, pp. 1913–1914 for the Pythagorean notion of the transport of the soul. I will come back to a more extensive discussion of this in Chapter 8.

46 For sources, see Jacobs, 1991 II, p. 313.

thoughts, rather than to seize upon non-Christian imagery. He also portrays Duivelaer's voice as a positive Christian variant of Horace's godless voice. Whereas the latter is heathen and seductive, the former is 'gesond, en klaar' ('healthy and clear') (l. 66).

The problem that Six focuses on in these texts is the same as in 'Op het blanketten van 't vrouwvolk in Spanje': the notion of the artist as a demigod who, with the aid of his imagination, tries to improve upon nature, God's sacred creation.[47] These poems are also characterised by the realisation that such an action implies a hubristic transgression against God's laws. Six tells us, however, that his poetic 'brush' lacks Horace's colours: 'I lack the pigments to paint with fine strokes'. He himself is not capable of performing that kind of magic.

Another aspect I will come back to later is the remarkable literary strategy that underlies both poems and that once again reveals the ambiguous and ambivalent character of Six's poetry. There is, indeed, more to say about these verses. It is striking that in both texts the poet spends a lot of time painting in quite some detail precisely what he proscribes. Through the rhetorical device of *praeteritio,* whereby one announces the intention not to mention something one names in the process of making, the poetic ornamentation of the *epithalamium* and the *laus urbis* is given plenty of play.[48] We have to take with a grain of salt Six's apologies to Duivelaer for his lack of poetic ability, just as we did in the poem I opened this chapter with, 'Huldekroon, aan den heer Geerard Bikker'. Through *praeteritio,* he succeeds in doing two things: honouring the bridal couple and the landscape of Oostkapelle in colourful poems of praise, while at the same time renouncing pagan poetry with its treacherous smells and colours.

'Depiction and Consecration of Roselle'

The last text – or, more correctly, the last group of texts – that I will discuss in this chapter brings us back to Six's Roselle. In 'Afbeeldinge en wydinge van

47 Rodenburgh, 1638, p. 8 (where he imitates Philip Sidney): 'Natuure verciert heur aerde nimmer zo rijckelijck, ghelijck zommighe Poëten die tapessieren, noch met zo schoone revieren, vrucht-baere boomen, wel-rieckende bloemen, heughelijcke lommeren, springhende watervlieten, en dierghelycke. Natuurens wereld is koper, die de Poëten een gouden afbeelden te zyn' ('Nature decorates her earth not so abundantly as some Poets present it, as though in tapestries, with such beautiful rivers, fertile trees, fragrant flowers, pleasant shades, rushing floods and the like. The world of Nature is copper, of which Poets make a golden image.').

48 As early as 1979, Schenkeveld-van der Dussen mentions this rhetorical figure in a discussion of 'Bruiloftsangh, aan Joannes Abeels getrouwt met Anna de Bra', but she does not devote any further attention to this in her study on Six ('Theorie en poëzie: een epithalamium van Six van Chandelier', in *De nieuwe taalgids*, 1979, p. 394, note 8). Six uses *praeteritio* on several occasions. I will discuss this figure of speech in more detail in Chapter 7, pp. 240–243, in considering the poem (also by Horace) from which Six derived this rhetorical figure.

Roselle, en haare bestraffinge' ('Depiction and Consecration of Roselle, and Her Punishment') (J59–64), Six takes the same iconoclastic path as he did for the two poems I discussed above. However, in this group of texts, he gives more play to his own persona and to his role as a travelling druggist-poet. The group of texts is the second-longest series of sonnets in the 'Klinkdichten' section of *Poësy*. The longest poem is 'Op het blanketten van 't vrouwvolk in Spanje', which we discussed earlier.

We can say, in view of the title, that this is once again a case of Petrarchan love poetry. In this series of sonnets, the druggist-poet is on one of his commercial trips, this time in Granada, Spain. The series deals with one of Six's favourite 'pastimes' when he is not in his native country, namely longing for Roselle. When he meets a sculptor of Catholic statues and learns that he was unemployed because the Catholic Church no longer needs images – after all, they were sacred and imperishable, the Calvinist ironically notes – Six hits on the idea of hiring the sculptor himself. He orders the Spaniard to make a statue of his Roselle, with a sceptre and crown as signs of her majesty, and with a matching cupid, the medium between the love poet and his lover: (J59, l. 7–14):

Snyd my een vrouw, van eenen gaaven berk,
Zyt seeker dat uw kost, noch loon zal spyten.
Beeld 't aangesicht, gelyk een frische maaghd,
Doe 't bloote haair, langhs 't halve rughkleed, daalen,
Maak dat se slinks een Kupidootjen draaght,
Sorgh dat se rechts mach met een scepter praalen,
Let dat haar kruin een Kooninghs kroone schraaght,
Omcier haar hals met parlende koraalen.

Cut a woman for me from a sound birch,
Rest assured that you will not regret the expenses and the earnings.
Depict the face like a healthy virgin's,
Make the uncovered hair fall down along the backcloth,
Have her carry a Cupid on her left side,
Make sure she flaunts a sceptre on her right side,
Have her head carry a Queen's crown,
Decorate her neck with pearly corals.

The altar Six creates for Roselle thus consists not only of words, but also of tangible materials. In this way, Six makes concepts he has taken from Petrarchan love poetry both plastic and concrete. Here Roselle is presented not as an earthly mortal, but as an idealised, imperishable work of art.

The series consists of six sonnets. The first is about the aforementioned encounter and the conversation with the sculptor. The second and third contain descriptions of the statue. We find out that Six has the statue dyed and gilded and then consecrated with incense. Six then tells us how he cuts the cupid from the statue, so that Roselle's image cannot be confused with images of Mary and the child Jesus, which are abundant in Spain. The fourth sonnet contains incitements to repentance and reflection. Just like the biblical Mary, Six's 'Mary' does not wear 'kooninghlyke klêen', 'kingly clothes'. We are told that it is impossible to capture her by describing her external splendour, because she is located in the heart of the poet. But the real regret comes only in the last two sonnets, in which Six presents a confrontation with the real Roselle. The fifth sonnet shows Roselle's reaction to Six after she has learned that he was worshipping her in Spain with the help of idolatry. Angrily, she expresses her horror. In the sixth sonnet, Six responds to her accusations. He wonders how an exalted woman such as Roselle can use insults so rudely, but he also asks her to forgive him for his sinful actions. The transgression that Six has committed, and that has already been presented as a theme in the title of the series, 'Afbeeldinge en wydinge van Roselle', is, of course, having ignored God's second commandment in the Calvinist Bible: 'Verbeeld, gebiedt Gods andere gebod, / Geen dingen, die om hoogh zyn, of beneeden' ('Do not – so demands God's second commandment – depict anything that is above or below') as we read in sonnet V (J63, l. 9–10). The worship of statues of saints, and the adoration of the altar and other objects, are essential parts of Catholic liturgy. In the eyes of Protestant pastors, Catholicism was nothing but idolatry. Believers should be in direct contact with God through prayer, according to the Protestant doctrine, not indirectly through priests or inanimate objects. Six's sin was to make his Roselle an object of devotion. As my summary of the contents also shows, the series is a chronological story. There is no room here for a comprehensive interpretation of the complete cycle of sonnets. I shall confine myself to the lines of verse that treat the role of drugs as colourants and fragrances.

Although the creation of the statue already takes place in the first sonnet, which describes how the sculptor makes the work, the creation of the devotional object takes place only in the second sonnet, in which Six has the statue 'painted and gilded' (l. 4), and in the third, when he consecrates the work of art with incense. Let us start with the second sonnet (J60). As soon as Six has the statue painted, it acquires the splendour and glory it is due. We then read that it even surpasses the famous statue of Venus (Aphrodite) in the classical city of Corinth in its beauty and exaltedness: 'Maar waarom moet Korinthen nu niet dulden, / Dit pronkbeeld my, in zoo een goed fatsoen, / Haar Venus lykt voor welke Achaje toen / Ten offer quam, met minnelyke schulden?' ('But why should Corinth not suffer this icon, in such a beautiful form, to resemble their Venus, to whom all of Achaea came to bring offerings, when their inhabitants had a debt to settle in the currency of love') (l. 5–8). Here we read that there is no reason why the Corinthians should deny that this statue of Roselle is even more beautiful than their statue of Aphrodite, to which all of Greece ('Achaje') made sacrifices in ancient times. We recognise this theme from my analysis of 'Op het blanketten van 't vrouwvolk in Spanje'. Just as the skin whitener makes the old Spanish woman seem younger, so the gold colours give the icon Roselle the necessary vitality and life force, the heavenly fire that Prometheus stole from the gods and that he used to breathe life into a man kneaded from clay. Here Six apparently bases himself on religious traditions that go back a long way: pagan statues of gods were indeed painted with beautiful colours and covered with holy oils.[49]

But Six's altar of love is not yet complete. At the end of the second sonnet, he says he has to think about what name to give the statue. The third sonnet (J61) then describes how the icon is 'baptised'. She would be called Mary, according to Six, but 'niet naa de Mary de Heemelkooningin' ('not after Mary, the Queen of Heaven') (l. 2), but after his beloved Roselle, whose name was also Mary in real life (l. 9–14):

Ghy zult den naam bekleên van myn meestres,
Wyl 'k van haar lief geselschap om gaa swarmen,
Zal sy in u ontsien zyn, als Godes.
Hier jonge tilt dat jongsken, uit heur armen,
En haal my voor een quartjen vyf of ses
Aan Wierook, om heur neusgat soet te warmen.

You shall bear the name of my mistress,
While I am far from her dear company,
She will be worshipped in you, as a Goddess.
Here, young lad, remove that little boy from her arms,
And get me Incense worth a quart
and five or six [maravedi] to sweeten her nostrils.

The capital letters (in the original) serve to emphasise the keywords in the poem: 'Goddess' and 'Incense'. Six asked a 'boy' (probably his own servant[50]) to remove

49 Schmidt 1924, p. 41. See, too, the description of the pigment cinnabar in Pliny XXXIII, 111–112: 'Verrius gives a list of writers of unquestionable authority who say that on holidays it was the custom for the face of the statue of Jupiter himself to be coloured with cinnabar, as well as the bodies of persons going in triumphal procession': [E]numerat auctores Verrius, quibus credere necesse sit Iovis ipsius simulacri faciem diebus festis minio inlini solitam triumphantiumque corpora; sic Camillum triumphasse' (Pliny, *Natural History*, IX, trans. by H. Rackham, 1934, p. 85).

50 Jacobs (1991 II, p. 60) explains that 'jonge', means 'loopjongen', 'errand boy'. Six had a servant on his travels abroad. See also 'Brief, aan Theodore Dodeur' ('Letter to Theodore Dodeur') (J252, l. 87).

the cupid/child Jesus, to avoid the resemblance with Catholic images, and to get some incense for a cheap price to inaugurate the icon – to 'sweeten her nostrils', as he put it (Fig. 5.4).[51] Thus Six makes it clear that the transformation is complete: the wooden block is *anthropomorphised.* It has human characteristics such as sense of smell. Although the sculptor has given form to the statue, it is thus the druggist who, with incense, has breathed life into this dead piece of wood. A mystery – a *sacramental* act – has occurred. The druggist-poet acts as a priest in a religious ceremony.

But as we have seen, in the last sonnet the wandering druggist-poet gets thinking. There follows an anti-climax, which retroactively reveals the ironic tone of the previous sonnets. In sonnet V (J63), Roselle scolds Six for his un-Christian action: 'Wat al verdriets deed deese kuur my lyden! / Foei schaam u ghy die Kristus letters spelt' ('How much sadness these whims gave me; shame on you, who spell the name of Christ') (l. 5–6). We recognise the strategy that Six uses in this group of texts from poems we have already looked at, such as 'Uitroep om hoornafsetters', where Six's narrative contained a turning point that changes the direction of the poem. The hallowed tone of the first sonnets is undermined by the arrival of the real Roselle, a really down-to-earth person who does not resemble at all Six's idealised image. This is shown especially by the description, in the last sonnet, of the language she uses. Here is Six's response to her impolite way of speaking (VI, J64, l. 1–6):

> Is 't ernst me me me Ioffrouw zoo te kyven?
> Heeft dan een duifje, als haagel blank van pluim,
> Met raaven swart, als roet, zoo bitter schuim
> Van gal gemein, dat nu komt booven dryven?
> Kan nu de tongh myns Engels quaade wyven
> Naabootsen, met een geemelyke luim?

> Do you, damsel, really mean to scold me me me?
> Does a dove, with snow-white feathers,
> Possess such bitter foam of vulgar bile – as black as raven and as soot –
> As the one that now comes drifting up?
> Can the tongue of my angel emulate
> Wicked women in a really foul mood?

51 The low value of the incense, a 'quartjen van vyf of ses / Aan Wierook' (l. 13–14) – 5 1/4 or 6 1/4 'maravedi'– raises the question of whether this is cheap (fake) frankincense. The irony is clear: this kind of adoration costs just a pittance. This mockery is in keeping with the satirical tone of the entire series of sonnets. Six is probably referring to the lowest coin in the Spanish monetary system, *maravedi.* I would like to thank Svein Harald Gullbekk for this information.

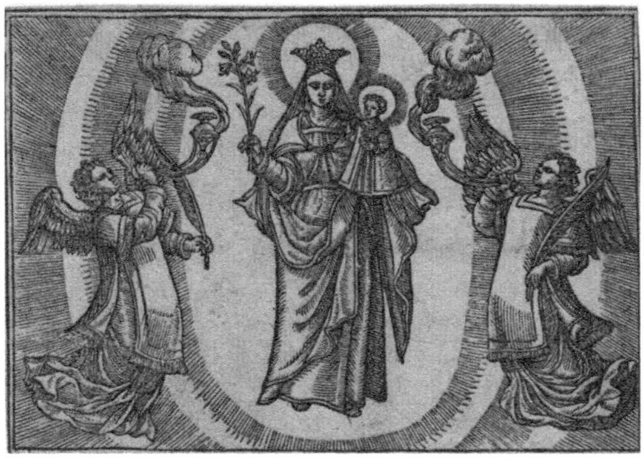

Fig. 5.4: Anonymous, *Mary with Child*, 1590–1599. Engraving. (© Rijksmuseum, Amsterdam).

According to Six, a wooden work of art could never reflect the real characteristics of Roselle. She swears like 'wicked women' and is full of 'bitter foam of vulgar bile' – bodily fluids that emphasise that we are dealing here with an earthy woman. She is *temperamental* in the original sense of the word.

To whom is this series of sonnets addressed? The many intellectual allusions in the text, such as the references to the survival of a pagan cult in the veneration of Mary, and the reflections on the true appearance of the biblical Mary do not belong to the *topoi* of early modern love poetry, but are commonplace in early modern Reformed, anti-Catholic literature. The worship of religious and non-religious statues is a theme of a French anti-Catholic treatise that was translated into Dutch. In this book the writer criticises a Jesuit theologian for allowing the worship of 'not only consecrated statues, placed in a church, but also statues that have not yet left the workspace of the woodcarver'.[52] Once again it is likely that the poem is not only meant for Roselle, but aimed at a larger group of readers, especially Dutch pastors who were concerned about the young druggist-merchant abroad. The temptations to which young Dutch travellers in the South were exposed had, on this view, more than just a sensual, earthy character. Counter-reformation propaganda, in which the worship of Mary and other ceremonies full of charming colours and scents played an important role, was aimed among other things at young, impressionable Protestants. An example is Reyer Anslo's conversion to

52 '[...] datmen de Beelden mach aanbidden, niet alleenlick dan, alsse ghewyet zijn, en geset in de Tempelen, maar oock datmense mach aenbidden in den winckel van een Beeldt-snijder', in Charles Drelincourt, *Cort-begryp van de dwalinghen der Roomsche Kercke*, translated by Abraham Pietersz Wilsenius; English translation and quotation from Els Stronks, *Negotiating Differences: Word, Image and Religion in the Dutch Republic*, 2011, pp. 129–135, quote on p. 134. *Cf.*, too, Romans 1:22 and 23.

Catholicism. Anslo was a friend of Six's, and was his travelling companion in Italy.[53]

A good indication of this is 'Brief aan Roselle' ('Letter to Roselle') (J198), which was written in rhyme and, just as the series of sonnets we looked at above, during a business trip to the South. Like the last sonnet, it contains a request for forgiveness from Roselle, who was waiting in the Netherlands. This time, however, it is not a question of excessive attention, but of a lack of it: Six admits that his trade interests kept on eating up his time. He nevertheless assures Roselle that he always thinks of her. After all, the Marian cult constantly reminds him of her (l. 5–8): 'Waar ik koopgierigh reis door landen, en door steeden, / Daar werd uw lieve naam, op kniejen aangebeeden, / Van alle menschen, als een Heemelsche Godin' ('Where I, eager to buy, travel through countries and cities, where your lovely name is offered up on bended knee, as a Heavenly Goddess'). The suspicion seems justified that this is not really about Six's love relationship with Roselle – the idea that a religious custom would remind him of her seems too artificial for that – but about Six's own faith, and that is addressed to Dutch pastors, and because of the resemblance of his beloved's real name to that of the 'Heavenly Goddess'.[54]

Then there is Six's own love poetry to Roselle: One could read 'Afbeeldinge en wydinge van Roselle' as a direct comment on the quasi-religious 'Op de schoonicheit van Roselle, aan de selve' (J27), a poem that Six probably wrote in his early years, and that we discussed at the beginning of this chapter. The earthy, choleric Roselle of 'Afbeeldinge en wydinge' contrasts sharply with the idealised image of the woman in this poem. Here, the cult of Roselle also takes the form of a sanctuary decorated with precious luxury goods. 'Toen lagh syn geest tot minnen ook te min / Al 't kindsche speeltuigh is verworpen met dat kooten' ('At that time his [Six's] spirits were too low for a desire to love. All these childish games are renounced with that fawning') (l. 66–67), Six writes in 'Het boek, aan den leeser' about verses that he wrote as a young man and with which he no longer wants to be identified.[55] 'Afbeeldinge en wydinge van Roselle', which deals explicitly with apotheosis in Petrarchan love poetry, can therefore be read as a reckoning with 'juvenile sins' such as 'Op de schoonicheit van Roselle'.

53 See 'Brief, aan R. Anslo, te Rome' ('Letter to R. Anslo in Rome') (J468). *Cf.* also the diary of Anslo's friend, Arnout Hellemans Hooft, who travelled in Italy in the same period as Six. He both went to the Catholic mass and kissed the Pope's feet: Arnout Hellemans Hooft, *Een naekt beeldt op een marmore matras seer schoon. Het dagboek van een grand tour (1649–1651)*, 2001.

54 It is also worth noting that cult objects were displayed in curiosity cabinets belonging to Protestants. The cabinet of Joan Breyne, for example, contained 'een geboutseert Venus-beeltje' ('a modelled idol of Venus'), 'twee porcelyne Maria-beelden' ('two porcelain statues of Mary'), and 'een Chinees wierookmonster van steen, heel raer' ('a Chinese incensory of stone, very rare'): *Catalogus van een groote partij extraordinaire curieuse Rariteyten* [...] *Joan Breyne*, 1693, pp. 7, 10, 13.

55 *Cf.* my interpretation of 'Het boek, aan den leeser' (J119) in Chapter 2, pp. 81–83.

Conclusion

Let us return to Six's disapproval of Vondel's 'colourful' poetry, with which I started this chapter. If we see this against the backdrop of the poems discussed in this chapter, we realise that Six's self-portrayal as a 'drab poet' is based on a well-considered authorial strategy. In the early modern period, the trade in drugs was synonymous with a wealth of colours and fragrances. Six develops literary strategies with a view to fostering a public image of himself as a reliable and level-headed merchant. It is therefore important to him to demonstrate a literary distance from the un-Dutch, aristocratic values that the expensive dyes associated with his profession represent. Six profiles himself as an intellectual merchant-druggist, someone who recognises and has mastered the transformative powers of cosmetics, whether in terms of the medical, moral or religious dangers associated with them.

The self-image he develops as a *flawed* poet is interesting in this context. His poetic 'brush' lacks the magical colours of Horace, as we have seen in 'Oostkappele, aan Abraham Grenier den jongen', but this does not prevent him – by means of the rhetorical device of *praeteritio* – from describing what colourful poems look like. The same goes for Six's wedding poem to Johannes Abeels and Anna de Bra, in which Six presented his poems as 'laffe rijmen' ('pallid rhymes'). In these texts, his image as a flawed rhymester thus serves as an alibi: despite the existence of these poems, he insists that he himself is not capable of performing this kind of magic. In 'Afbeeldinge en wydinge van Roselle', in which Six directly confronts the religious pretensions of the Petrarchan praise poem, and criticises the dehumanising effect of incense, we see a particular elaboration of this 'flawed poetics'. Six's reaction to Roselle's angry reprimand in the last sonnet in the series is interesting: he has no rational explanation for his sinful acts, but responds with a stuttering 'me me me' (VI, J64, l. 1). Roselle's frenzied swearing and this stuttering answer serve as a contrast to the Neoplatonic doctrine of harmony in Renaissance love poetry. We do not expect to find this kind of temperamental woman or this kind of 'flawed' language in the euphemistic love poems of early modern poets such as P.C. Hooft. It would be hard to imagine a greater contrast with Hooft's beloved, 'Mithra Granida'.[56] But that does not mean that the image of women that finds expression in Six's poetry is 'realistic' or 'feminist' in the modern sense of the word. Farah Karim-Cooper shows how, according to literary works that were opposed to cosmetics, women 'had a responsibility to help preserve the national identity because of the centrality of their role in the household'.[57]

56 'Mithra Granida' is the quasi-mythological name that P.C. Hooft uses for his wife, Christina van Erp. 'Mithra' refers to a Zoroastrian sun god; 'Granida', to a Persian princess.

57 Karim-Cooper, 2006, p. 41. A good example of this, which takes place specifically in a kitchen, is in 'Geusemirakel' ('Geuzen Miracle') (J426), where Six portrays a bold, down-to-earth Dutch maid, immune to any form of Catholic 'superstition'. See, too, Six's portrait of the woman as the active one in sexual

According to the view of art expressed in this series of sonnets, and in 'Op het blanketten van 't vrouwvolk in Spanje', we could link this ideal of flawed poetics with the notion of authenticity, and perfect, divine poetics with artificiality. I will come back to these issues in the following chapters, where I will discuss the concept of the poet as the possessor of divine power, the idea of the Pythagorean transport of the soul, and colours and smells as bearers of transformative, deifying properties.

Another point I will elaborate on in the following chapters is Six's dramatic and theatrical poetry: rather than promulgating Calvinistic arguments against the worship of saints and statues, he embeds these beliefs in a theatrical and fanciful story, with a central place for himself as a vulnerable, sinful human being. Sacramental uses of material objects will also be at the centre of the last two chapters of this part of the book. I will go into more detail regarding the aspects I mentioned above. First, though, I would like to consider another kind of ornamentation: gunpowder as it was used during festive processions. That is the theme of the next chapter. That said, I will also discuss other uses of gunpowder, such as for ammunition and even as a medicine.

intercourse in 'Boerde, aan den selven' ('Mockery, to the Same Person') (J407). *Cf.* also the chapter 'The heroic housewife', in: Schama, 2004, pp. 398–429, and the criticism of Schama in Lia van Gemert, 'The Power of the Weak Vessels: Simon Schama and Johan van Beverwijck on Women', in: Els Kloek, Nicole Teeuwen & Marijke Huisman (eds.), *Women of the Golden Age: An International Debate on Women in Seventeenth-Century Holland, England and Italy*, 1994, pp. 39–53.

6. Drugs as explosives

Abstract
In this chapter I focus on gunpowder, both in the sense of materials for warfare, and fireworks for public celebrations. The Dutch word for gunpowder, *buskruit*, proves the close connection with the topic for this study, *kruid*, 'spice'. I show how in his poems Six distances himself from gunpowder by demonstrating a punishment on the 'Dutch body', both on his own body and 'the body' of the city of Delft. I argue that this is the theme of two poems Six wrote on accidents with his loaded pistols, and a poem he wrote to the explosion of the gunpowder depot in Delft in 1654. But in this Chapter too, we learn to know Six as a pragmatic poet. I show how glorifying poems to the Orange Prince Frederick Henry were furnished with references to gunshots and fireworks.

Keywords: Jan Vos, gunpowder, fireworks, saltpetre, gunpowder explosion in Delft in 1654, Frederick Henry

Jupijn zal op 't geluidt van huilen, schreeuwen, gillen,
En donderen, verbaast van zijne zetel zien,
En vraagen of'er, om de werreldt te gebiên,
Een nieuwe Jupiter zijn godtheidt komt braveeren:
Dan geeft men deeze stof, daar 't oorlog by zal zweeren,
De naam van bussekruid, jaa booskruidt in de strijdt.

Jupiter will, because of the sound of crying, shouting, screaming,
And thundering, look in surprise. from his throne,
And ask whether, in order to rule the world,
A new Jupiter is coming to defy him as a god:
Therefore, this substance, by which war will swear,
Shall be given the name of 'gunpowder', even 'wicked powder' in battle.
– Jan Vos[1]

1 *Medea* (1667). The quotation is from W.J.C. Buitendijk, *Jan Vos' toneelwerken*, 1975, p. 420.

Spaans, R., *Dangerous Drugs: The Self-Presentation of the Merchant-Poet Joannes Six van Chandelier (1620–1695)*. Taylor & Francis Group, 2020
DOI 10.5117/9789462983543_CH06

Gunpowder

The previous chapters have given us a good picture of the use of the 'pharmaceutical' vocabulary used in the poetry of Joannes Six van Chandelier. This is reflected in the *ornatus*, embellishing metaphors that are full of references to seventeenth-century fragrances and dyes. As can be seen from my interpretations, multifunctional drugs cannot be regarded in an unambiguously positive way as poetic ornaments. And this is how the masking and alluring effects of cosmetics come up for discussion. But what is most striking are the medical-scientific arguments against drug use. Drugs were conceived of as substances that heated up the body and aroused dangerous desires. And from a religious perspective, we are also warned against their transformative powers as manipulators of the human body, God's sacred work of creation. The drugs and powders in Six's poetry are thus ambiguous substances. The drug that best demonstrates this ambivalence is probably gunpowder. It was used for festive fireworks, and in firearms, but also as a medicine. For this reason it was a popular metaphor in both art and literature. Moreover, in early modern times it was regarded as a wonderful new substance; by contrast with exotic items such as incense, gunpowder was not known in classical times. We should also mention here the interest of alchemists and 'chymists' in pyrotechnics – the 'art of fire'. Chymists believed that pyrotechnics could reveal the secrets of nature through the art of distillation. Probably more than other chemical products, gunpowder was intertwined with the pursuit of transformation and perfection. And as we shall see below, Six relates the invention of gunpowder to alchemy.[2]

Gunpowder did not leave Six van Chandelier unmoved – despite the image he used of himself as the lowly 'black rooster' of Dutch poetry. Six's poems about the Anglo-Dutch naval wars are full of references to modern warfare, where gunpowder was accorded a central position. The contents of these poems show that Six's commercial practices were severely affected by the English blockades and the hijacking of Dutch merchant ships.[3] He therefore took part enthusiastically in the propaganda against the English. For example, 'Geluk, aan den Weleedlen Jakob van Wassenaer [...]' ('Success, to Jakob van Wassenaer, Esquire [...]') (J358), written on the occasion of the appointment of Jacob van Wassenaer Obdam as admiral in 1653, during the First Anglo-Dutch War, trumpets the praises of the Dutch navy and its strength. We read that, thanks to his 'kryghsdeughd' ('virtue as a warrior') (l. 53), Van Wassenaer deserves a place in the firmament as a 'bright new star' (l. 59) next

2 Cis van Heertum, *Alchemie aan de Amstel: Over hermetische geneeskunst. Catalogus bij een tentoonstelling in de Bibliotheca Philosophica Hermetica*, 2012.

3 'De waarom, van myne vrymoedige reise, naa Engeland' ('The reason For My Self-Confident Journey to England') (J404), l. 10–11.

to that of Hercules, the son of Jupiter; and that, thanks to the 'donder, en kryghs blixemweeder' ('thunder and lightning of war') of his military fleet, 'Neerlands hoogen ceeder' ('the tall cedar of the Netherlands') is experiencing a miraculous revival, according to this very literal commendation of the naval hero (l. 60–64):

Zoo siet men Neerlands hoogen ceeder,
Door donder, en kryghs blixemweeder,
Veel hooger met syn takken gaan,
Dan Boomen, die op Liban staan.

In this way, one sees the tall cedar of the Netherlands,
Through the thunder and lightning of war,
Go much higher with its branches
Than the Trees that are in Lebanon.

Van Wassenaer is 'medicinally loaded' with miraculously explosive powers, as it were, for his battle with the English. The Van Wassenaer family was considered to be the oldest and noblest family in the Republic, with an uninterrupted lineage that could be traced back to a Batavian commander.[4] Van Wassenaer therefore represents the continuation of fearlessness, the hallmark of the lowly, simple Batavian people. In a fiery discourse, Six praises Van Wassenaer's 'aadeldom' ('nobility') (l. 53) as the virtue of a warrior. It seems, then, that in times of crisis, the poet evidently does not follow all that closely his literary self-presentation as a level-headed druggist.

Medea's new weapon

Other poems in *Poësy*, however, attest to a more problematic approach to the use of gunpowder. The druggist-poet also includes explosives in texts in which he examines himself. I will look at three texts here: 'Bussekruid vervloekt. Aan myn moeder' (J383) ('Accursed Gunpowder. To My Mother'), 'Op het barsten van myn pistool, teegens buskruid' ('On the Firing of My Pistol, against Gunpowder') (J338) and 'Buskruids donder, en blixem, te Delft' ('The Thunder and Lightning of Gunpowder, in Delft') (J396). I will then look at drugs as a decoration used in city parades. This is the theme of several texts Six wrote for the collection *Amsterdamsche Vreugdtriomfe* (*Joyful Triumph in Amsterdam*) (1660), which appeared in 1659 on the occasion of the visit to Amsterdam of Amalia of Solms-Braunfels, the widow of Prince Frederick Henry, and her daughters and sons-in-law. But first, a few words on the function of

4 Jacobs, 1991 II, p. 636.

gunpowder as both an efficient *topos* and a material in the Dutch Republic. Once again the glassmaker and playwright Jan Vos comes to our aid here. In some of his texts, gunpowder plays an important role – not only as a poetic ornament, but also as a key concept in his particular poetics, his conception of the writing of literature (Fig. 6.1). I will go into this in more detail here, because it sets out views that were held about gunpowder in the Dutch Republic.

The preface to Vos's *Medea* (1667) is a plea for the renewal of the theatre. The poet rejects the classical laws of theatre and argues that 'nature' and 'experience' can serve as new guidelines for the writing of dramatic texts. The preface can be regarded as an elaboration of Vos's poetics. By 'nature', Vos means two things: the talent of the playwright, but also the disordered reality of the seventeenth century. As he saw it, the literary theories of authorities such as Aristotle and Horace were no longer compatible with the new perception of reality, and could therefore no longer be regarded as guiding principles for literary production. Noteworthy in the context of this argument is Vos's emphasis on the conduct of war by the Dutch navy, in which he sees proof of modern, seventeenth-century 'nature'. As far as 'experience' is concerned, Vos refers to new inventions of his time, including gunpowder. 'Who invented the large and small blunderbusses, which are loaded with saltpetre, iron and lead, slay fewer people, and produce greater power than the weapons with which Alexander conquered the world?' Thus the rhetorical question is: Were these modern inventions known to the ancient Greeks and Romans? No, these were invented by the geniuses 'of the most-recent centuries'.[5] The examples are not randomly selected. For sixteenth- and seventeenth-century humanists, gunpowder, the compass, and the art of printing were proof that their own time was at the same level as classical antiquity, or even surpassed it.[6]

Vos put his progressive thoughts about literature into practice in theatre. Explosives play a central role in one of the most important scenes in *Medea*. When Medea is with Proserpina (Persephone), the goddess of the underworld, she asks about her most dangerous poison. Instead of giving Medea a traditional potion, as in the classical myth, Proserpina brings out a 'futuristic' invention: gunpowder. In a panegyric to her magic powder, Proserpina lets us know that, in 26 centuries' time, people will invent gunpowder.[7] The playwright tells us that, only then, in the distant future, will humanity experience the power of this terrifying substance. When people use gunpowder, he says, even the god Jupiter will be surprised by

5 'Wie vormden de groote en kleene donderbussen, die van salpeeter, yzer en loodt bezwangert, minder volk vermoorden en grooter krachten baaren dan de waapenen daar Alexander de werreldt meê verwon?', Buitendijk, 1975, pp. 364–365.

6 Sipko Melissen, 'De heedendaagse Goude-eeuw', *Spektator*, 1981–1982, pp. 37–38.

7 Vos dates the myth of Medea back to around 1300 BC: Buitendijk, 1975, p. 420.

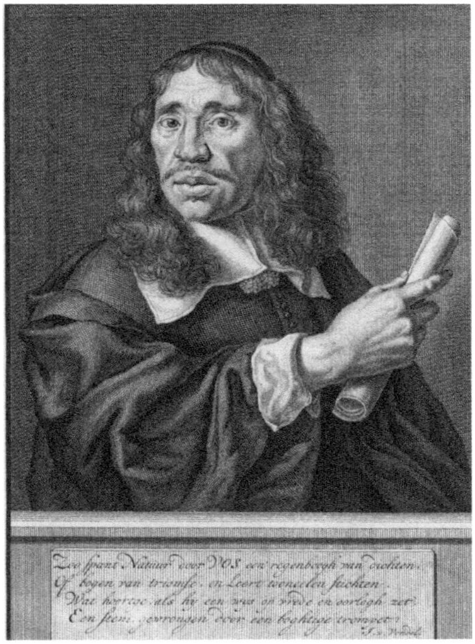

Fig. 6.1: Andries van Buysen (Sr.), *Portrait of the Poet Jan Vos*, 1726. Engraving.
(© Rijksmuseum, Amsterdam).

the genius of the earth's inhabitants. Whoever is in possession of this 'wicked powder' is a new supreme god, a new Jupiter (see the quote at the beginning of this chapter). Gunpowder is also found elsewhere in Jan Vos's *oeuvre*, such as – and this is no surprise – in his praise of Dutch admirals and their victories at sea. In 'Zeekrygh tusschen De Staaten der Vrye Neederlanden, / En het Parlement van Engelandt' ('Naval War between the States of the Free Netherlands and the Parliament of England') – a poem in the form of a dialogue between two gods, Jupiter and the river god Meuse (a personification of the Dutch Republic) – Vos presents Admiral Tromp as an earthy Jupiter, with a divine thunderbolt in his possession like that of the heavenly god. The supreme god Jupiter is amazed at the strength of his cannons:[8]

Toen d'opper Jupiter het donderen der vlooten,
En 't blixemen vernam, riep hy verbaast: heeft d'aardt
Een andre Jupiter? Ik hoor zijn donderklooten,
En zie zijn blixemen. Wie heeft dien godt gebaart?
Ik, riep de Maas; 't is Tromp: hy poogt ons vry te houwen.

8 Jan Vos, *Alle de gedichten*. Part 1, 1662, p. 324.

When the supreme Jupiter noticed the thundering of the fleet,
and the lightning, he shouted in surprise: Has the earth got
Another Jupiter? I hear his thunderbolts,
And see his lightning. Who has given birth to this god?
I, shouted the Meuse. It is Tromp: he is striving to maintain our liberty.

With both his descriptions of the chaotic reality of modern warfare and his expressive, 'pyrotechnic' idiom, Vos tells the reader what kind of divine powers Dutch naval heroes have at their disposal.

This 'explosive' language can also be found in a number of texts that Vos wrote for city festivals and Joyous Entries, and in the context of important official events such as the conclusion of peace treaties and royal weddings.[9] This is not about gunpowder as a terrifying modern weapon, but as a fiery spectacle at festivities, whether in the form of gunpowder for the city guard or of fireworks. Vos was appointed by the city government as the organiser of 'performances on stage, arches of triumph, joyous entries and triumphal chariots'.[10] We see him in this role at the inauguration ceremony of the new Bailiff of Muiden, Gerard Bicker, which he organised together with other poets, and which was accompanied, among other things, by a procession of theatrical chariots on which various allegories and mythological scenes were enacted. On the same day that Bicker was installed as Bailiff of Muiden (5 May 1649), poems and descriptions of the performances were presented in the Amsterdam theatre to celebrate the event.[11] In his 'Blyde Inkomst van den Eed. Heer Geeraardt Bikker [...]' ('Joyous Entry of the Noble Mr. Gerard Bicker [...]'), Vos describes, for example, how 'donderbussen braakten vuur en vlam uit meetaale kaaken' ('blunderbusses vomited fire and flame out of metal jaws') in honour of the young patrician. And we also read: 'Het vuur van yver is niet dan door tijdt te blussen' ('Nothing but time can extinguish the fire'). Vos's praise poem adopts the same tone as do those by Vondel and Six on the same occasion as the one I discussed in the preceding chapter. But Vos's visual language is more radical – or, if you like, more explosive. Vos adorns Bicker with his own kind of ornamentation: explosive cosmetics.

The trade in saltpetre and sulphur

Let us turn now to gunpowder as a material. Was gunpowder one of the commodities of the seventeenth-century druggists? The etymology of the Dutch word 'buskruit'

9 *Cf.* Snoep, 1975; Eberhard Fähler, *Feuerwerke des Barock. Studien zum öffentlichen Fest und seiner literarischen Deutung vom 16. bis 18.* Jahrhundert, 1974, pp. 77–133.

10 'Vertooningen op toneelen, zeegeboogen, blyde inkomsten en staacywagens', Vos, 1662, I, p. 577.

11 Vos, 1662, I, p. 596. For more details about the ceremony, see Snoep, 1975, p. 82.

gives us a hint that it was. It is a composite word; the first part derives from 'buks', which is related to the English 'box'; the second, from 'kruid' ('spice' or 'herb').[12] Other names for explosives in Six's *oeuvre* confirm the pharmaceutical link to the substance: 'musketkruid' ('spice of the musket') ('Dank, aan Manuel Spranger. Voor kaaviaar') (J135, l. 22) and 'geswaavelt kruid' ('sulphured spice') ('Tempel, aan den kooningh van Spanje') (J246, l. 61). In the seventeenth century, the boundary between 'buskruit'/'kruit' and 'kruid' was less clear than it is today.

In addition, gunpowder was discussed in early modern pharmacopoeias, together with the ingredients from which it was made: the mineral *simplicia* charcoal, saltpetre, and sulphur. These were substances to which several useful properties were attributed, usually of a medicinal nature. Van Beverwijck writes, for example, about these last two: the 'smelly odour' of sulphur is among other things, 'helpful for those with cold Brains, and who are much tormented with Sinking [fluids]', while saltpetre is 'suitable for all kinds of fevers, internal Inflammations, Pleurisy, Squinancy, all kinds of Blockages.'[13] And gunpowder itself was also used for therapeutic purposes: Van Beverwijck tells us that many soldiers mixed it with vinegar and used it as an antidote to the plague.[14] Thus, in the seventeenth century, explosive substances were actually used as medicines for internal use.

Saltpetre and sulphur were probably for sale in Six's shop, and gunpowder may have been too. In any case, Six had connections that had apparently focused on the trade in gunpowder, including Caspar van Ceulen, whom we remember from my discussion in the last chapter of 'Bruiloftnacht van Kaspar van Keulen, en Katarina Opmeer' (J131). The groom was part of the international trading company 'Jeremia e Gasparo van Collen', one of whose specialties was its trade in gunpowder. In a poem published in 1660 in *Amsterdamsche Vreugdtriomfe*, 'Prinsselijk inhaal, t'Amsterdam [...]' ('Princely Welcome in Amsterdam [...]') (J612), Six goes into remarkably specific detail in telling us about the fireworks at the ceremony in question: 'dat Meulekruid van Krook' (l. 53), he writes, referring to gunpowder from the factory of Abraham P. Croock, a producer of and dealer in gunpowder. According to the Ledger of the Wisselbank, Six received money transfers from Croock. It is probable, then, that he sold him saltpetre and sulphur.[15] Six would have got the main constituent of gunpowder, saltpetre (75 percent of the mixture), from

12 See 'buskruit' in the WNT.

13 'De stinckende reuck [...] behulpsaem voor de gene, die kout van Herssenen zijn, ende veel met Sinckinghen ghequelt werden'; 'bequamelijck ghebruyckt in alderhande Koortschen, inwendighe Ontstekinghen, Pleuris, Squynancy, in alderley Vertstoppinghen', *Schat der ongesontheyt*, 1656, pp. 44, 45 and 57.

14 *Heel-konste, ofte derde deel van de Genees-konste*, 1656, p. 148.

15 Jacobs, 1991 II, pp. 455, 825, Elias, *Vroedschap*, 1903–1905, 1, pp. 464, 644. See the Ledger of the Wisselbank, Amsterdam City Archives. The money transfer between Six and Croock took place June 1672, but it could be that Six did business with Croock earlier, too. Six's account for the years 1655–1666 are missing in the Amsterdam City Archives.

Bengal. As I mentioned above, the brother of the druggist-poet, Joost or Justus Six, was stationed there as an assistant with the VOC. When Six mentions in a poem the kind of drugs he deals in, he talks about 'Spices of Ganges' ('Aan Raimond de Smeth') (J70, l. 10). At the beginning of the seventeenth century, saltpetre was one of the most important commodities on VOC ships.[16] If saltpetre and sulphur, or even gunpowder, were for sale in 'De Vergulde Eenhoorn', then, for an individual such as Six, with his self-critical spirit, these sought-after but dangerous exotics would have been a problematic aspect of his profession.

Staged self-injuries

Poësy expresses not only praise for the power of gunpowder, but also contempt. This is evident from the poems I will discuss in this chapter. 'Bussekruid vervloekt. Aan myn moeder' and 'Op het barsten van myn pistool, teegens buskruid' describe events that seem actually to have taken place in Six's life. They recount two accidents with loaded pistols that befell Six on his commercial trips. As we can see from its title, 'Buskruids donder, en blixem, te Delft' is about the famous explosion of the gunpowder depot in Delft on 12 October 1654.

Given the content of 'Bussekruid vervloekt. Aan myn moeder' (J383), the first accident likely occurred when Six was on a business trip in Spain, probably around the turn of the year 1649–1650. The report tells us that, before Six entered the city of Granada, he shot his gun – apparently on the orders of the city guard – because one could enter the city only if one was unarmed.[17] The shot backfired and nearly hit him in the head. The realistic tone of the description is striking, not only in terms of the representation of this event itself, but also in terms of the everyday details that Six gives. In this way he describes the tinnitus in his ear that the accident has caused him (l. 17–18): 'Al is 't een week geleên, syne ooren blyven suisen. / Al wat hy hoort, gelykt een waaterval van sluisen' ('Even though it was a week ago, his ears keep ringing. All that he hears resembles a torrent of locks being opened'). But this realism does not mean that Six did not have a greater purpose in writing this poem. At the end of the text, our attention is shifted from the external circumstances of the accident to its cause, the gunpowder. Six curses the inventor of the substance (l. 31–36):

16 For Joost Six, see Jacobs, 1991 II, p. 280, and the sources he lists there. The place where Joost Six was stationed, Pipely ('Voorwind, naa nieuw Batavie, aan 't Schip de Paarle [...]') ('Tailwind, to the New Batavia, for the Ship De Paarle [...]') (J374, l. 76), was a major port of export for saltpetre: vocsite.nl/geschiedenis/handelsposten/bengalen.html (consulted 18 May 2019). For the Dutch trade in saltpetre, see Rutten, 2008, p. 56; Israel, 1989, p. 256.

17 Jacobs, 1991 II, p. 674.

Verdoemlik loot, en bussekruid,
Gemaakt om menschen te vernielen,
Wat schryft ghy al millioenen zielen,
Op reekningh van dien kloosterguit?
Een doodslagh zal men op des menschen ziel verhaalen,
Hoe kan die Munniks ziel zoo grooten schuld betaalen?

Accursed lead and gunpowder,
Made to destroy people,
How many millions of souls do you record
On the account of that villain of the monastery?
That man's soul will be charged with manslaughter,
How can the Monk's soul pay such a debt?

The 'villain of the monastery' is a reference to a monk from Freiburg, Germany, who was involved in alchemy and who, according to legend, had invented gunpowder.[18] The text seems too well thought through to be a poem about some random event. Did the accident with the gun give Six a good opportunity to show his aversion to this dangerous drug? Typical of our travelling Calvinist is his mention of the inventor's Catholic origin. With these considerations in mind, we will move on to the next text.

In 'Op het barsten van myn pistool, teegens buskruid' (J338), the accident takes place aboard a ship. According to A.E. Jacobs, it happened during Six's first commercial trip to England, which took place in 1654 and 1655.[19] The incident repeats itself: the gun unexpectedly goes off in Six's hands, and the bullet shoots backwards, barely missing his head. The text is almost a hundred lines long, but the description of the incident comprises just ten lines. Our suspicion is confirmed: it is not just about the depiction of an accidental event: Six uses the event to convey a deeper message. Most of the poem is a summary of the history and effects of gunpowder, from ideas about lightning dating from classical times – gunpowder was, as is also clear from my discussion of Jan Vos's poems, known as the earthly equivalent of lightning – to the invention and use of gunpowder in Six's own time. Six relies also on contemporary theories on lightning. According to early modern science, there were substantial, and not merely surface, similarities between these two phenomena; it was thought that saltpetre was involved in thunderstorms.[20] The fact that the ingredients sulphur and saltpetre

18 James Riddick Partington, *A History of Greek Fire and Gunpowder*, 1960, pp. 91–93; Jacobs, 1991 II, p. 675. See also the quote from 'Op het barsten van myn pistool, teegens buskruid' below.

19 Jacobs, 1991 II, p. 599.

20 See Van Beverwijck's explanation of lightning and gunpowder, *Heel-konste, ofte derde deel van de Genees-konste*, 1656, p. 147. And see Sven Dupré, Dedo von Kerssenbrock-Krosigk & Beat Wismer (eds.), *Art and Alchemy. The Mystery of Transformation*, 2014, p. 107.

(l. 37–38), and another substance, nardus (l. 65), are named, shows once again that a craftsman is speaking here. The devastating effects of the explosive are the *leitmotif* in this encyclopaedic account. According to the opening of the text, gunpowder embodies a rebellious, blasphemous fire – a view that is supported by a story from antiquity, the myth of the Greek king Salmoneus, who wanted to imitate thunder but was severely punished by Jupiter for doing so (l. 13–30).[21] Six emphasises that only certain artists, whom he calls 'geniuses', have been allowed to copy divine things. One of these, he tells us, is the Greek painter Apelles, who painted lightning so well that no one dared to look at the painting without wearing a laurel wreath (according to Pliny, laurel wreaths protected the wearer against thunder and lightning) (l. 7–12):[22]

Die Fenix, aller schildren wonder,
Houdt d'eer, hy 't rollen van den donder,
  Als die, uit dikke wolken, straalt
  Met barstingh, zoo heeft afgemaalt,
Dat niemand, sonder lauwerieren,
Het oogh dorst wenden, naa die vieren.

That Phoenix [Apelles], the wonder of painting,
Is famous for having painted
The rolling of the thunder,
When it, from thick clouds, radiates with bursts,
So that no one, without laurels,
Dares to turn the eye to that fire.

Six lets us then know how gunpowder is made. At first, people experimented with sulphur and saltpetre in order to discover new medicines. But they soon realised the true character of the new invention. Six insists that those who praise the creator of gunpowder are mistaken: Whoever the inventor, the monk of Freiburg, really was – a 'black Dane' (a word play on the name Berthold Schwarz) or a chemist, Konstantin Anklitzen – he is nothing but a 'son of Pluto' (l. 33–36). Six then tells us that gunpowder came into the hands of the Pope and that Catholics, by strengthening the power of the explosive, turned it into a dangerous weapon. His view is that, while science has never produced anything perfect before, the question arises as to whether this has now been done. For such an unparalleled weapon as gunpowder has never been invented before (l. 45–65): now even the Pope can make 'de werld doen springen / Met alle werreldlyke dingen, / Voor d'aankomst van den jonghsten

21 See Jacobs, 1991 II, p. 600, as well as *Salmoneus* (1657), a tragedy by Joost van den Vondel.
22 See Jacobs, 1991 II, pp. 599–600.

dag' ('make the world explode, with all earthly things, even before the coming of Judgment Day') (l. 83–85). This encyclopaedic review is followed by a brief account of the accident involving Six's own pocket gun (l. 88–98).

Six's theoretical discussion of gunpowder seems to be based on an axiom by the Persian doctor-philosopher Avicenna (Ibn Sina, 980–1037, a name that is mentioned several times in *Poësy*): 'art is weaker than nature'. In his works, Avicenna looks at the connections between technology, alchemy, art and nature, and concludes that people are unable to copy things created by God. His argument is related to the notion of human weakness – that people's creative capacity cannot match God's.[23] We recognise this point from the preceding chapter. The debate over the opposition between natural and artificial was central to the series of sonnets 'Op het blanketten van 't vrouwvolk in Spanje', and was accompanied by a warning against the Prometheus' hubris. It now seems that the 'boundary lines' were crossed. Technological developments have come so far that people's creative powers surpass God's. The reader will not have missed the message of the argument: both the apocalyptic consequences, outlined above, of the use of gunpowder and the story of Six's own accident make it emphatically clear that this is a substance that Six does not wish to be associated with.

The detailed narrative of the origin and use of gunpowder should be re-examined in the light of the poet's profession. This is also evident from the specialised information in the text. What does the travelling trader in drugs hope to achieve with the publication of this text? By making a distinction between morally defensible and objectionable products in a drugstore, Six wants to show that he is an honest merchant, trading exclusively in products that promote the prosperity and health of his country. Activities associated with gunpowder – 'Ketteryen' ('heresy') (l. 67) as the poet calls them – are described as Papist practices: a monk invented the explosive, and Catholics developed it further.[24]

The Delft thunderclap

In 'Buskruids donder, en blixem, te Delft' (J396), Six once again curses gunpowder. The poem is about a notorious accident in Delft, the explosion of the gunpowder depot there on 12 October 1654 (Fig. 6.2). Once again we are dealing with a text that, on its first reading, gives the impression of being a spontaneous, immediate reaction to an event, but which, on closer inspection, turns out to be a carefully

23 Lawrence M. Principe, *The Secrets of Alchemy*, 2013, pp. 47–49; William R. Newman, *Promethean Ambitions: Alchemy and the Quest to Perfect Nature*, 2004.

24 The fact that Dutch merchants not only sold wood and grain, but also weapons and ammunition to Spain, makes the ethical implications of these poems even stronger (Mooij, 1999, p. 21). Was Six himself involved in this trade?

thought-through composition. Like the last poem, this text is full of allusions to mythology and classical antiquity. Already in the opening lines, Six links gunpowder to paganism, pointing to the similarity between the city name Delft and the name of the most famous oracle of all antiquity: that of Delphi.[25] Six argues that the explosion does not have a rational cause, but is rather the result of the struggle between God and the devil (l. 1–14):

Het Delfsch Orakel, dat vlak stom
Geworden was, voor sestienhondert jaaren,
Toen onder 't blinde heidendom
Een suivre maaght Gods Woord begon te baaren,
Die loogenmond, met zulken prop,
Van eeuwen, als met yser, toegeklonken,
Borst, binnen Delft, hooghmoedigh op,
Uit eene delf, met assche, puin, en vonken.
Die duivel blies een sprenkel vuur,
In 't waapenhuis, van Staatenkruid, beleegen,
Socht, door den onderaardschen muur,
Een bresche, en tocht, langhs doemelyke weegen.
Dat vlamsiek kruid, vol domme kracht,
In vlam, brak uit, en rukte 't al in stukken.

The Oracle at Delphi, who fell
Quite speechless sixteen hundred years ago,
When, in the time of blind paganism,
A pure virgin gave birth to the Word of God;
That lying mouth that was blocked
With a solid plug, as with iron, so it would stay that way for centuries.
It burst arrogantly forth in Delft,
Out of a pit with ash, debris and sparks.
The devil blew a spark of fire
Into the arsenal, filled with gunpowder from the States [the Netherlands],
[Which] sought, through the subterranean wall,
An opening and a passage along accursed pathways.
That inflammable drug, full of foolish power,
Broke out in flames and tore everything to pieces.

25 See the same play on words in Jan van Hout: Johan Koppenol, *Leids heelal: Het Loterijspel (1596) van Jan van Hout*, 1998, p. 201.

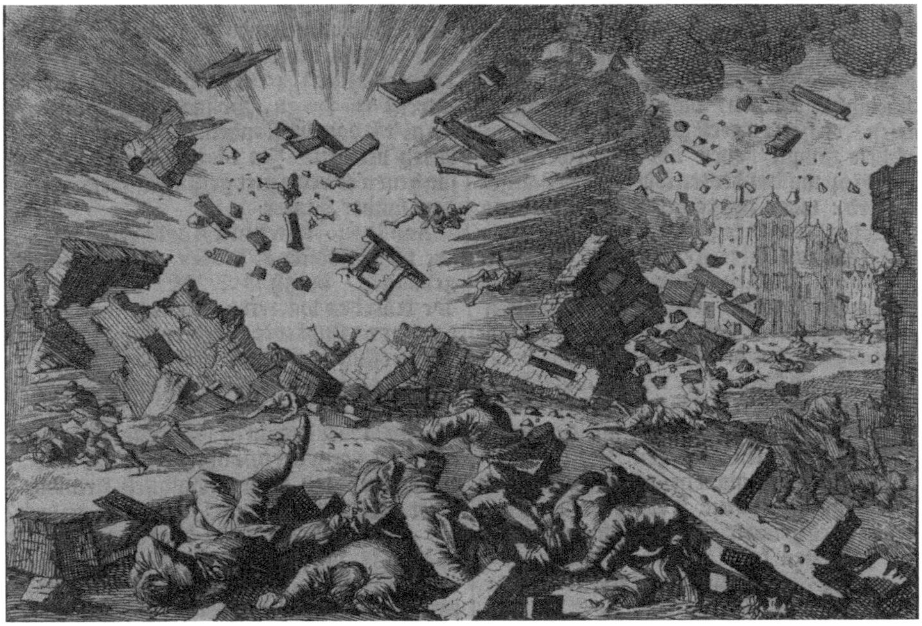

Fig. 6.2: Caspar Luyken, *The Delft Thunderclap*, 1698. Etching. (© Rijksmuseum, Amsterdam).

The Oracle of Delphi fell silent when Jesus was born, Six tells us, thus drawing a contrast between the false, pagan virgin Sibyl and the Christian Virgin Mary.[26] But Delphi's priestess, who tells only lies, has actually not gone completely quiet. Although the crevice was closed with a 'prop', the gases underneath continued to gather lies for centuries. And finally, thanks to the devil, these ever-increasing inflammable forces came into contact with the gunpowder depot in the city of the same name, where the fumes have ignited the gunpowder. Six believes the explosion resulted from a resurgence of superstition. Behind 'loogenmond' – which means both 'fire mouth' and 'lying mouth' (*loog* is an old Dutch word for 'flame')[27] – is the image of a priestess who was intoxicated by fumes emanating from a crevice as she proclaimed her oracles (Fig. 6.3). Thus, Six ascribed the prophetic statements of the priestess, not to divine inspiration, but to the inhalation of infernal vapours – pyro-intoxication, as it were, caused by mineral gases.[28] The gases that have risen from the earth are thus a materialisation of paganism. The following lines (15–48)

26 For early modern discussions on the Delphic Oracle, see Anthony Ossa-Richardson, *The Devil's Tabernacle: the Pagan Oracles in Early Modern Thought*, 2013; Paul Faure, *Magie der Düfte: eine Kulturgeschichte der Wohlgerüche – Von den Pharaonen zu den Römern*, 1993, pp. 163–165.
27 *Cf.* 'loog'[2] in the WNT.
28 Rodenburgh sees the priestess of Delphi as an example of *vates*. See Chapter 3, note 31. The passage can thus be read as a critique of the concept of the divine poet. In Chapter 8, I will have more to say on

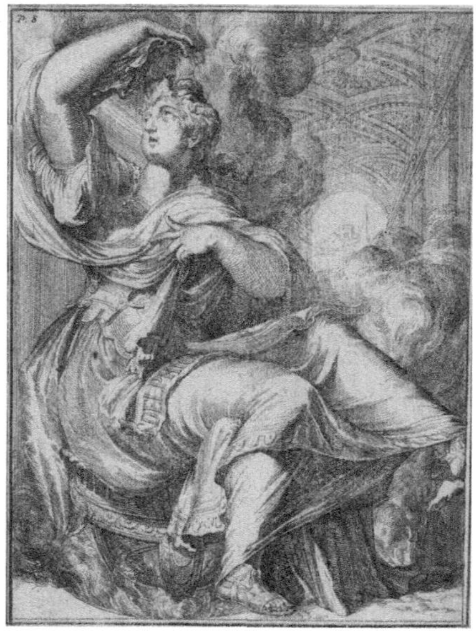

Fig. 6.3: Romeyn de Hooghe (attributed to), after Romeyn de Hooghe, *Sibyl of Delphi*, 1688. Engraving. (© Rijksmuseum, Amsterdam).

are full of references to apocalyptic prophecies and themes, and describe how the residents of Delft experienced the explosion: as the end of the world.

This time, too, the poet does not remain in the background as an anonymous narrator, but places himself, as we have grown to expect from him by now, in the middle of the story. At the time of the explosion, he tells us, he was on a business trip to England, and he was already strolling through the peaceful streets of London and over its bridges, having discussions with a colleague. There, however, the river was still coloured red by the blood of Charles I, who had been executed, an event that took place almost five years before the explosion – and which appears to have held great symbolic significance for Six.[29] In this situation, the two men hear the great explosion (l. 57–64):

poetic inspiration as intoxication. *Cf.* also 'Aan den brandenden Vesuvius' ('To the Burning Vesuvius') (J83), where Six links fire that comes up from inside the Earth to the devil.

29 The image of the Thames filled with blood is remarkably common in Six's poetry. *Cf.* 'Uitvaard van Marten Harpertse Tromp, ridder, L. admiraal van Holland, en Zeeland &c ('Funeral of [...]') (J352), l. 24). In 'De gekneusde hoogmoed des heerschaps van de Zee' ('The Bruised Pride of the Dominion of the Sea') (J618), which Six wrote in June 1666 (17 years after Charles I's beheading), on the occasion of the Four Days' Battle near North Foreland, he still refers to the Thames as 'den bloedstroom' ('the blood stream') (l. 58). For the biblical story of the blood-red river, see Exodus 7:14–25, and Rev. 16:4.

Terwyl wy streeden, mond, met mond,
Of 't waater, dat daar onder door loopt bruisen,
Naa zee toe, rood geleek, of blond,
Zoo voelden wy 't gedruis, in d'ooren, suisen.
Elk vraaghde ontset, van welke kant
Komt deese schoot des donders aangetoogen?
't Is helder weer, op 't naaste land,
Aan Zee, is wis een kruidslot opgevloogen.

While we were arguing, face to face,
As the water of the Thames that rushed beneath us,
Towards the sea, seemed red, or white,
We felt the bang whizzing in our ears.
Each [of us] appalled: from which direction
Has this thundercrack come?
The weather in the neighbouring country is clear, on the other side
of the Channel; a gunpowder depot has gone up in smoke for sure.

Shortly afterwards, a messenger comes to relay the news to Six and his companion: the gunpowder depot in Delft has exploded, and the city has been destroyed as though a war had raged. But there was a bit of luck, he continues: the rather fragile tomb of the House of Orange in the Nieuwe Kerk has miraculously escaped damage. On this basis Six concludes the poem with a statement that leaves no doubt about his political leanings (l. 105–108): 'Eer zal de druk verlooren gaan,/Dan dat de Faam vergeeten zou te melden/Der Princen gaadeloose daân,/Waard voor gestelt in 't boek van Batoos helden' ('The printed word will fade before Fame forgets to herald the matchless deeds of the Princes, which are worth recording in the book of the Batavian heroes').

Whereas Six linked the diabolical character of gunpowder in the previous two poems to the inventor's Catholic hubris, he now associates the explosion of the gunpowder warehouse in Delft with the rebellious English. The *topos* of a blood-red river, taken from the story of Egypt's plagues (Exodus 7:14–25), refers to punishments that are imposed on a people who oppose God's will. The entire poem is permeated with sin and guilt. God's punishment for England anticipates His reprisals against the Netherlands. Six's intention becomes clear if we consider when the poem was produced: during the First Stadtholderless Period (1650–1672). Six sees the fact that the tomb of William of Orange, a 'Protestant saint', remained untouched, as a sign from God. Given that the country was then without a prince from the House of Orange, which advocated a much more Calvinistic policy than the so-called States Party, the republican faction in power in the First Stadtholderless Period, it is no coincidence that it is precisely in the Dutch Republic that pagan lies have exploded. Six thus interprets the explosion as God's punishment for the Netherlands. In contrast to the first two poems, in which only the microcosm of the merchant – his own body – is discussed, this text has a larger theme: a collective punishment for the 'body' of Delft.

Although it is not the main subject, the reader is given indications as to why Delft has called God's wrath upon it. The play on the words 'Delft' and 'Delphi', from the beginning of the aforementioned passage, is given a third layer of meaning in line 8. I believe that the reference to 'Delf' here is twofold. First, it refers to the underground depot, the 'delf', in which the Delft gunpowder was stored. And second, it means a group of early modern drugs, the 'minerals' (in Dutch, 'delfstoffen') saltpetre and sulphur.[30] Six thus makes a connection between the devilish character of these drugs and the underground. Pluto, who in the previous poem still figured as the supreme being of the underworld, is also the god of riches, because mineral wealth was found underground. It should not be forgotten that gunpowder, which had a lot of functions, was also used for fireworks – that is, for ornamental purposes. It is likely, then, that Six denounces the role that the gunpowder depot played as a repository of earthly riches. When the poet, in 'Buskruids donder, en blixem, te Delft', mentions another city that has been destroyed by a large stockpile of gunpowder, he talks of the 'kruidslot' (l. 64) of that city. 'Slot' translates as 'closed place', in the sense, here, of 'depot', but another meaning is 'castle', which as we know is a symbol of earthly luxury.[31] These observations point to a connection between Six's vision of the explosion in Delft and the criticism of opulence and abundance in the Netherlands as a trading power. Delft has exceeded the amount of wealth permitted – and is therefore punished by God.[32]

As we have seen, it is striking how Six reinserts himself into the middle of the story. In addition to the foregoing argument, I will also discuss the subject of transgression with regard to Six's own body, the microcosm. We read that he and

30 'Delf' was also the old name of Delft, used by Vondel among others. See 'Op het Onweder van 's Lants Bussekruit te Delft', in: J.F.M. Sterck *et al.* (eds.), *De werken van Vondel. 1645-1656*, vol. 5, 1931, pp. 821–823, where Vondel also plays with the double meaning of 'Delf'. According to Schenkeveld-van der Dussen (2007, pp. 164–165), Six's text forms a contrast to Vondel's poem on the explosion.

31 *Cf.* the Calvinistic criticism of tall buildings, which is more explicitly expressed in other texts. See, for instance, 'Toorenbouw, aan de graavers' ('Tower Construction, to the Diggers') (J122). And see the subterranean as an expression of *avaritia,* such as in 'Gierigheits woninge en gestaltenisse' (J99). *Cf.* Pliny, XXXIII, 1: Metals are 'diligently sought for in the bowels of the earth in a variety of ways. For in some places the earth is dug into for riches, when life demands gold, silver, silvergold (amber) and copper, and in other places for silver luxury, when gems and colours for tinting walls and beams are demanded [...]': 'Tellurem intus exquirente cura multiplici modo, quippe alibi divitiis foditur quaerent vita aurum, argentum, electrum, aes, alibi deliciis gemmas and parietum lignorumque pigmenta'. In Pliny, *Natural History*, IX, trans. by H. Rackham, 1952, p. 3).

32 Many of the arguments used by Six in this poem can be found in the sermon *Delfschen donder-slagh ofte Korte aensprake aen de bedroefde gemeente van Delf* (*The Thunderclap of Delft, or a Short Speech to the Miserable Community of Delft*) (1654) by pastor Peter de Witte.

his travelling companion feel 'bang whizzing in our ears' (l. 60) because of the explosion in Delft. We recall 'Bussekruid vervloekt. Aan myn moeder', in which Six reported the tinnitus that he had from the accident with his pistol (l. 17–18): in keeping with my interpretations of poems such as 'Dankoffer, aan gesondheit' and 'Uitroep om hoornafsetters', I wonder whether this observation should not also be read as a scene in which the poet stages an exposure of dangerous substances. Lectures given by the Reformed theologian Gisbertus Voetius to his students reveal a deep ambivalence to hearing as well as sight; he believed that all sensory stimuli can lead people away from God.[33] Wittewrongel's discussions on the dangerous influence of outer beauty also include sound impressions. In a discussion about whether musical instruments should be allowed during urban parades, he refers to the 'ornamentation and entertainment of the external senses, in particular the eyes and ears'.[34] The theologian might just as well have added the experience of fireworks. The banging and thunder of fireworks will have enchanted the early modern spectator no less than their brilliance and lustre.

It is therefore once again a question of controlling the physical limits of dangerous foreign drugs. Six confesses in the poems we have looked at above that he has lost this control when it comes to gunpowder. He is, so to speak, doing penance by staging a punishment of his own body. 'Bussekruid vervloekt. Aan myn moeder', 'Op het barsten van myn pistool, teegens buskruid', and 'Buskruids donder, en blixem, te Delft' can therefore be understood as expressions of Protestant self-flagellation. And wittily enough, this does not take the form of the atrocities of modern warfare, but – in accordance with Six's 'realistic' poetics – of an everyday event, namely tinnitus.

Literary rockets

Six's attention to explosives is also reflected in other texts in his *oeuvre*. In an anthology that appeared after *Poësy*, *Amsterdamsche Vreugdtriomfe* (*Joyful Triumph in Amsterdam*) (1660), there are poems by Six that once again draw a parallel between poetic words and the power of gunpowder. Following on from the foregoing analysis, I will now turn my attention to this group of texts. In them, a view of gunpowder emerges that does not correspond to the self-critical attitude in the three poems we have discussed.

Amsterdamsche Vreugdtriomfe appeared on the occasion of a visit to Amsterdam by Amalia of Solms, Frederick Henry's widow, with her four daughters and two of her sons-in-law. These were thus central figures from the House of Orange, who

33 Els Stronks, *Negotiating Differences: Word, Image and Religion in the Dutch Republic*, 2011, pp. 132 and 133.

34 'Cieraat ende vermaeck van de uyterlicke sinnen, insonderheyt de oogen, ende de ooren', Wittewrongel, 1661 II, p. 1146.

were no longer in a dominant position but who were invited to Amsterdam by the burgomasters in 1659 as a conciliatory gesture. The occasion for the visit was the marriage, which took place in the same year, between Henriette Catharina of Nassau, a princess of Orange, and John George II of Anhalt-Dessau. The organisation of their Joyous Entry was in the hands of the aforementioned poet and playwright, Jan Vos. The noble procession was welcomed by triumphal chariots with allegorical, geographical and royal *tableaux vivants* on them – from Unity, Gratitude, Amsterdam, the Seven Provinces, the ancestors of William III, and so on. These were then also shown in the theatre. In the evening there was a feast at the Town Hall, and a spectacular fireworks show on the water in front of the Kloveniersdoelen.[35] In addition to poems of praise by Jan Vos himself and other literary stars of the Golden Age, such as Vondel and Huygens, five poems by Six van Chandelier were included in *Amsterdamsche Vreugdtriomfe*.[36] I will comment on two of them, namely 'Prinsselijk inhaal, t'Amsterdam, van mevrouwe, Ameelia, Oudprincesse van Oranje &c. En doorluchtigheeden van dat huis, van Anhalt, en Nassouw' ('Princely Welcome in Amsterdam of Mrs Amelia, Former Princess of Orange etc., and Illustrious Persons of That House, of Anhalt, and Nassau') (J612) and 'Vierpylen, opgeschooten onder het prinsselyk aavondmaal' ('Rockets Set off during the Princely Supper') (J613). As can be seen from the title of the latter text, the poets present were so overwhelmed by the festive fireworks that they dedicated separate poems to them. Along with Six's poems, the books include Joost van den Vondel's 'Op het Triomferende vierwerck' ('On the Triumphant Fireworks'), in which Vondel praises 'hoe in 't velt / Der lucht *Oranje* wiert gespelt / Uit letteren van vier en vlammen' ('how *Orange* was spelled in the heavens with letters of fire and flame') (l. 9–11). The fireworks that were set off in the evening, which are beautifully reflected in the water, have a stunning effect on the spectators: 'Men zagh, in 't schijnen van de maen, / Het vierwerck, als een wonder, aen' (l. 13–14) ('The fireworks were seen, in the shining of the moon, as a miracle').[37] In Six's 'Vierpylen', at the centre of which is the feast at the Town Hall, the amazement at the wonderful power of the fireworks is at least as great. The poem takes the form of a dialogue between Jupiter and Venus. The chief deity notices a fire that does not come from his heavenly quarters. It is not a natural but an artificial phenomenon. Jupiter is deeply impressed. He realises that the sparks and blasts even surpass the divine fire of Prometheus. So this time we do not see an angry Jupiter who punishes *hubris* among people by sending nemesis as he did in the myth of the Greek king Salmoneus, who appears in 'Op het barsten van myn

35 See Jan Vos, 'Beschrijving der Vertooningen op de Staacywaagens [...]' (Vos, 1662 I, pp. 613–625). And see Frijhoff & Spies, 2004, p. 448; Snoep 1975, pp. 83–86.

36 Jacobs, 1991 II, p. 823.

37 In J.F.M. Sterck *et al.* (eds.), *De werken van Vondel. 1656–1660*, vol. 8, 1935, pp. 720–721. The poem is printed on pp. 107–110 of *Amsterdamsche Vreugdtriomfe* (1660).

pistool, teegens buskruid'. On the contrary, in his admiration Jupiter invites the other gods to come and celebrate this phenomenon with a feast in heaven. At the end of the text, Six describes how the immortal heavenly inhabitants – enthusiastic as they are about the commitments that were made in Amsterdam, both between the burgomasters and the House of Orange and between the bride and groom – drink nectar from a 'diamante schaal' ('diamond bowl') (l. 62–63).[38]

What does Six mean when he equates the fireworks at the feast in honour of the bridal couple with the thunder and lightning of the gods? In telling us that the 'heavenly adornment' of the feast has divine support, the poet signals quite clearly that the couple themselves are of divine origin: Johan van Anhalt is 'een Brandeburger Mars'; Henriette of Nassau, 'een Pallas' (l. 29–30).[39] As a supporter of the House of Orange, he is thus according it divine legitimacy. We must not forget that all of this was taking place in the First Stadtholderless Period. As D.P. Snoep puts it, it was 'particularly curious that in the midst of an official anti-Orange and anti-monarchical trend in the city of Amsterdam and in the States of Holland, this demonstration in favour of the House of Orange could take place'.[40] Six's high-flown, dramatic poetry full of mythological allusions and 'pyrotechnic' metaphors must also be understood in this light. They not only serve as literary ornamentation; they have a political purpose, which is to propagate Orangism. Despite the non-Sixian tone of the poem, it cannot be ruled out that the druggist-poet felt a certain pride in the wonderful spectacle of the fireworks. Gunpowder still exuded something exotic and mysterious, even supernatural. The presence of this kind of miracle product in the Republic was thanks to those who traded in drugs.

As we noted above, in 'Vierpylen, opgeschooten onder het prinsselyk aavondmaal' we cannot find any evidence of the pronounced critical attitude towards gunpowder that we saw in the poems we looked at earlier. In Six's second poem in *Amsterdamsche Vreugdtriomfe*, 'Prinsselijk inhaal, t'Amsterdam [...]', we are given an explanation. This text contains interesting details on the new phase in the poet's life at that time. In the opening lines, he says that he leads an ascetic life on his estate in the Diemermeerpolder. He lives alone with his books (he probably means his psalms), drinks bottles of water imported from Spa, and enjoys the therapeutic,

38 The Town Hall as the divine temple and altar of the Republic, see Joost van den Vondel, 'Op den princelijcken genadepenning. Aen de doorluchtigste Mevrouwe Douagiere Amelia, Princes van Oranje en Nassau, &c'. In J.F.M. Sterck *et al.* (eds.), *De werken van Vondel. 1656–1660*, vol. 8, 1935, pp. 725–726.

39 This mythological symbolism is also present in the *tableaux vivants* and in the poems by the other contributors, but the Orange-friendly Six pays more attention in his verses to the House of Orange than do the other poets. For the careful treatment of Orange propaganda during these parades, see Snoep 1975, pp. 77–90. In the performances Jan Vos put on on the occasion of the Peace of Westminster in 1654, for example, there were no references to the House of Orange.

40 Snoep, 1975, p. 86.

sensory impressions of the season: the singing of birds and the smells and colours of nature.[41] Earlier, the poet described the implied opposite of this existence, the unhealthy, alienated life of the city, in 'Nooddruft is genoegh' and 'Dankoffer, aan gesondheit'. These autobiographical details are interesting for us; Six shows that his cure in Spa has had an effect on his spleen disease, and that he has adapted his lifestyle in line with the medical advice from 'Dankoffer, aan gesondheit'. He has even begun to lead the healthy, arcadian existence of which he spoke in 'Wilde tuilken, aan Raimond Smeth'.[42] Yet a longing for the city arises in him when he discovers the wonderful sounds of Amsterdam (l. 1–8):

Wat gebalder, wat gedonder
   Dreunt, en daavert, uit de stad,
   Stoort myn stilte, op 't vyvers pad,
Waar ik boek, en Spaa houde, onder
   Dryerhande sinplaisier,
In een lucht van lieve geuren,
Van een perk vol bloemekleuren,
   En der vooglen soet getier?

What roaring, what thundering
Rumbles and shakes in the city,
[And] disturbs my silence on the path along the edge of the pond,
Where I spend my time with a book and Spa water,
Enjoying the pleasures of three senses:
In an air of sweet scents,
Of a bed full of floral colours,
And the sweet singing of the birds?

The text dramatises how Six responds to an impulse. He learns what is going on: the visit to Amsterdam by a number of important figures from the House of Orange is being celebrated with a spectacle and fireworks, says a neighbour. This arouses both excitement and curiosity in the poet, who then runs to the city to be present for the spectacle. The following verses contain descriptions of the various explosive adornments at the ceremony: first the fireworks and then the gunfire. The spectacle fills Six with national pride. He allows that the impressions the artificial colours and sounds of the fireworks make are even more impressive than the smells and colours he enjoyed three months before, at the beginning of the summer (l. 45–57):

41 The festivities took place at the end of August 1659 (Jacobs, 1991 II, p. 823).

42 See Chapter 4, pp. 132–133.

O wat blonk hier eene lent,
Voor dry maanden al verdweenen,
Van den hoofde, tot de teenen,
Als een bloemgard ongeschent!
Al de veelerleije naamen
Van koleur, aan pluim, en zy,
Uit de linteweevery,
Mochten Flooraas ryk beschaamen.
Al dat Meulekruid van Krook,
Dat gebalder, dat gedonder,
Leek my soeter, en gesonder,
Dan onsichtbre bloemenrook,
En bly schaatrend voogelsingen.

Oh, what a spring shone here,
Gone, now, three months ago,
From head to toe,
As an unspoiled flower garden!
All of the many names
Of colours, in the form of feathers
And woven silk ribbons,
Would put the realm of Flora to shame.
All that gunpowder from Croock,
That roaring, that thundering
Seemed sweeter and healthier
Than the invisible smell of flowers
And the happily chattering birdsong.

The self-critical druggist, who earlier denied that gunpowder had any therapeutic effects, now avers and even praises those therapeutic effects. Six even experienced the fireworks at the royal party as 'sweeter and healthier' than his salutary stay in the countryside. Avicenna's warning against the hubris of art is evidently worth less in a time of crisis. The passage quoted is a testament to professional pride: 'Krook', or Abraham Pietersz. Croock, the supplier of the fireworks for the festivities, was, as we noted above, a colleague of Six's.

Six continues with this theatrical staging of his own enthusiasm: he emphasises to his readers that, even though he is not among the members of the city guard, and although he is known as a rhymester, he can write exalted poetry – poems that 'spew fire and flames' (l. 89–101), like the poem of Vondel:

Staa ik mee niet onder schutters,
  Die hunne offerhanden doen,
  Noch zo is mijn boesem koen
Dat te volgen, en wat nutters.
  Al uw donders rollen heen,
Met de snelbesweeke winden,
Wat myn rymboek in zal binden,
  Wed ik niet zo snel verdween.
Ik, gewoon op rym te dichten,
  Kan ook geeven vuur en vlam [...]

Even though I am not standing among the members of the city guard,
Who are delivering their offerings,
My breast is nevertheless eager
To follow them, and usefully.
All your thunder rolls away
With the whipping winds.
All my rhymes, which my book of poetry will bind,
Will not disappear that fast, I'll wager.
I, who am accustomed to writing in rhyme,
Can also spew fire and flames [...]

Six is keen to honour the members of the House of Orange with the 'buskruit' of his 'book of poetry'. He wants to give them an offering of fire, as it were, as if they were human gods from some ancient cult. And he wants 'kort, maar braaf verhaalen / Al het godlik seegepraalen' ('to tell briefly, but bravely, about all the divine triumphs') (l. 102–103) by Frederick Henry, the illustrious stadtholder from whom the royal guests in Amsterdam are descended. The rest of the text is a tribute to the power of this prince. Trade flourished under him, and there was peace with the other European powers. At the end of the text, Six tell us that Frederick Henry is therefore an example for future leaders of the Republic. Like Six's other poems in *Amsterdam's Vreugdtriomfe*, 'Prinsselijk inhaal, t'Amsterdam' has a clear goal: the poet encourages readers to remember bygone times of cultural and economic prosperity. The parallels with the preceding poem are clear. Six praises the Prince of Orange, telling us that, even though he is dead, he 'nu betreedt robyne velden, / Die 's nachts lichten, met geblik' ('He enters the fields of rubies, which light up, flickering, at night') (l. 39–40). This glorification is an *imitatio* of the so-called Roman imperial cult. Frederick Henry is depicted as a constellation of stars: thanks to his politics, the Republic has reached a Golden Age.[43] Once again, it is assumed that gunpowder possesses powers both magical and medicinal. The Prince of Orange appears in the form of a constellation, as a heavenly equivalent of the earthly fireworks during the festivities.

It is thus no coincidence that Six contributed to this anthology. Our druggist-poet felt chosen to do this. His skills in poetry and pyrotechnics make him a natural partner of Jan Vos at the Festival for the House of Orange. Six had a good reason in 1659 to remember Frederick Henry's glorious reign. His business had suffered during the First Anglo-Dutch War. The Republic's global dominance as a trading power had shown its first cracks: by 1654, it had already lost its possessions in Brazil. His texts show that Six was conflicted when it came to the struggle between those siding with the States and those on the side of the House of Orange. But although he felt a connection with the former as an Amsterdammer, he leaves no doubt as to whose side he is on when push comes to shove. It was his Calvinistic faith that carried the most weight.[44] Only a new Prince of Orange can unite the country in this time of crisis, is Six's implicit message.

Conclusion

The view of gunpowder we find in the *Amsterdamsche Vreugdtriomfe* is surprisingly positive. It is quite distinct from the representation of gunpowder in the other texts we have looked at in this chapter, as well as from the critical attitude towards drugs that we have seen in the other chapters so far. As I have argued, however, the non-Sixian language in the poems I have discussed should be interpreted against the political background of the time. As we have seen, in the opening lines of 'Prinsselijk inhaal', Six presents his new-found lifestyle as an arcadian existence. The rural life that he temporarily leaves in this poem – curious as he is about the spectacle in Amsterdam – implies that he has distanced himself from the glitter and glamour of urban life. He has renounced fiery and expensive drugs in favour of healthy Spa water that costs nothing. The fact that he is now returning to the splendour of his old merchandise should thus, as I see it, be seen as a merely temporary interruption of his arcadian lifestyle. It is the political situation that has forced this interruption on him. Excited, he decides to take part in the fireworks shows put on by Jan Vos.

43 Although the Republic, unlike many other European countries, did not have a court culture, in praising the House of Orange, Dutch Renaissance poets made use of courtly concepts and ideas: See Melissen 1981–1982, p. 42. For drugs as a means of deification, and for the Roman imperial cult, see Chapter 7.

44 *Cf.* 'Amsterdamsche rondheit' ('The Frankness of Amsterdam') (J382).

Gunpowder is proving to be a panacea – a miracle cure that is capable of conjuring up a new Golden Age across the Republic. The druggist-poet leaves us in no doubt that he still has his skills: 'I, who am accustomed to writing in rhyme, can also spew fire and flames'. Professional pride in his trade as a druggist wells up in him. The flourishing period under Frederick Henry would not have been possible without the achievements of Dutch merchants, especially those involved in the profitable gunpowder trade.

Once again, then, this chapter shows us Six as a pragmatic poet. But we also see his self-presentation as a sober, self-critical druggist, even as a self-flagellating merchant. Here, too, there are some external factors that we must take into account in Six's literary representation of gunpowder. As we have seen, it is no accident that the identification of explosives with the Pope took place during one of Six's commercial trips to areas that Dutch moralists considered to be dangerous to the well-being of their homeland: the Catholic South of Europe. The same applies to the thunderclap in Delft, which was linked to the rebellious British. But despite this relativising conception of drugs, the chapter follows up on the discussions from earlier chapters on the natural versus the artificial, and the concept of human weakness versus the pretensions to divine knowledge and creativity. These discussions are also reflected in the last two chapters of the main part of this book. First, I will look at the ceremonial language of Six's poems of praise for people of high standing – royals. Here, drugs are presented as a means to deification. I will also discuss Dutch imitations of the cult of the Roman Emperor in more detail. Chapter 8 then revolves around the influence of drugs on the poet's own body.

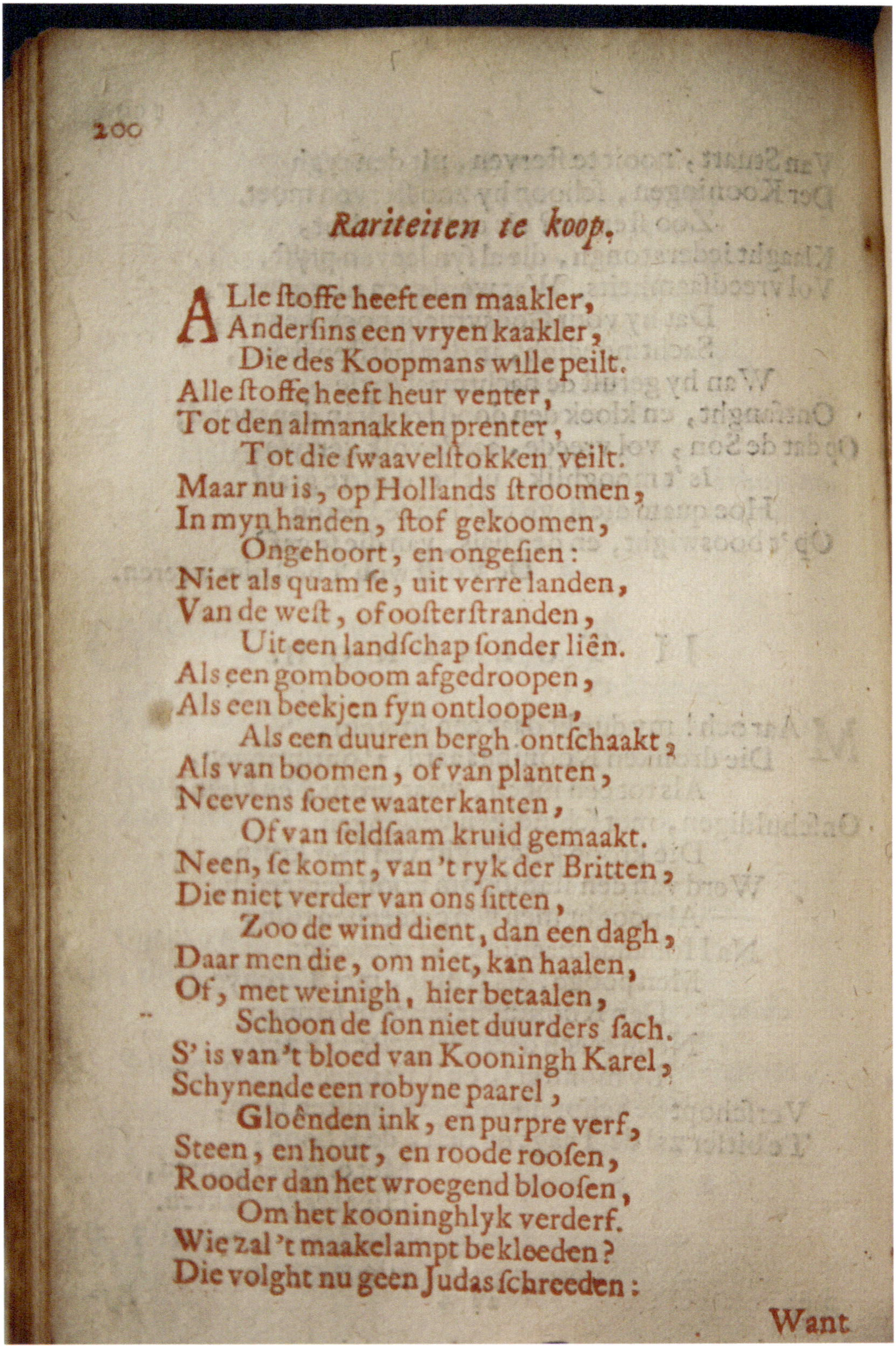
200

Rariteiten te koop.

ALle ſtoffe heeft een maakler,
Anderſins een vryen kaakler,
Die des Koopmans wille peilt.
Alle ſtoffe heeft heur venter,
Tot den almanakken prenter,
Tot die ſwaavelſtokken veilt.
Maar nu is, op Hollands ſtroomen,
In myn handen, ſtof gekoomen,
Ongehoort, en ongeſien:
Niet als quam ſe, uit verre landen,
Van de weſt, of ooſterſtranden,
Uit een landſchap ſonder liên.
Als een gomboom afgedroopen,
Als een beekjen fyn ontloopen,
Als een duuren bergh ontſchaakt,
Als van boomen, of van planten,
Neevens ſoete waaterkanten,
Of van ſeldſaam kruid gemaakt.
Neen, ſe komt, van 't ryk der Britten,
Die niet verder van ons ſitten,
Zoo de wind dient, dan een dagh,
Daar men die, om niet, kan haalen,
Of, met weinigh, hier betaalen,
Schoon de ſon niet duurders ſach.
S' is van 't bloed van Kooningh Karel,
Schynende een robyne paarel,
Gloênden ink, en purpre verf,
Steen, en hout, en roode rooſen,
Rooder dan het wroegend blooſen,
Om het kooninghlyk verderf.
Wie zal 't maakelampt bekleeden?
Die volght nu geen Judas ſchreeden:

Want

Plate 1: First page of 'Rariteiten te koop', Joannes Six van Chandelier, *Poësy*, 1657. (© Privately owned).

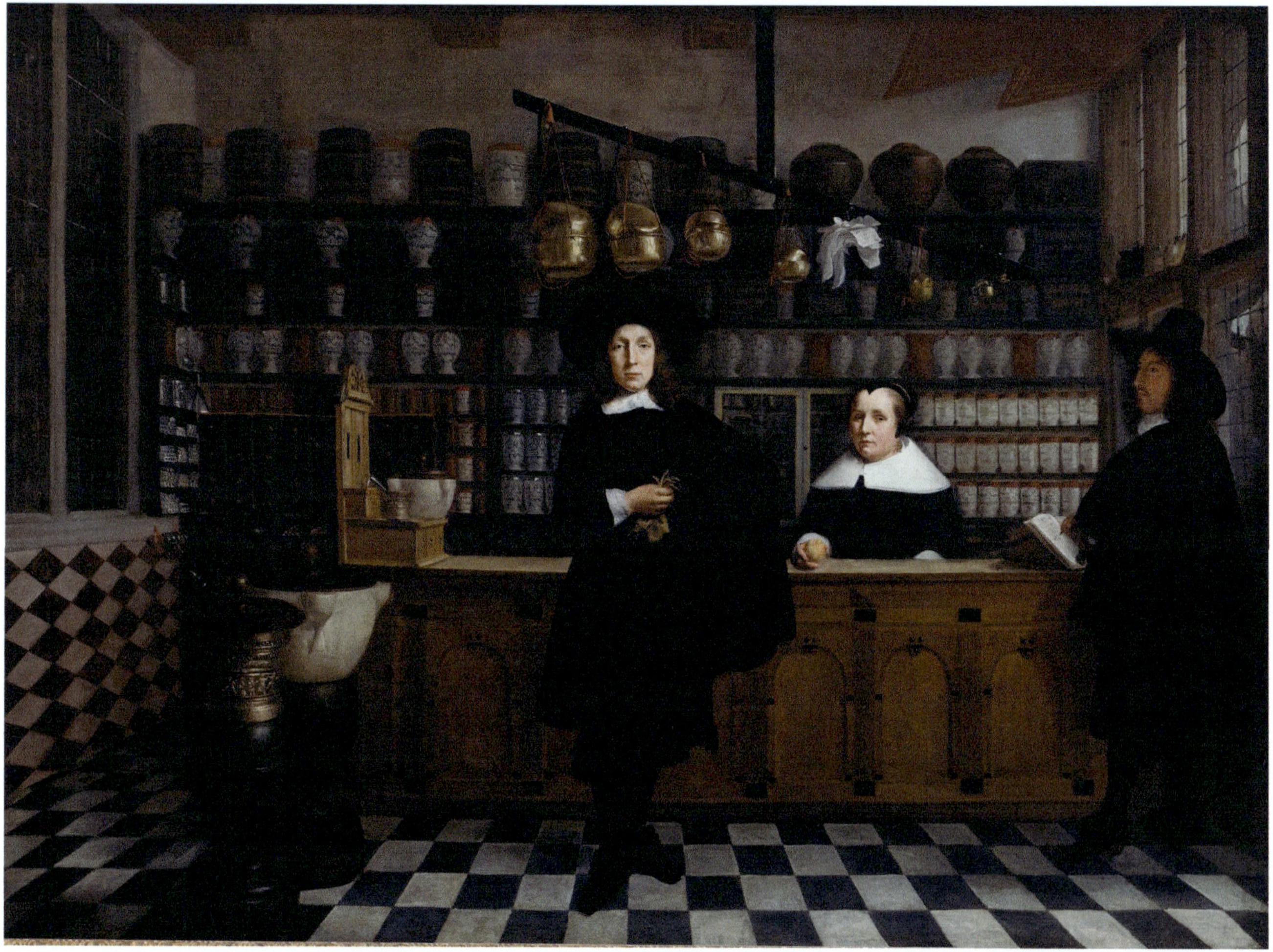

Plate 2: Unknown, *Dutch apothecary or drug store from the 17th century*. The druggist stands in the front, and to the right probably his mother, with an orange in her hand. The scene could have been Six's 'De vergulde eenhoorn'. 1686.
Oil on panel. (© Apotekarsocieteten, Stockholm).

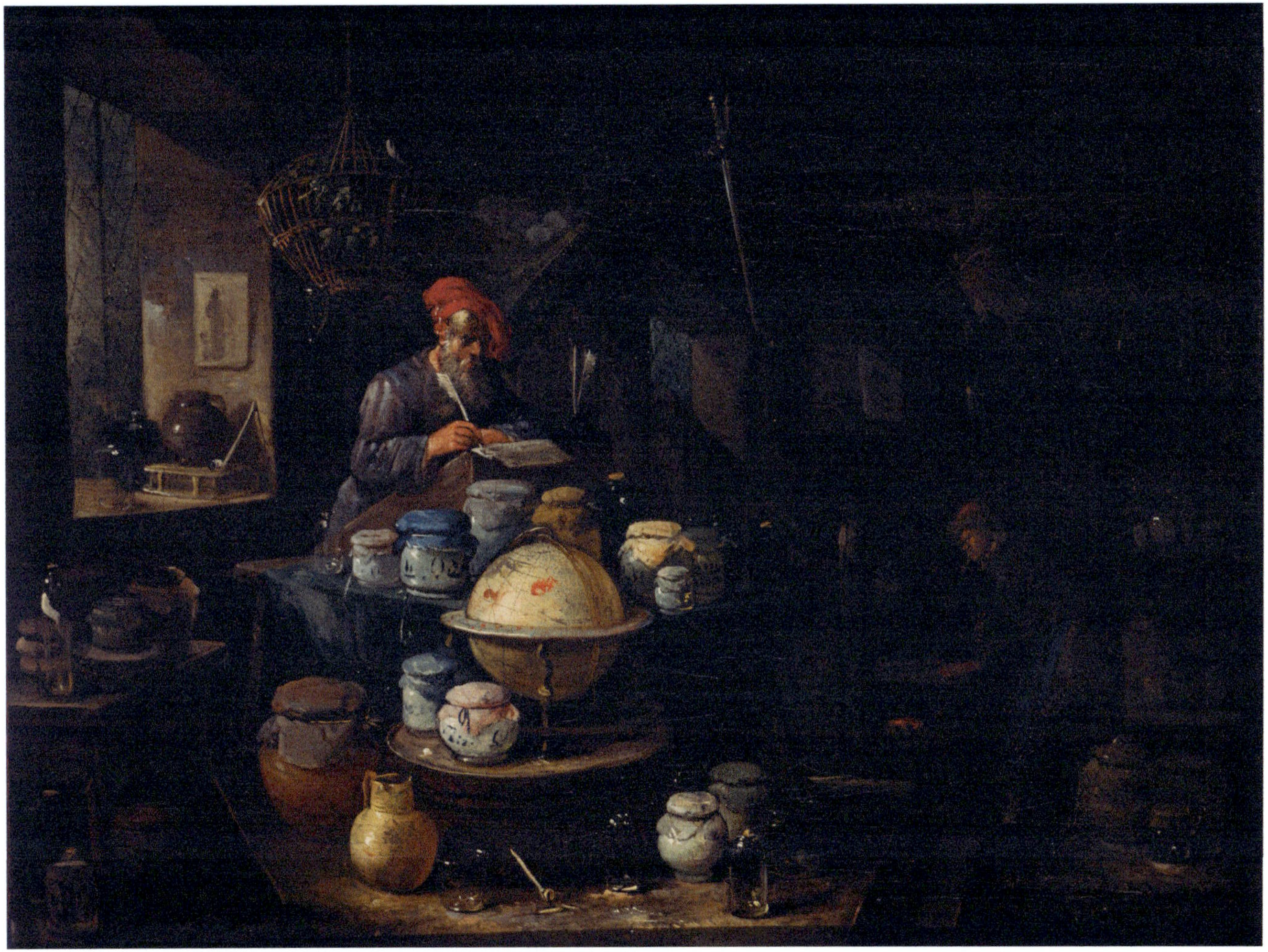

Plate 3: Egbert van Heemskerk, *An Alchemist in His Study*, 17th century. Oil on canvas. (© Science History Institute, Philadelphia).

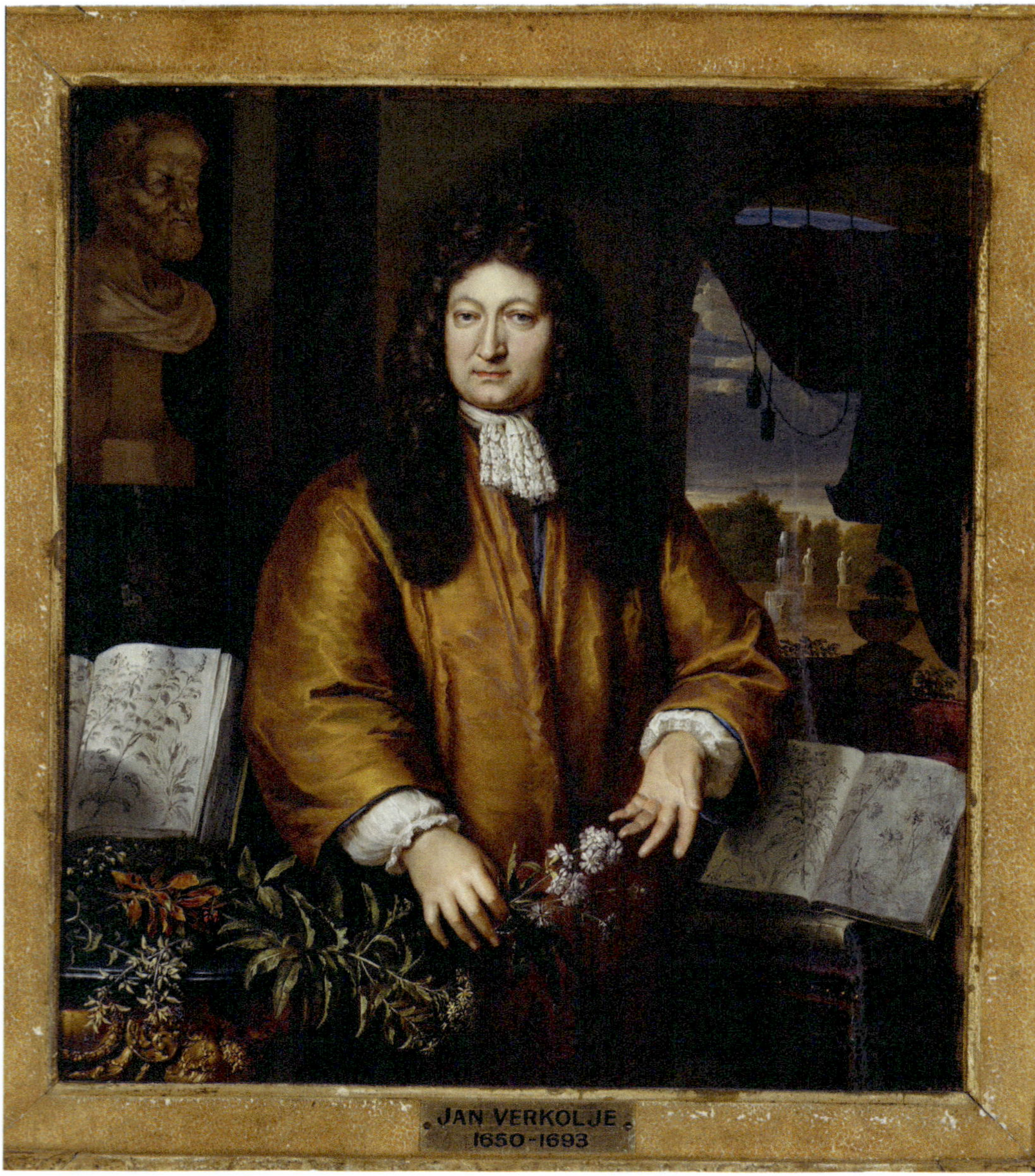

Plate 4: Gerard Hoet, *Jan Commelin*, c. 1680. Oil on canvas. (© Amsterdam Historical Museum).

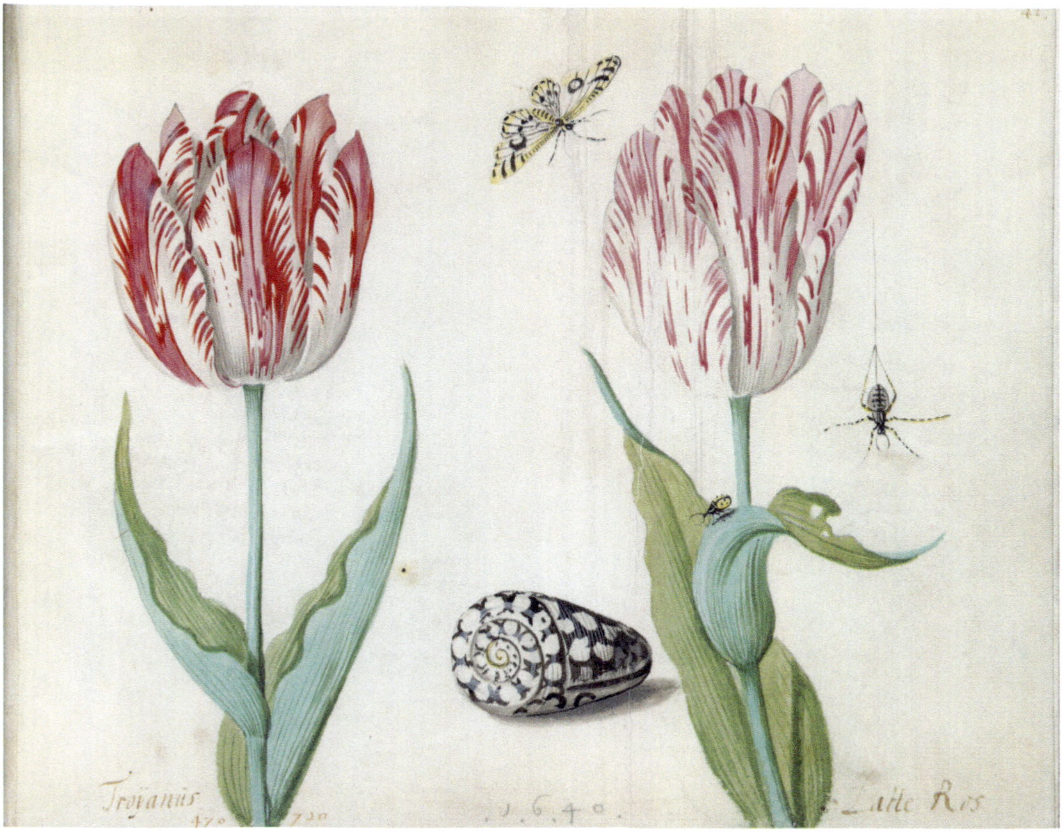

Plate 5: Jacob Marrel, *Two Tulips with Shell , Butterfly, Spider and Ladybug,*, 1640. Brush on parchment. (© Rijksmuseum, Amsterdam).

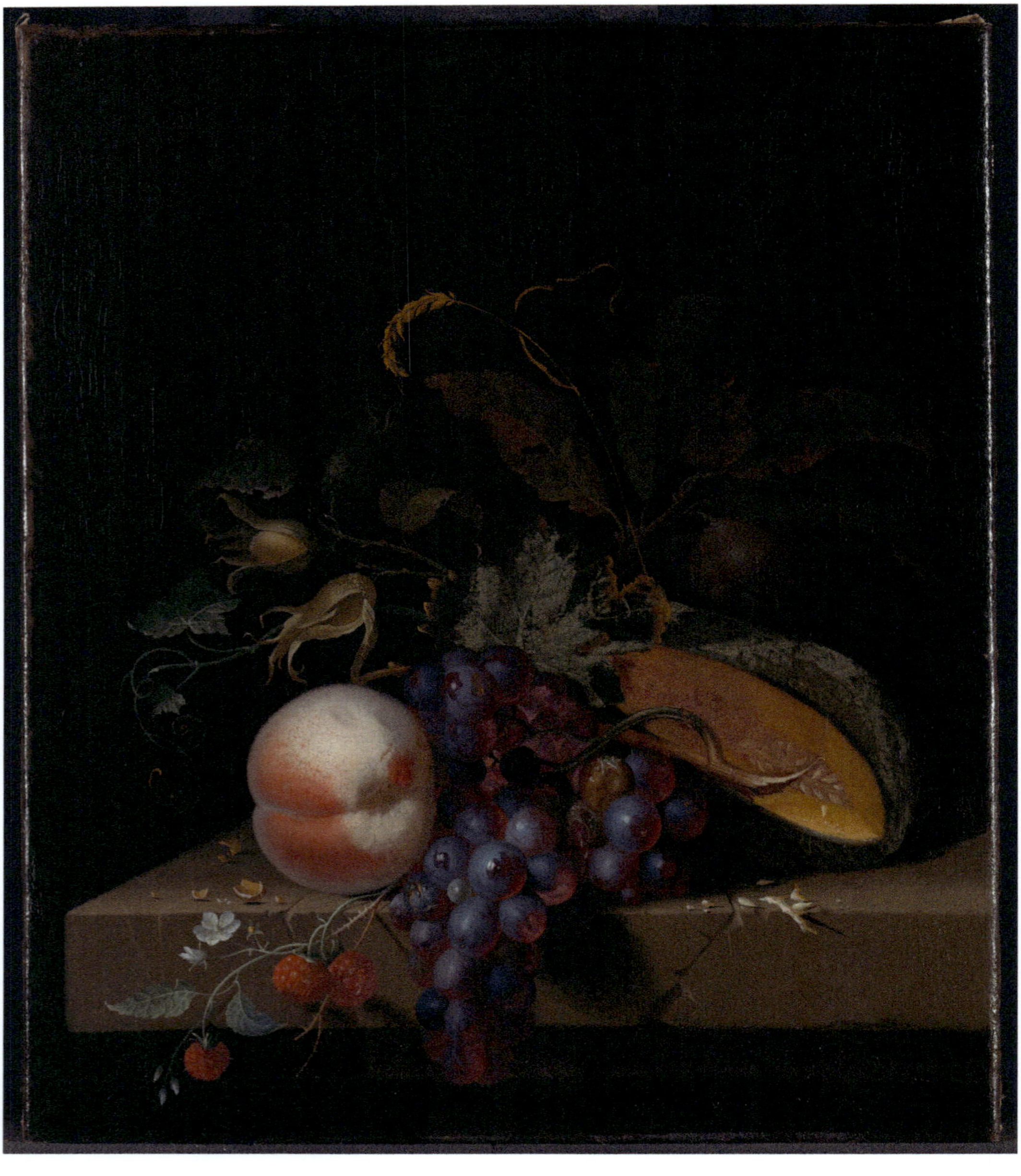

Plate 6: Pieter Gallis, *Still Life with Fruit*. Both peach and melon are depicted in Six's 'literary still lifes'. 1673. Oil on canvas. (© Rijksmuseum, Amsterdam).

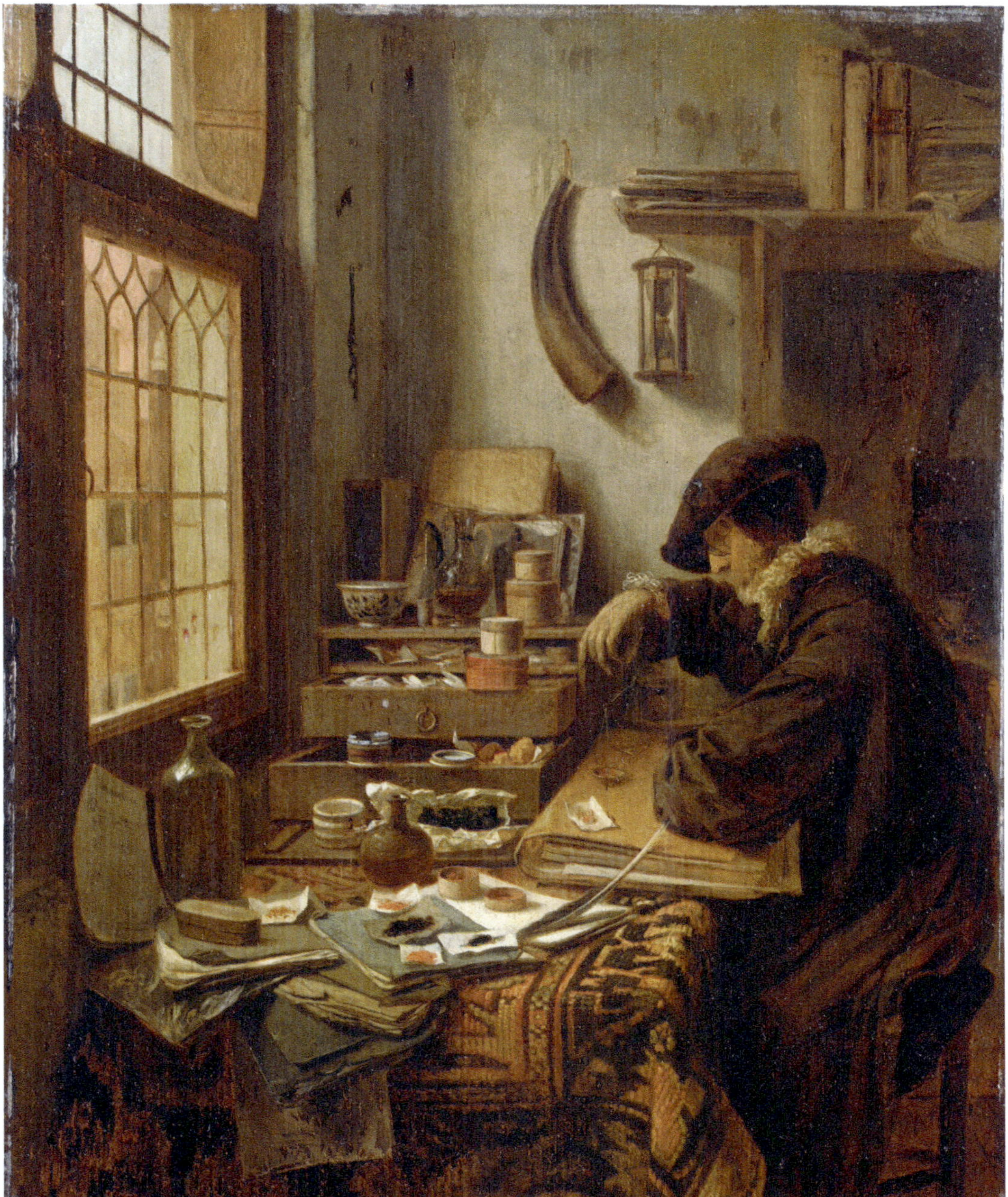

Plate 7: Job Adriaensz. Berckheyde, *The Merchant of Colours*, c. 1670–1690. Oil on panel. (© BPK Bildagentur / Museum der Bildenden Kunste, Leipzig / Ursula Gerstenberger).

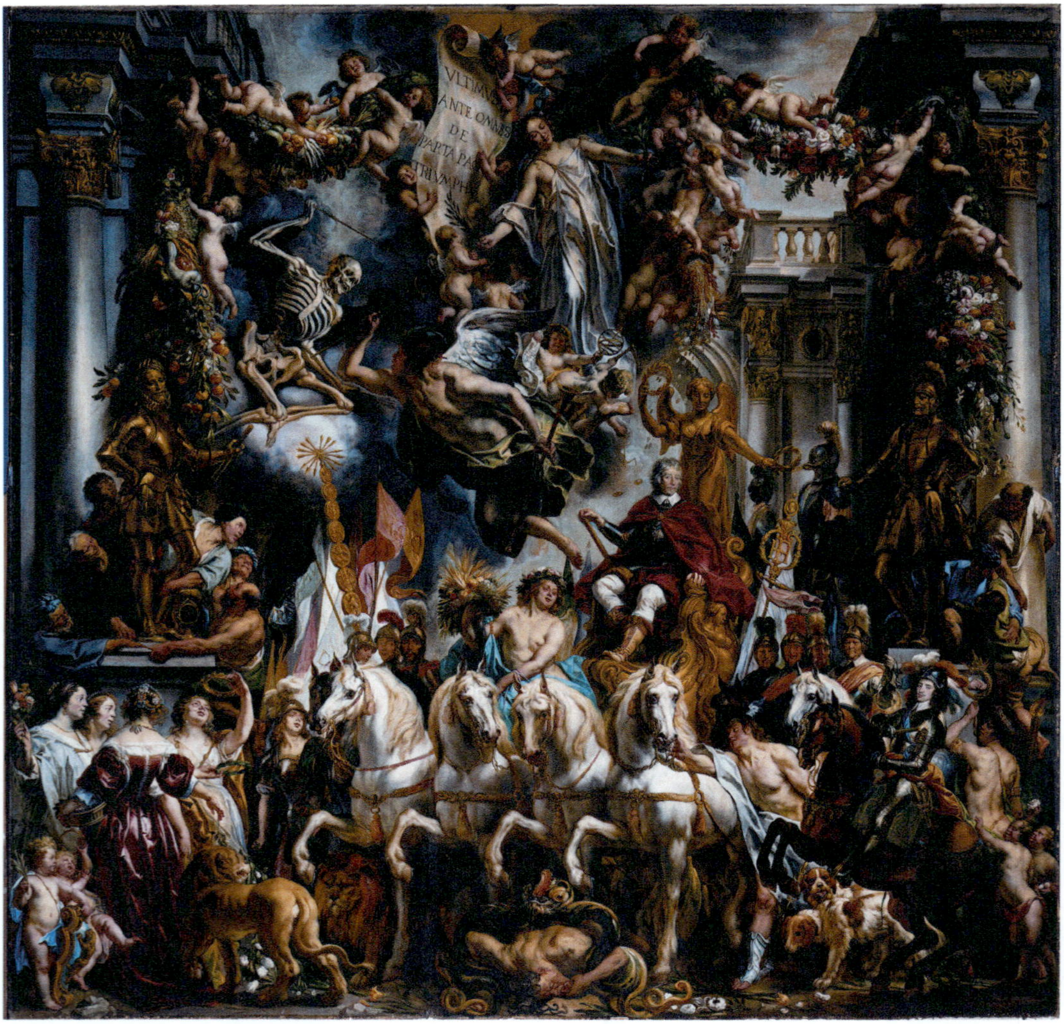

Plate 8: Jacob Jordaens, *Triumph of Frederick Henry*, 1651. Oil on canvas. (© Koninklijke Verzamelingen, The Hague / State of the Netherlands. Photographer: Margareta Svensson).

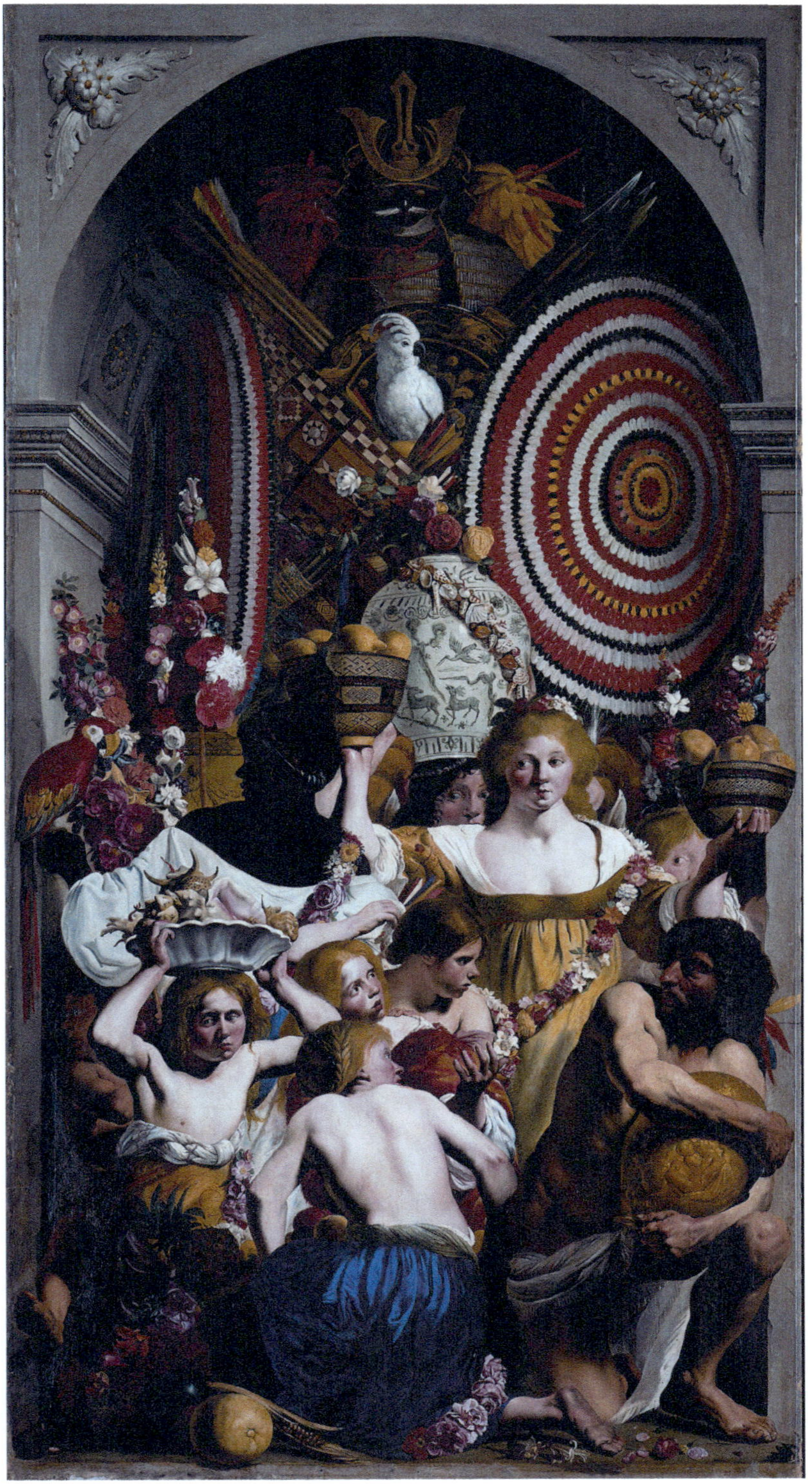

Plate 9: Jacob van Campen, *Part of the Triumphal Procession, with Gifts from the East and the West*, 1651. Oil on canvas. (© Koninklijke Verzamelingen, The Hague / State of the Netherlands. Photographer: Margareta Svensson).

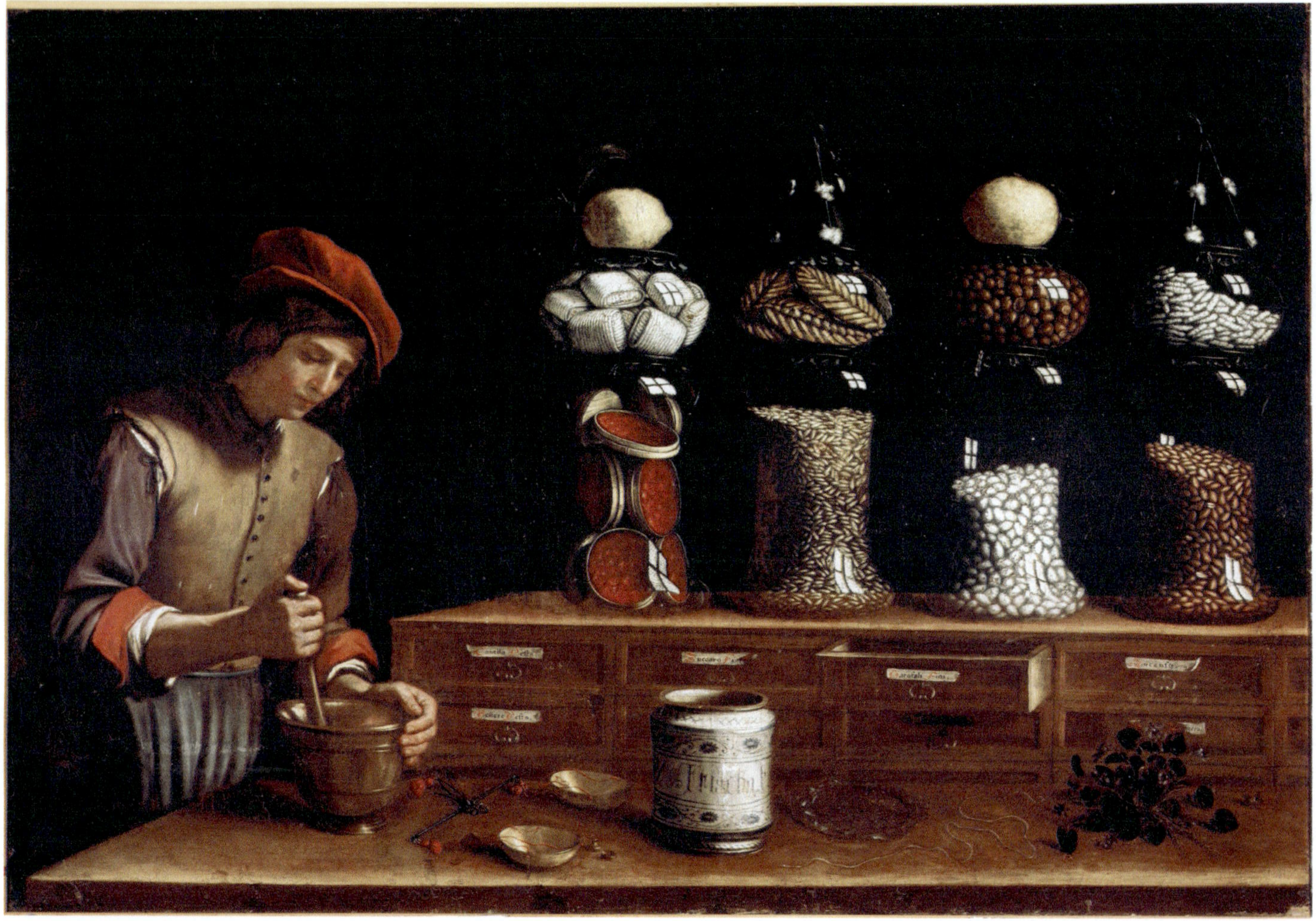

Plate 10: Paolo Antonio Barbieri, *The Spice Shop*. The apothecary is making theriac. 1637. Oil on canvas. (© Bridgeman Images).

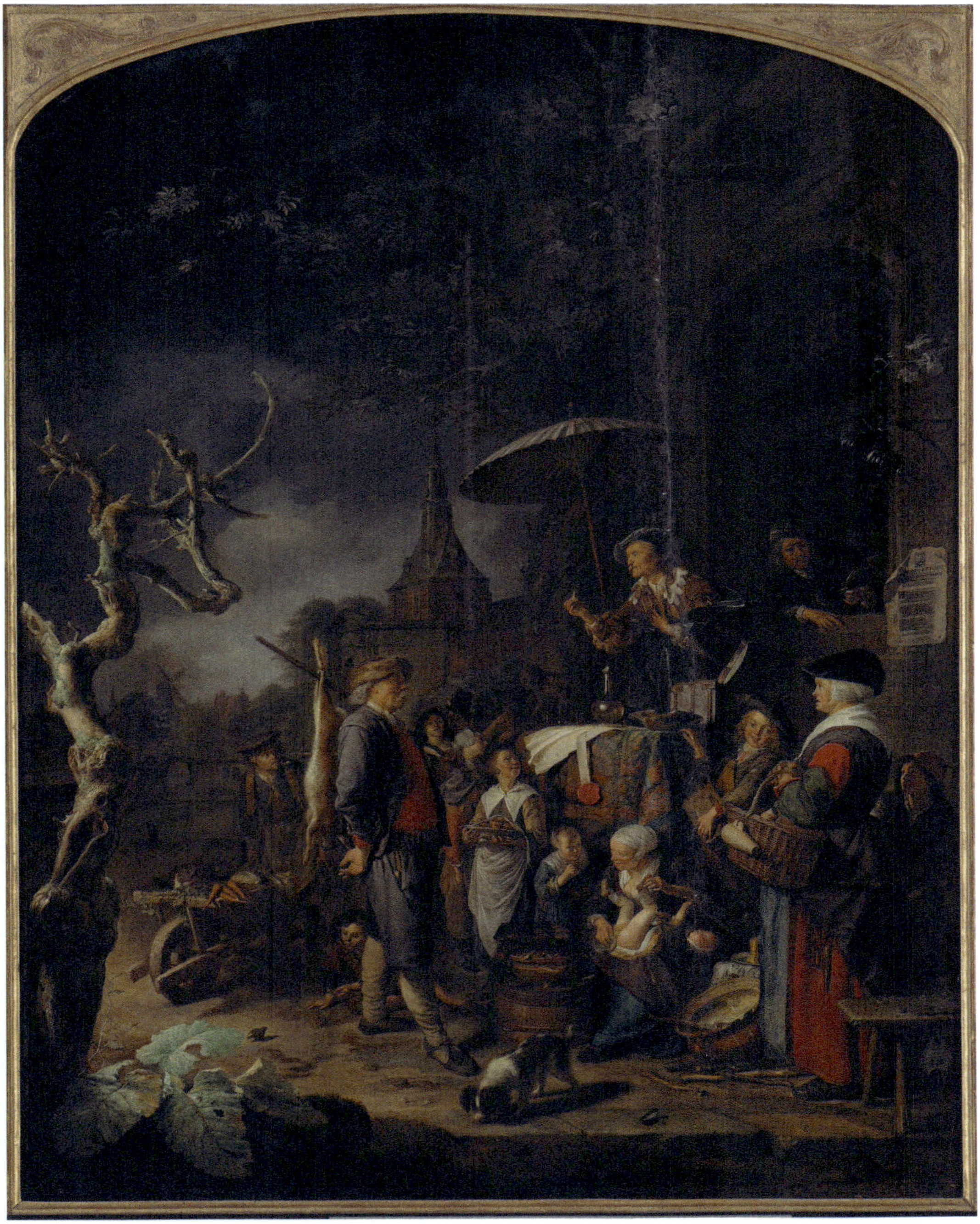

Plate 11: Gerard Dou, *The Quacksalver*, 1652. Oil on panel. (© Museum Boijmans Van Beuningen, Rotterdam. Loan: Stichting Museum Boijmans Van Beuningen / photographer: Studio Tromp, Rotterdam).

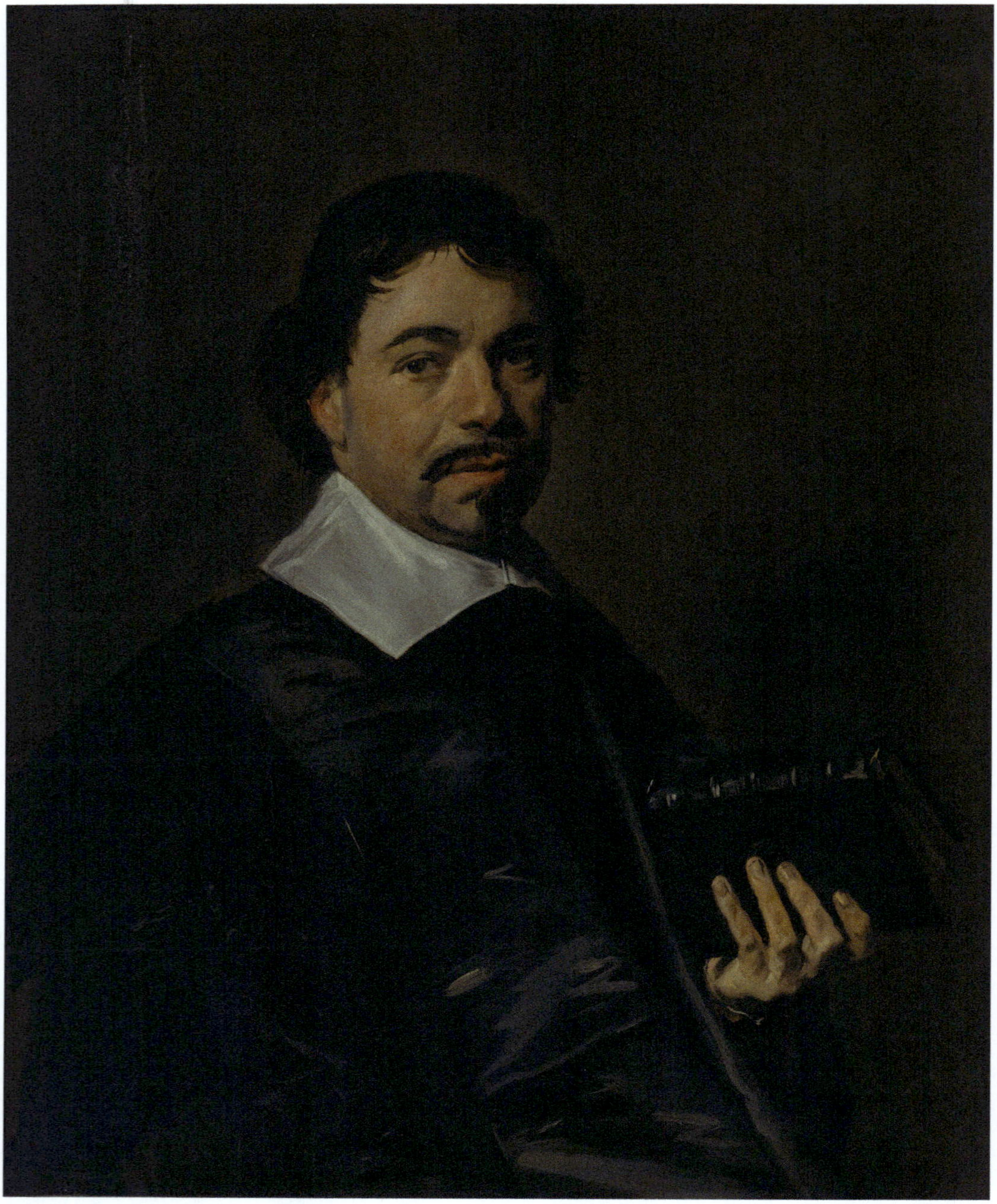

Plate 12: Frans Hals, *Portrait of Johannes Hoornbeeck*, 1645. Oil on canvas.

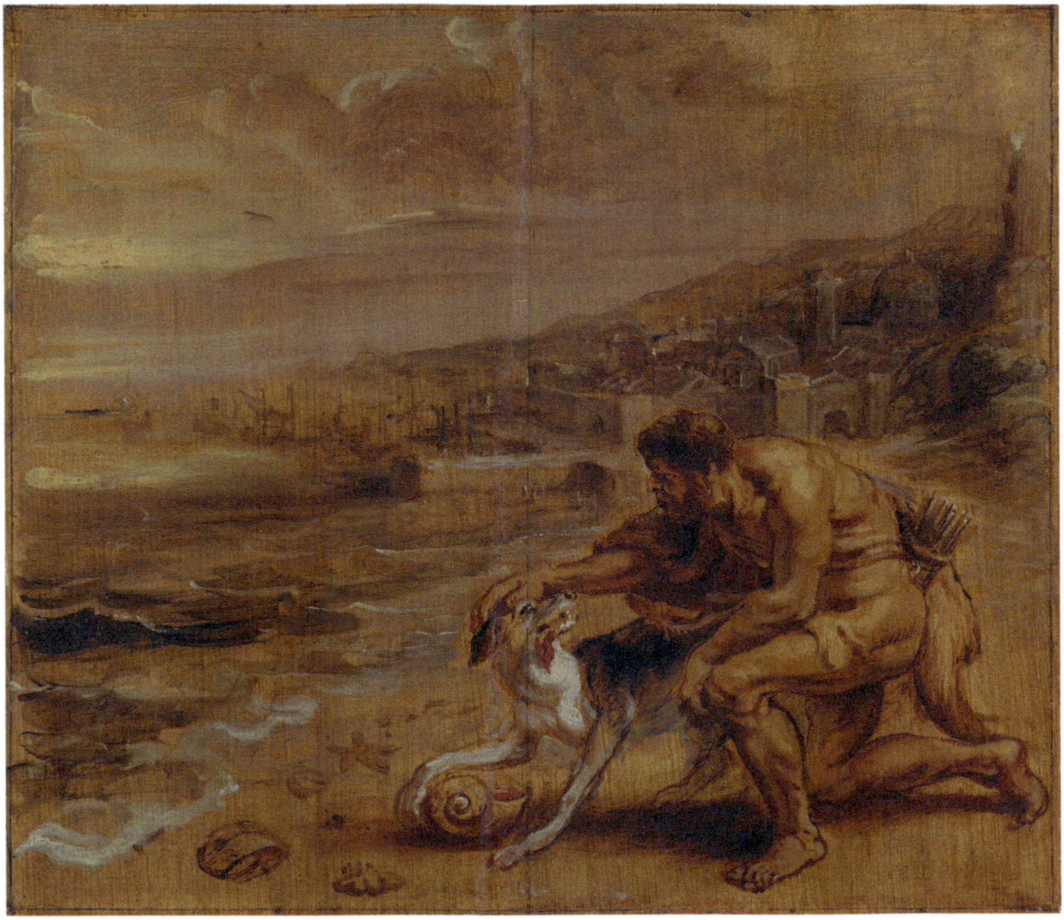

Plate 13: Peter Paul Rubens, *The Discovery of Tyrian Purple*. According to the myth, Hercules and his dog were walking on the beach on their way to court a nymph named Tyro. The dog bit a sea snail, and the snail's blood dyed the dog's mouth. Seeing this, the nymph demanded a gown of the same colour, and the result was the origin of purple dye. C. 1636. Oil on panel. (© Musée Bonnat-Helleu).

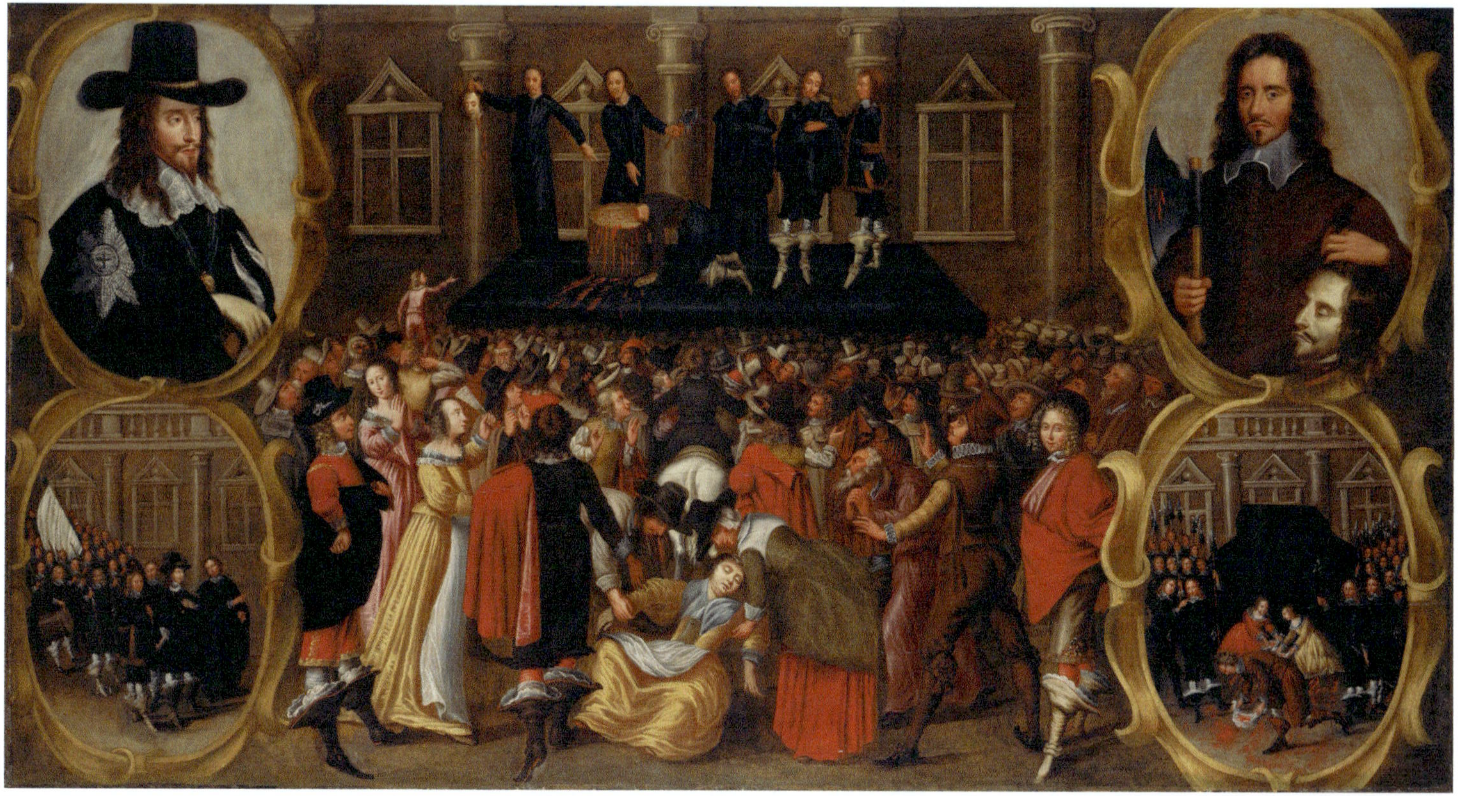

Plate 14a: Unknown, *Charles I, 1600–1649. Reigned 1625–1649 (The Execution of Charles I)*, c. 1649. Oil on canvas. (© National Galleries of Scotland. On loan from Lord Dalmeny since 1951).

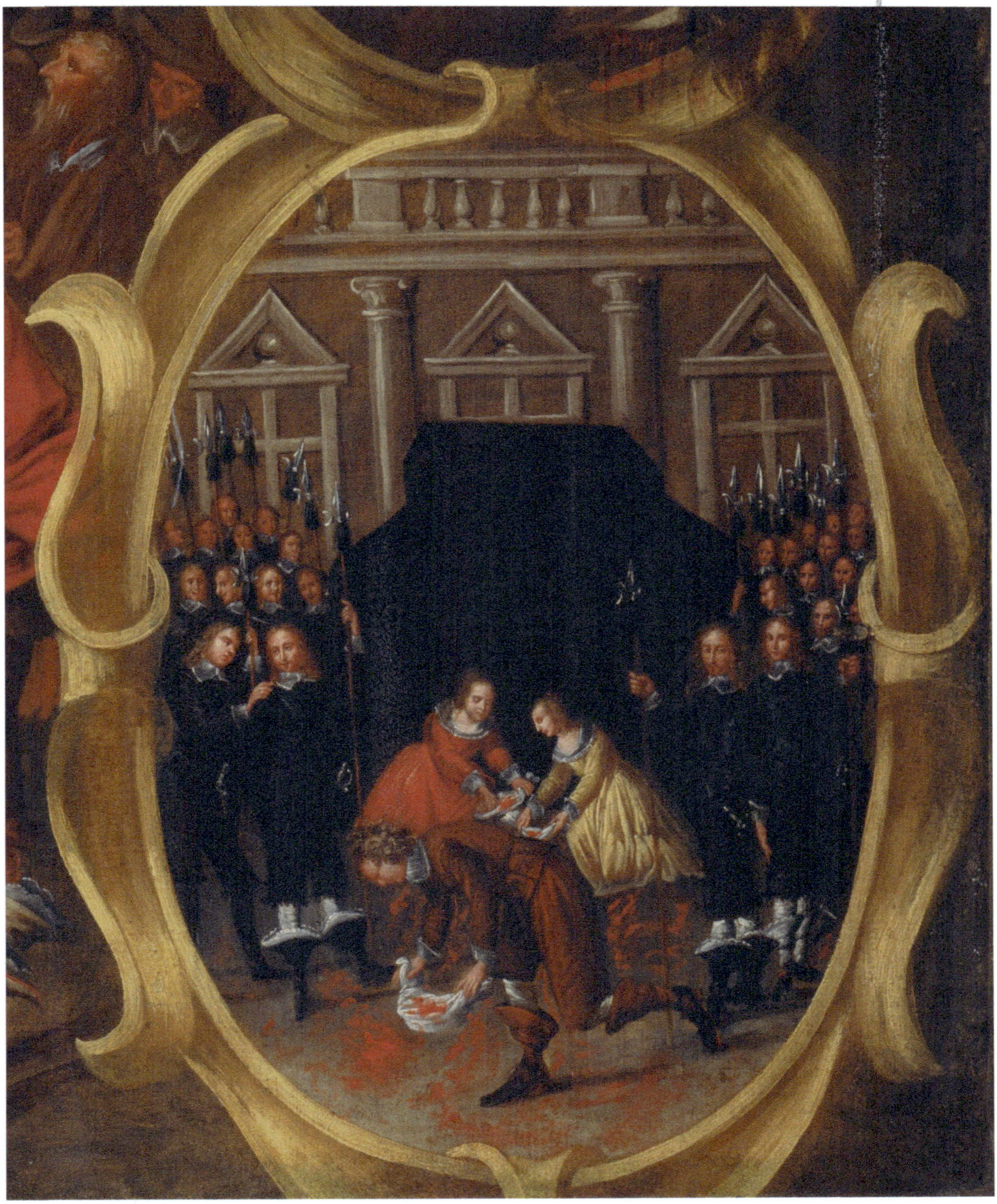

Plate 14b: Detail of Unknown, *Charles I, 1600–1649. Reigned 1625–1649 (The Execution of Charles I)*, c. 1649. Oil on canvas. (© National Galleries of Scotland. On loan from Lord Dalmeny since 1951).

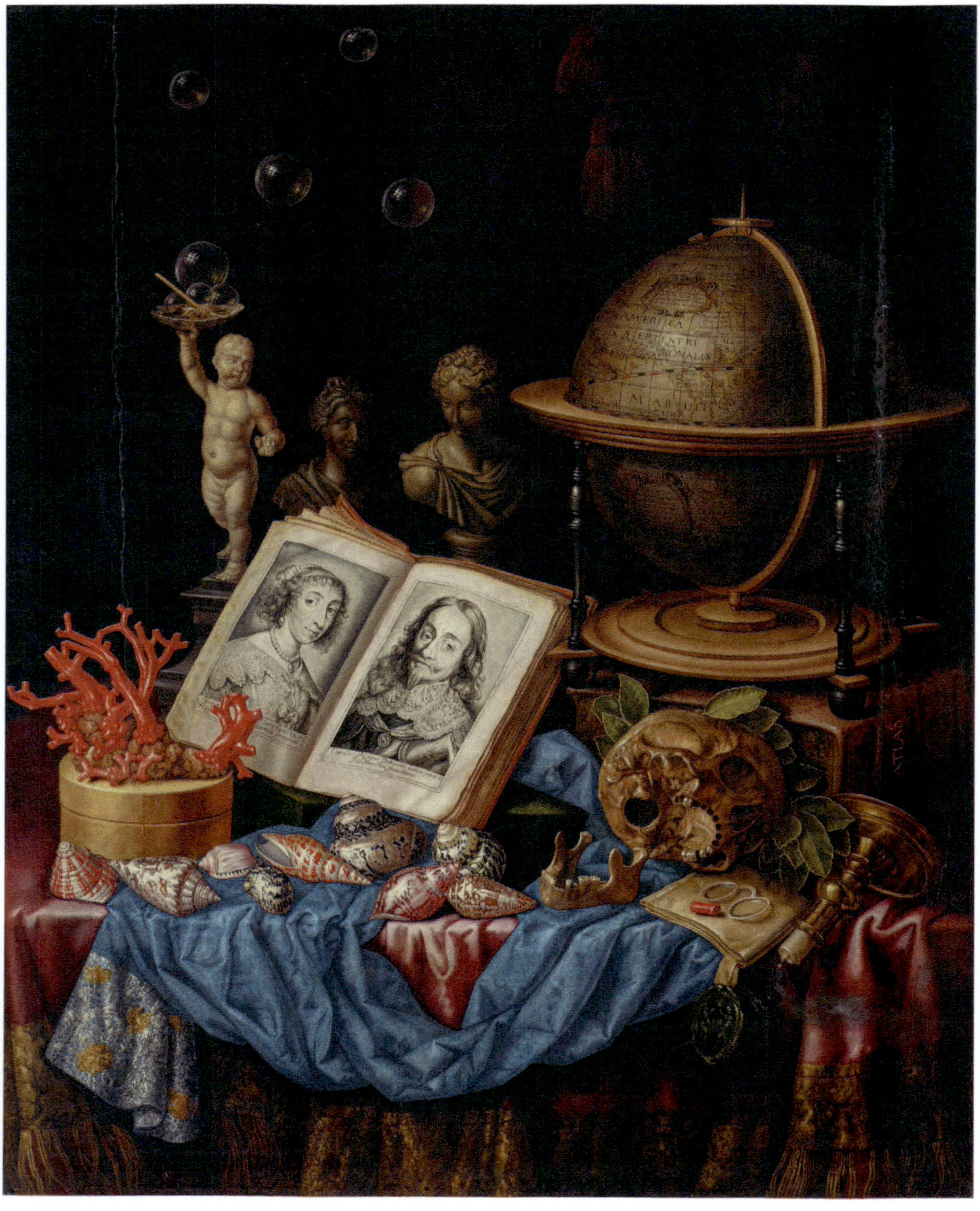

Plate 15: Anonymous, *Allegory of Charles I of England and Henrietta of France in a Vanitas*, after 1949. Oil on canvas. (© Birmingham museum of Art).

7. Drugs as Sacred Offerings

Abstract

In this chapter I discuss ceremonial uses of drugs in the poetry of Joannes Six van Chandelier. I focus on drugs as holy offerings – both in the literal and figurative senses – in Joyous Entries by political leaders into cities. I discuss two groups of texts: a series of praise poems Six wrote to Frederick Henry, Prince of Orange, on the Treaty of Münster (1648), in which Six presents the antidote theriac as an offering and a source of inspiration; and a series of poems that Six wrote on the Joyous Entry of Queen Mariana and King Philip IV to Madrid in 1649. Here, incense and olive oil are presented as sacraments for the royals. I show how Six associates the alleged apotheosising power of drugs with idolatry and pride.

Keywords: Joyous Entry, apotheosis, theriac, olive oil, Philip IV and Mariana of Spain, emotions

> Incense and myrrh from Saba, once used by pagans as sacrifices to their gods, served here as incense offerings to the goddess of France.[1]
>
> – Joost van den Vondel

A Dutch Golden Age[2]

Colours and fragrances occupy a large place in the early modern Royal Entry, also known as a Triumphal or Joyous Entry. We see this in the development of Orange propaganda in the Republic of the mid-seventeenth century. Art in the Netherlands was influenced by the new court culture that Frederick Henry had

1 'Het wieroock, en de Myrrhe van Saba, eertijds van de Heidenen den Goden geoffert, dienden hier voor reuckoffer aen de Godin van Vranckrijck', J.F.M. Sterck *et al.* (eds.), *De werken van Vondel*, vol. 3, 1929, pp. 629–630.

2 A shorter version of this chapter has been published as an article: 'Exotica, ornaments and idolatry in the poetry of Jan Six van Chandelier (1620–1695)' In: *De Zeventiende Eeuw. Cultuur in de Nederlanden in interdisciplinair perspectief*, 2016, pp. 115–136.

Spaans, R., *Dangerous Drugs: The Self-Presentation of the Merchant-Poet Joannes Six van Chandelier (1620–1695)*. Taylor & Francis Group, 2020
DOI 10.5117/9789462983543_CH07

become acquainted with in France. A culmination of this baroque style can be found in the mythological-allegorical décor in the Oranjezaal of Huis ten Bosch, designed by Frederick Henry's widow, Amalia of Solms. She was inspired by similar series that Rubens had made for various royal courts in Europe. The paintings depict a Royal Entry, in which the Prince of Orange is celebrated as a Prince of Peace. The political background to the décor is the Peace of Münster, the end of the 80-year struggle for freedom from Spain (1568–1648), to which Frederick Henry made a major contribution. The largest painting in the Oranjezaal, 'Triumph of Frederick Henry' (1651), by Jacob Jordaens, can be seen as a rebirth of the Roman imperial cult, where the Roman Triumph played an important role (Plate 8). Frederick Henry appears as a Roman *triumphator*: he comes riding through a triumphal arch, and all the established attributes of the classical triumphal procession are present. The prince wears the red imperial toga, the *toga picta*. He is celebrated as the bearer of peace and prosperity, symbolised by olive branches and the cornucopia above him. The artwork is flanked by canvases by other painters, depicting other interesting scenes. The painting by Jacob van Campen depicts part of the triumphal procession (Plate 9). We see colourful, exotic fruits, and birds and shells from the East and West Indies that are dedicated to the Prince of Orange, while the painting by Pieter de Grebber shows a white ox on its way to the Capitol, where it will be sacrificed to Jupiter. In the background sits Jupiter with his attribute, lightning. Other paintings depict the nine Muses and Apollo in his sun chariot.[3]

The display of flowers and fruits was meant not only as a random selection of exotics from the Dutch East and West Indies. Like the other paintings, Van Campen's picture is an *imitatio* of an important element of the Roman triumph. According to Pliny, in some triumphs, exotic fragrant trees from the countries that had been conquered were shown during the procession, together with other spoils such as luxury artefacts and slaves. But not all products were the spoils of war. Some were also given as gifts to the Romans by kings in foreign lands. What these exotic objects had in common was the royal provenance that ancient sources attributed to them.[4] The exotica refer to the beginning of a period of prosperity: a new *aetas aurea* – a Golden Age – about which Virgil wrote in his *Bucolica*. The Roman emperor Augustus hoped to make this dream come true by extending

3 D.P. Snoep, *Praal en Propaganda. Triumfalia in de Noorderlijke Nederlanden in de 16de en 17de eeuw*, 1975, pp. 77–82; Margriet Eikema Hommes, *De Oranjezaal in Huis ten Bosch. Een zaal uit louter liefde*, 2013; Frijhoff & Spies, 2004, pp. 98–100. See also Beatrijs Brenninkmeyer-de Rooij, 'Vergoddelijkte vorsten', in: *Openbaar kunstbezit. Kunstschrift*, 1981, pp. 46–50; Brinkkemper & Soepnel 1989, pp. 31, 38–39.

4 Pliny XII, 20 and 111. See Laurence Totelin, *Botanizing Rulers and Their Herbal Subjects: Plants and Political Power in Greek and Roman Literature*. In: *Phoenix*, 2012, pp. 122–144; Ida Östenberg, *Staging the World: Spoils, Captives, and Representations in the Roman Triumphal Procession*, 2009, pp. 91–127, pp. 168–188. For the link between exotics and royal provenance, Östenberg, 2009, p. 94.

his *Imperium Romanum* to *Arabia Felix*, the legendary 'Happy Arabia', a land of incense and an important transit country for exotica and spices. In this, he and other Roman emperors were inspired by Alexander the Great who, according to Pliny, had conquered Arabia for its frankincense (Fig. 7.1). When the wars with Spain and Gaul came to an end, a monumental altar was erected in Rome, *Ara Pacis Augustae*. This place of honour was dedicated to Pax, the Roman goddess of peace, and decorated with images of the imperial family's virtues and with mythological scenes, including one representing the myth of the Golden Age. The representation of exotic sacrifices is thus a manifestation of the political power of the Prince of Orange. It is an imitation of the *Divus Augustus*, and the Peace of Münster represents a Dutch *aetas aurea*, an early modern Dutch representation of the *Pax Romana* – a *Pax Hollandica*.[5]

However, the display of exotica evoked associations, not just with imperial power in the Roman Empire, but also with moral decadence. When Manlius Vulso celebrated a triumph in 186 BC, 'the beginnings of foreign luxury were brought to the city by the army from the East', according to Livy.[6] Other authors in Ancient Rome also identified the introduction of foreign luxury goods to triumphs as a key moment of the change in Roman morals. Dionysius of Halicarnassus claimed that the triumph of his day had 'departed in every respect from the ancient tradition of frugality'. It was then, he writes, that Roman banquets began to feature 'lute girls and harpists, and other seductive dinner party amusements'. We have seen similar points made in previous chapters.[7]

The mythological-allegorical imagery was also expressed in the literature of the Dutch Republic, and the Orange-friendly poet Six van Chandelier is no exception. In Six's poetry, we also see an ambivalence about the Royal Entry, the early modern version of the Roman Triumph. He himself erects *literary temples* in honour of his God of Orange. This is evident from a series of panegyrics that he wrote on the occasion of the Peace of Münster in 1648, and that I would like to discuss in this chapter. In 'Vreughdesangh, oover den eeuwigen Vreede, met Spanje' ('Song of Joy on the Eternal Peace with Spain') (J219), Six asks: 'O saalige eeuw, in onsen tyd, /

5 Pliny XII, 62. For the concept *aetas aurea*, see Vergil's eclogue IV. The poem originally tells us about the fulfillment of a Golden Age on Roman soil, but the idyllic condition also includes exotic plants: 'Assyrian spice shall spring up on every soil'. See also Schmidt, 1924, p. 64; Faure, 1993, p. 234. The significance of the Roman imperial cult for Dutch Joyous Entry, see Snoep, 1975. On the poetry of princely deification addressed to Frederick Henry regarding the concepts of the Prince of Peace and the Golden Age, see Melissen, 1981–1982, pp. 30–60.

6 Livy 39.6.7: 'luxuriae [...] peregrinae origo ab exercitu Asiatico inuecta in urbem est'. Quotation from: Parker, 2002, p. 57. *Cf.* Pliny XXXIII, 148–149.

7 Dionysius of Halicarnassus, *Roman Antiquities*, 2.34.3. For this and other statements see Mary Beard, *The Roman Triumph*, 2007, pp. 161–163.

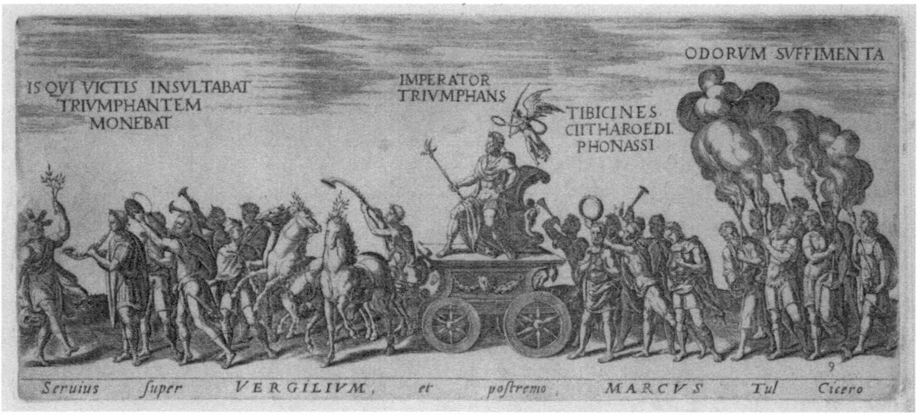

Fig. 7.1: Onofrio Panvinio, after Jan Snellinck (I), after Maarten van Heemskerck, *Triumph Procession with Incense*, 1618. Engraving. (© Rijksmuseum, Amsterdam).

Die geener Vaadren goud benyd! / Wat Godheit zal men offerdraagen, / Voor deese staage sonnedaagen?' ('O blessed century in our times, which does not envy the gold of the Ancestors [*i.e.*, the *aurea aetas* of Antiquity]! To which Deity shall we make a sacrifice [as thanks] for these long summer days?') (l. 69–72): The 'deity' that deserves to be glorified is of course Frederick Henry. Another example is 'Lauwer en olyfkrans om 't Princenhoofd' ('Laurel and olive wreath around the Prince's head') (J277). Why dedicate '[e]en tempel, en altaar, van wierookgeur gelicht' ('a temple and altar of uplifting incense') (l. 2) to a pagan god such as Janus, when one can honour a real deity such as Frederick Henry, Six asks, and then tells us how he himself can honour his 'holy head' (l. 5) '[o]p perkament, omkranst, met groenend lauwerier, / En oligroen' ('On paper, wreathed with green laurel and olive branch') (l. 6). The parchment on which such an exalted hymn is written is 'onsterfelyk papier' ('immortal paper') (l. 8).

The new baroque style is also prevalent in Six's contributions to *Amsterdamsche Vreugdtriomfe* (1660), the series of poems that he wrote following a visit to the city by some members of the Orange family, and which I discussed in the previous chapter. In 'Schuldoffer, aan mevrouw Ameelia, oudprincesse van Oranje, &c.' ('Offering Prompted by Guilt, to Mrs Amelia, Former Princess of Orange, etc.') (J614), Six addresses the widow Amalia of Solms and her Huis ten Bosch directly. The text opens with a somewhat jaunty confession from the merchant-poet, who is travelling abroad. He admits that he has been negligent in singing of domestic marvels, especially of the palace of Princess Amalia (l. 1–36). He admits in bombastic terms that he '[n]iet eens het Godlik aangesicht / Van haare Son heb aangebeên' ('has not even worshipped the Divine sight of her Sun') (l. 51–52). He throws himself at her feet as if he were a subject of a queen of the East, and, he promises, will repent by making an offering at her divine altar: 'Ik vinden zal het hoogh altaar, / In uw palleisen, en aldaar / Het wierook van den stroom Permes / Opoffren, aan Mevrouw Princes' ('I shall find the high altar, in your palace, and there offer incense from the flood Permessus to Madam Princess') (l. 61–64).[8] Six's panegyric must of course be understood ironically.

Sacrifices to the gods

This study has identified Six's affinity with a strict Protestantism. One would expect that texts by the self-aware Calvinist would contain few references to the worship of pagan gods. Terms such as 'priest', 'altar', 'sacrifice', 'oil' and 'incense' – to which we have already found many references in Six's poetry – were viewed with suspicion by Calvinist pastors. One reason for this lies in the general Christian aversion to the wealth of pre-Christian religion. Appeals to the imperial cult of Ancient Rome served as an important argument against the use of incense in churches: once Roman emperors began to declare themselves gods, it became customary to burn incense in front of an image of the emperor. And as is known from the history of the Roman Empire, the duty of burning incense was used as a test of loyalty to the emperor. Christians refused to participate in what they regarded as the worship of a pagan god. The early Church Fathers were therefore clear in their condemnation of incense, which they regarded as part of the trappings of idolatry – as 'food for demons', in Origen's words. These arguments were important to reformers in the early modern period such as Calvin, when they omitted incense from Protestant religious services.[9] What is interesting in this connection is that the term 'druggist' is explicitly associated with pagan abundance in early modern theological works. The prophecy of Ezekiel describes how the Jews will be abducted and taken to Babel (Babylon), 'a city of merchants' (Ezekiel 17:4). According to the comments on the *Statenvertaling*, 'merchants' refers to 'spice merchants or druggists', and Babylon was a famous commercial city: 'because it was full of all kinds of spices, drugs, and precious wares, providing not only necessities and amusement, but also luxury and lavishness'.[10] Another reason can

8 The Permessus was a stream rising in Mount Helicon, which was sacred to Apollo.

9 For classical and early modern arguments against incense, see David Robertson, 'Incensed over Incense: Incense and Community in Seventeenth-Century Literature.' In *Religion and Writing in England, 1558–1689*, 2009, pp. 389–409.

10 'Kruydeniers, ofte, droogisten'; 'om datse vol was van allerley specerijen, drogen, ende kostelicke waren, dienende niet alleen tot nootdurft, ofte vermaeck, maer oock tot leckernije, ende overdadicheyt', see comment 13 to Ezekiel 17: 4. 'Babel' is a *topos* in the poetry of Six, both referring to the Calvinist criticism on tall buildings, as in 'Toorenbouw, aan de graavers' ('Tower Construction, to the Diggers') (J122), and to

be found in Protestant theology. According to the New Testament, the contract between God and people involving the offering of sacrifices is dissolved: Jesus Himself became a sacrifice. He is also king, priest and prophet – the three functions that anointing with holy oils was part of. Christ is the divine fragrance; the word 'Christ' itself means 'anointed'. He sacrifices himself and makes God benevolent.[11] Precious, fragrant substances in the Bible should therefore be understood only figuratively, as symbols of the pleasant, wholesome body and blood of the Son of God, who died for our sins. A crucial Bible passage in this respect is James 5:14, in which healing with oil is the theme. The Calvinist commentators emphasise that the oil has no 'hidden power', but should be seen as an 'extraordinary sign' of the miracle of God. The 'altar', the 'priest', and the 'offering' were rejected as non-Christian concepts.[12] The pulpit and the preacher were introduced in their stead. The preacher is not a mediator between God and people, but should rather be seen as a teacher.

Nevertheless, one would think that, since many Calvinists were Orange supporters, they would not have made a fuss about the cult around their princes of Orange. But they did – especially the orthodox among them. When in 1660 the burgomasters asked for money for the Royal Entry for which *Amsterdamsche Vreugdtriomfe* was written, the famous doctor and burgomaster Nicolaes Tulp asked that 'such pagan gods and goddesses on triumphal chariots as in the past year on the festivities of the House of Nassau drove through the city' stay away this time. By 'the past year', Tulp means another royal visit to Amsterdam: in 1659, Amalia was given a state welcome in the city, on the occasion of the marriage of one of her daughters.[13] Tulp's criticism most likely also included poems of praise full of mythological embroidery written to the widow of the Prince of Orange.

disobedience to God in general, as in 'Aan myne vrienden' ('To My Friends') (J84) and 'Brand van Aken' ('The Fire of Aken') (J462). *Cf.* the reference to 'Babel' in Dutch art, Koenraad Jonckheere, 'An Allegory of Artistic Choice in Times of Trouble: Pieter Bruegel's Tower of Babel,' *Nederlands Kunsthistorisch Jaarboek*, 2014, pp. 151–177.

11 Faure 1993, p. 266. See also Song of Songs 3:6 and Hebrews 9-10, with accompanying comments.

12 'Verborgene kracht', 'extra-ordinaris teecken', comment 51. See also comment 16 to Mark 6:13; and comment 15 to Hebrews 23:10. The term *heilig* is essential in this context: The concepts of *heil*, 'medical health' or 'spiritual salvation', and *heilig*, 'holy' point to the close relationship between religion and medicine. *Heil* and derivations from it are found in *Poësy*, in which it is clear that they refer to both *medical* and *spiritual* well-being. See for example 'heilinge' ('healing') in 'Trouwen raad om naa het Spa te koomen [...]' (J112), l. 31; and 'heilbre' ('wholesome') in 'Aan Simon Dilman geneesheer t'Amsterdam' (J116), l. 11. *Cf.* Alfred Schmidt, *Drogen und Drogenhandel im Alterum*, 1924, pp. 39–49. See also the terms *heilmiddel* and *heiland*, the latter meaning both 'saviour' and 'healer'.

13 'Sulcke hydense goden en godinnen op triumpwaegens, als in den voorleeden jaere op de festoyeringe van 't huys van Nassouw door de stadt reeden'. Quote taken from Hans Bontemantel, *De regeeringe van Amsterdam, soo in 't civiel als crimineel en militaire (1653–1672)*, 1877, vol. I, p. 491, note 2.

We should therefore expect that there might be few references to the classical gods in Six's texts, as is the case in the poetry of his fellow Protestant poets Joachim Oudaen and Jeremias de Decker, who develop an anti-classical programme in their texts, and who, unlike their fellow poets, stayed away from such pagan triumphal ceremonies. Oudaen's 'Godsdienst- en het godendom ontdekt: Aan de Hedendaagsche Dichters' ('Religion and the Idolatry of Gods Disclosed: to the Poets of the Present Day'), which I mentioned in the introduction, discusses this new language of the high Parnassus:

Hoogverheve Heerlykheden,
Als ten hemel opgevaren,
Ingevoert, en aangebeden;
G'eert met Tempels en Altaren,
Daar men 't bloed der offerbeesten
Zag in volle stroomen vlieten,
D'eed'len wynen, op uw feesten,
Deed uit gouden koppen gieten,
Daar u ryk'lyk mocht gebeuren
Wierook, Ooster-kruideryen,
Oliën, en dierb're geuren,
Om uw' Godheen in te wyen;[14]

Lofty Majesties,
Who seem to have ascended to heaven,
Introduced and adored:
Honoured with Temples and Altars,
Where one saw the blood of the
Sacrificial beasts flow in full streams,
And the noble wine, on your feast days,
Pour out of golden cups,
The Incense, Spices of the East,
Oils and expensive fragrances
That were conferred sumptuously upon you,
In order to consecrate your Divinity.

We would expect Six to do just as Oudaen did and reject this cult of 'lofty majesties'. But the poems mentioned above present a different picture. In Six's case, the use of solemn language is often accompanied by numerous references to classical

14 Joachim Oudaen, *Gedichten*, vol. 1, 1712, pp. 190-192.

mythology. The frequency of the word 'gods' illustrates this; a quick analysis shows that it occurs 45 times in *Poësy*. For comparison's sake: in *Poëzy* (1684) by 'the son of Vondel', Joannes Vollenhove, a book of about the same size, it occurs 34 times.[15]

This chapter is about the literary representation of exotic drugs as 'offerings' to royalty at civil ceremonies and Joyous Entries. This does not necessarily mean ceremonies that would actually have taken place. For example, the paintings in Huis ten Bosch do not refer to a specific triumphal procession, because the Peace of Münster came about only one year after Frederick Henry's death. And of course, this does not mean that the mythological embroidery was limited to Huis ten Bosch – the Republic was characterised less strongly by courtly culture than were other European countries – but the new baroque impulses also influenced urban culture. The Amsterdam Town Hall was seen as an urban counterpart to the Oranjezaal. In quasi-religious language, Vondel calls the building ''s lants hooghste altaer' ('the land's highest altar') (l. 8) in 'Op den princelijcken genadepenning. Aen de doorluchtighste Mevrouwe Douagiere Amelia [...]' ('On the Princely Medal of Mercy. To Mrs Dowager Amalia of Solms-Braunfels [...]'). The Town Hall is thus depicted as the Republic's Capitol.[16] In the city, poets were, as we have seen, responsible for organising triumphal chariots of allegorical and historical 'tableaux vivants'. The Dutch 'city poet' thus shared to some extent the elevation and solemnity that would otherwise be the hallmark of the European 'court poet'.[17]

In this chapter, attention has shifted from the poet-druggist as a make-up artist and as a pyrotechnician to the poet-druggist as a priest and master of ceremonies. I am picking up again here the thread of 'Afbeeldinge en wydinge van Roselle', in which Six transforms his love into an immortal 'Goddess' by means of holy sacraments. The question is how Six handles texts full of mythological embellishments. In this chapter, I will argue that ceremonial uses of drugs are a problem for Six's self-presentation as a sober Protestant. I will discuss two groups of his texts in which he criticises the role of the Renaissance poet as a priest in civil ceremonies. I will first analyse the series of poems of praise that Six wrote to Frederick Henry, Prince of Orange, on the occasion of the Treaty of Münster (1648), where the poet presents the antidote theriac as an offering and a source of inspiration for the celebration of the

15 The singular 'god' is also common, but I have examined only the frequency of the plural forms 'gooden', 'goon' and 'goôn', because they specifically indicate polytheistic belief. The pastor-poet Vollenhove states in his book that he is publishing his wedding poems with reservations, especially the section that contains references to pagan gods: these poems are the 'immature fruits of his youth', he says, and the classical gods should be read as symbols of virtues – Venus as love, and so on – just like in the poems of Hooft and Vondel, see *Poëzy*, 1686, pp. 409–411. *Cf.* also the use of mythological language in *De Ystroom* (1671) by Joannes Antonides van der Goes, another 'son of Vondel', and the argumentation of the poet in the introduction to the work.

16 Compare, too, the Joyous Entry of Gerard Bicker, which I mentioned in Chapter 5.

17 Frijhoff & Spies, 2004, pp. 432–445. *Cf.* also Jan Vos as a city poet, in: Geerdink, 2012, pp. 47–72.

Peace. At the beginning of this chapter we saw a number of examples of apotheosis in the poems of praise from this series. I will then discuss a series of poems that Six wrote on the occasion of the Joyous Entry of Queen Mariana of Austria, the second wife of Philip IV, on 15 November 1649. He wrote it during a commercial trip in Spain, in which some druggists' goods, incense and oil are presented as sacraments for the wedding. Six's praise poems to the Spanish king and queen provoked negative reactions in the Republic. In two poems in *Poësy,* Six comments on this criticism, and clarifies his view on the apothesising power attributed to drugs. In one of these texts, Six refers to a third civil ceremony, which took place almost 10 years earlier: the Joyous Entry of the French queen mother, Maria de' Medici, to Amsterdam in 1638. These texts will also be discussed because they clarify Six's ironic position towards pharmacy and poetry as apotheosis.

Songs of Joy

As we have seen, there never was a Triumphal Entry by Frederick Henry through Amsterdam. But there were solemn ceremonies on the occasion of the Treaty of Münster in 1647 and 1648. Already in 1647, when the negotiations between the Republic and Spain concluded successfully, Vondel's play celebrating the peace, *Leeuwendalers,* was performed. The official proclamation took place on 5 June 1648. It consisted of a series of symbolic spectacles performed on Dam Square and again in the theatre over the next few days, and included a fireworks display in the evening. Besides the elder poet Samuel Coster, two young fellow poets of Six's, Jan Vos and Geeraardt Brandt, were responsible for the design of the spectacles. These three provided the triumphal chariots with accompanying poems in which the Princes of Orange and the burgomasters of Amsterdam were compared to historical and mythological figures.

Six also participated in the celebration of the Peace. As we have seen, he wrote a series of praise poems that were published in the pamphlet *Vreughde-Zangen / Over den eeuwigen / Vreede, / Tusschen / Spangien / En de Vereenighde / Nederlanden: / Daar by noch andere invallingen van den Rijmer, voor en omtrent 't sluyten der selver Vreede* (*Songs of Joy About the Eternal Peace, Between Spain and the United Netherlands: In Addition to Other Whims of the Rhymester, for and about Concluding That Peace*) (1648). The pamphlet appeared without the author's name, but the prose introduction to the work, 'Toewydinge aan de vreegodinne' ('Devotion to the Goddess of Peace'), and the last poem are signed with Six's initials, I.S.V.C.[18] The

18 The pamphlet was printed in 1648 't' Amstelredam, Voor Joost Hartgers, Boeck-verkooper in de Gast-huys-steegh, bezijden 't Stadt-huys, in de Boeck-winckel'. Joost Hartgers was related to Six, see Appendix II.

following year, all eleven poems in the pamphlet were included in the collection *Olyf-Krans Der Vreede, Door de Doorluchtigste Geesten, en Geleerdste Mannen, deezes tijds, Gevlochten* [...] (*Olive Garland of Peace Braided by Illustrious Minds, and the Most Learned Men of This Time* [...]) (1649), together with works of praise by a number of other writers, Vondel's *Leeuwendalers*, and two poems by Vondel and Reyer Anslo about the construction of the new Town Hall. When Six published *Poësy* in 1657, he also included most of his *Vreughde-Zangen*, but he did not keep to the original order, and made significant changes to some of the poems. My interpretations are based on the revised versions that were included in *Poësy*.[19]

Catholic, Remonstrant and Calvinist poets took part in the *Olyf-krans der Vreede*; the only ones who showed restraint in the face of peace were fierce Calvinists, who opposed a peace with the Catholic Spaniards, whom they saw as deceitful. One might wonder whether Six belonged to this group. But new prospects for trade were apparently more important to the merchant-poet than any resentment he might once have felt towards Spain. This is evident from 'Beraad, of het niet goed waar vreede met Spanje' ('Consideration of Whether a Peace with Spain Would be a Good Thing') (J213), where Six asks these rhetorical questions: 'Waar 't schaade dat de bloedge deegen lagh? / Dat 's handelaars profytelyke vlag / Voer sorgeloos, voor roovers nacht, en dach?' ('Would it then be detrimental if the bloody sword were laid down? If the profitable flag of the trader could sail without worries for pirates, day and night?') (l. 65–67). Participating in the festivities was an opportunity for Six to commit himself to Dutch power politics in a period marked by a struggle between Orange and States supporters. According to J. de Gier, Orange propaganda is more readily discernible in Six than in the verses of the other poets.[20] However, I am interested in the associations that the peace celebration created with pagan processions and thus Six's ironic self-profiling as the poet-priest of Amsterdam. He thematises his roles as both a provider and a consumer of exotic offerings.

Here I focus on the two most striking texts in Six's group of texts: 'Toewydinge aan de vreegodinne' ('Devotion to the Goddess of Peace') (J218), the prose introduction to the series of praise poems, and 'Hooghloffelijke gedachtenisse, van ['Most Laudable Memory of'] Freedrik Henrik, Prince van Oranje' (J215). 'Toewydinge aan de vreegodinne' presents us with one of the most precious medicines, the classic wonder drug theriac. At the beginning of the text, Six says, with a certain embarrassment, that he is contributing to the celebration of the peace between the Republic and Spain. He says he does not feel comfortable in the exalted company of the goddess of peace. Pax, who is 'schooner dan de sonne, booven de maane,

19 Frijhoff & Spies, 2004, pp. 432–444. For the changes Six made, see Chapter 1, note 79.

20 J. de Gier, '"Den krijg is uitgebannen." De Vrede van Munster in de poëzie'. In H.H.J. van As *et al.* (eds.), *Vrede, vrijheid, vaderland*, 1998, pp. 151–171.

starren, en alle Heemelsche cieraaden' ('more beautiful than the sun, more than the moon, the stars, and all the Heavenly jewellery') (l. 4–5), arouses ecstasy among the poets who feel called to honour her. Those poets who are chosen sparkle in her splendour, and the goddess of peace fills them with heavenly powers, so that they experience a holy unity with cosmic harmonies – 'sielbetoovrende maaten, en toonen' – 'rhythms and tones to enchant the soul' (l. 13). Six describes this mystical unification ironically: the great poets 'lodderen en dartelen, in de spiegelende Sonneschyn' and 'ontvonken en swellen in hunne keelen' ('delight and frisk about in the reflected Sunshine [...] ignite and swell in their throats') (l. 9–10): however, Six goes on to explain that he does not belong to that group of poets. Two types of poets can be distinguished among the crowd of worshippers: noble nightingales and bastard birds. Six counts himself among the latter (l. 14–19). Since he is one of the simple rhymesters, he also uses a source of inspiration that originates in the world of this kind of charlatan (l. 19–23):

> En dierhalven gevoelende in my rysen een krachtige gest
> van nieuwen Triaakel, gelyk ik daagelyks handel, dewelke geensins
> naauw wil zyn beslooten, zoo moet ik uitbarsten om locht te scheppen,
> genoodsaakt niet min vroolik, als met eerbiedinge, voor uwe
> Goddelyke voeten te verschynen, met deese myne offerhande.

> And for that reason, when feeling a powerful yeast of a new Theriac rising up in me, like the one I trade in daily, and that in no way will be bottled up within me, I have to erupt in order to draw my breath, forced as I am – no less cheerful than respectful – to appear at your Divine feet with this, my offering.

The rhymester hopes that his poems of praise ('my small piece of work'), written in a theriac-induced intoxication, will be appreciated by the goddess, and that, if they go up in smoke on the goddess's sacrificial altar, she will find the smell pleasing. Six then compares himself to the classical poet Marsus: although his work is not as 'wydloopende' ('long-winded') as Marsus' epic poem on the war against the Amazons, he hopes that the goddess will receive his poetic gift (l. 24–26). His series of poems is thus presented as a perfumed sacrifice to the gods (l. 27–32):

> Ai! versmaad se niet: maar ontfangh dit klein werksken, wanneer het
> aan de vlamme gegeeven, door synen rook, en reuk, neevens die van
> zoo veel duisend pektonnen, zal beneevelen uwen Heemelschen
> throon, om als wierook uwe neusgaaten lieffelyk te bewaassemen. Zoo
> langh ik leeve, en uwer gunste deelachtigh ben, zal ik niet naalaaten
> uwen Tempel, en Altaaren te eeren, en onderhouden.

> Oh! Do not scorn it; but receive this, my small piece of work, when it is given to the flames, with its smoke and smell, next to the smoke of the pitch barrels, it shall bemist your Heavenly throne, in order, as incense, to befog lovely your nostrils. As long as I live and am blessed with your favour, I shall not fail to honour and maintain your Temple and Altar.

What does Six mean here? His hyperbolic description of the goddess of peace and the fact that he presents himself as a bastard bird do not sound strange to us. This depiction is based on Six's rhymester poetics. He is half-poet, following Persius' example (I will come back to this in the following chapter). This 'confession' thus has a satirical meaning. First, Six is doubly ironic in his reference to Marsus. The poet Marsus is only known by name; almost all his poems, like his *Amazoniad* – an epic poem on the war against the Amazons, the famous warrior women – are lost. And when it comes to the 'long-winded' style of Marsus, Six is alluding to a satirical epigram of Martial, where Martial writes that 'Persius scores more often in his single book than trifling Marsus in his whole of his *Amazoniad*'.[21] Further, Six acts against the social hierarchy of classical Renaissance poetics: Ronsard criticises the rhymester as 'un Charlatan vendeur de triacles', and this criticism is repeated in Vondel's identification of rhymesters with 'quacks peddling their jars'. Six is probably also referring to another literary-theoretical work: Theodore Rodenburgh, in his apology for the Amsterdam chamber of rhetoric *Eglentiers poëtens borst-weringh* (*The Battlement of the Eglentier's Poets*) (1638), speaks of the contrast between 'rymers' and 'bastards-Poëten' on the one hand and the inspired 'Poëten' on the other. These bastard Poets have no access, he tells us, to the 'power of a Celestial breath', which creates a poetry that transcends nature.[22] Six thus jokingly admits that he himself is a rhyming quack, stupefied by a nostrum and not by divine inspiration. He turns Ronsard's literary ranking on its head. Six tells the reader that, contrary to all prejudices, his position is better than that of the inspired poets with all their high social and religious pretensions.

But this explanation assumes a similarity between rhymester and druggist, and as we have seen, the ambivalent concept of 'druggist' does not guarantee simplicity and humility. The trade in drugs evoked associations with the strange and the exclusive in early modern times. I suppose the same applied to theriac.

21 Martial, *Epigrams*, vol. I, translation by D.R. Schackleton Baily, 1993, p. 301. Six also refers in another poem to the obscure poet Marsus, see Schenkeveld-van der Dussen, 2007, pp. 207 and 236.

22 'Krachte van een Hemelsche azem', Rodenburgh 1638, pp. 11 and 45, and see Schenkeveld-van der Dussen, 1983, p. 310. Rodenburgh is a poet Six probably knew not only through books, but also through his family. In Rodenburgh's *Eglentiers poetens borst-weringh* (p. 288), a wedding poem is published on the occasion of the marriage of Hendrik Kemp and Catharina Juliens. The latter is an aunt on Six's mother's side, see Schenkeveld-van der Dussen, 1983, p. 311.

'Moeten dan gedichten iemand zyn *toegewydt* [my italics]' ('Do poems need to be *devoted* to anybody'), reads the opening of 'Toewydinge aan de vreegodinne'. This once again draws attention to the religious foundation of the act of poetic devotion and glorification, and makes the reader wonder whether theriac might have another function than a joking allusion to Ronsard's socio-literary hierarchy. In the seventeenth century, theriac was by no means known as a 'bastard agent'; it was an expensive, exclusive substance. Six does not speak of a theriac from charlatans, but of 'new theriac [...] like the one I trade in daily'. He thus refers to his own experience with the medicine. According to early modern pharmacopoeias, 'new theriac' meant Venetian theriac, a medicine imported from that Italian city, which Six visited on business (Plate 10). It was the most important centre of theriac production during the Renaissance. In classical times, it was a legendary medicine, and in the Renaissance, it was considered the very best of all medicines. Venetian theriac contained 81 ingredients, most of them of exotic origin, including opium, certainly the most psychoactive substance in it.[23] As we have seen, Six himself emphasises what he saw as its mysterious healing properties.[24] The exclusive status of the miracle cure led to cheap forgeries, which were sold by theriac merchants at markets and fairs – the quacks with whom Ronsard compares the rhymester. Theriac is also among the exotic drugs that Johan van Beverwijck discusses in his plea for Dutch medicines (p. 7). In Six's text, theriac does not fare well either. In spite of the exclusive status of the drug, as a poetic source of inspiration it is not sound. The 'strong fermentation' in the body, which 'in no way will be bottled up within me', makes the rhyme 'erupt in order to draw my breath'. The inspiration does not come from outside, as it does in Rodenburgh's 'Celestial breath', but from within, as an internal pressure that results in an 'eruption'. Six also writes that the poems he wrote under the influence of theriac 'bemist' the heavenly throne of Pax as incense, and 'bewaassemen' ('befog') her nostrils.[25]

The terminology is interesting: the concept of 'wasem' ('vapour') appears in early modern medical treatises on the nature of passions, dizziness and drunkenness in the human body. In early modern medicine, these were various forms of

23 Freedman, 2008, p. 68; Beecher, 2002, p. 245; Wennekes, 1996, p. 204. The firm of Six van Chandelier would, as mentioned in Chapter I, probably have imported opium from Bengal.

24 Chapter 4, p. 118. *Cf.* also Donald Beecher, 'Ficino, Theriaca and the Stars', in: Michael J.B. Allen, Valery Rees & Martin Davies (eds.), *Marsilio Ficino: His Theology, His Philosophy, His Legacy*, 2002, pp. 243–256. What is interesting in this context is that Ficino mentions theriac in a chapter (XXI) on 'the Power of Words and Song for Capturing Celestial Benefits and on the Seven Steps That Lead to Celestial Things', pp. 355–361.

25 The Renaissance humanist Ficino described poetic inspiration as a physiological process, but the glowing spirit that would bring a poet into contact with the soul of the world and thus create an ingenious *imaginatio*, is missing from Six's ecstasy. Six's rapture ends in a 'bewaassenen'. I will come back to the concept of fermentation in the next chapter.

'razernij' – a medical term that encompassed various phenomena such as anger, insanity and delight.[26] Johan van Beverwijck explains drunkenness in the section entitled 'Sieckten des Hoofts' ('Illnesses of the Head') of his *Schat der ongesontheyt.*

> One finds also a Frenzy without Fever, to which DRUNKENNESS belongs, and which, like the other types, has its own causes. For as with Fevers where hot Vapour from corrupted Humours rise in the Head, and tangle up Sickly Spirits, in the same way hot Vapours from the Stomach, when filled with Wine or something of the sort are sent to the Head, where they damage the Imagination and the Mind and confuse its Workings.[27]

We also read that the humoral vapours that rise to the brain, 'those from wine drift up there, and cannot escape', cause hallucinations in the drunkard. The passage quoted is about the effect of wine on the human body, but the physician attributes the same effect to different types of drugs: 'seed of hemp', 'fragrant spices', 'nutmegs' and 'tobacco'. 'Opium can do the same', says the doctor.[28] In my opinion, this medical reality lies at the root of the poetic madness in 'Toewydinge aan de vreegodinne'. By means of a self-diagnosis, the druggist thus makes a medical criticism of the concept of heavenly inspiration. The oracular language in his poems is occasioned, not by divine revelation, but by a pathological confusion caused, in turn, by the effect of theriac on his body.

Six as an imitator of Horace

The introduction thus presents Six as a rhymester who does not feel at home in the role of 'poet-priest' for a civil ceremony. Is the series of praise poems intended as a satire on the apotheosis of Frederick Henry as a prince of peace? We can get a better grasp of the matter if we take a quick look at perhaps the most telling Orange hymn

26 Johan van Beverwijck, *Schat der gesontheyt*, 1656, pp. 87–114. See also the description of *Insanae Nuces* ('Mad plums') in Carolus Clusius, *Exoticarum libri decem*, 1605, Chapter 24: see Kaspar van Ommen, *The Exotic World of Carolus Clusius (1526-1609)*, 2009, pp. 59–60.

27 'Men vint oock Rasernye sonder Koortse, waer toe behoort de DRONCKENSCHAP / op de eyghen manier als de andere haren oorspronck nemende. Want gelijck in de Koortschen uyt bedorve Vochtigheden heete Dampen in 't Hooft opvliegen, die de Zielijcke Geesten ontstellen: soo werden oock uyt de Maegh, als sy met Wijn, ofte diergelijcke vervult is, warme Dampen nae 't hooft gesonden, die de Inbeeldinge, en 't Verstant beschadigen en hare Werckinghen verwarren', 'die van de Wijn aldaer op-waessemen, ende niet uyt konnen geraken', p. 88.

28 'Zaet van kennip', 'wel-ruyckende kruyden', 'noten muscaten', 'taback', 'Het selfde kan oock doen opium', *Schat der ongesontheyt*, 1656, p. 29. *Cf.* also Wittewrongel's discussions of different types of 'drunkenness': 1660 II, pp. 1094–1096 and 1105.

in *Vreughde-Zangen*, namely 'Hooghloffelijke gedachtenisse, van Freedrik Henrik, Prince van Oranje' (J215), in which Six invokes the genius of the late Orange Prince. The concept of the imperial cult can readily be found in the text. Not only does Frederick Henry belong to the ancient, noble family of Nassau, which produced an anointed Roman-German emperor (l. 5–8). The Prince of Orange is even portrayed as a synthesis of three imperial giants: Trajan, Julius Caesar and Alexander the Great (l. 9–11). Moreover, as a new Augustus, he introduced a Golden Age, an era of peace and prosperity, and expanded the territory of the Dutch empire (l. 29–31).

However, what arouses our interest is the striking confession of the poet at the beginning of the text: he falls short when it comes to the language of the Parnassus, in which this kind of praise song is written (l. 13–21):

> Maar groote Vorst, o voorste van ons land,
> O Sonne, die van wysheits straalen brandt,
> Wie derft een riet, met swaavelpoêr, bestreeken,
> Om uw wat lichts te geeven, flaauw ontsteeken?
> Myn vleuglen, van wat sacht gegooten was,
> Sien om, bevreest, na Ikars val, en plas,
> En raân niet, met den aarend, snel te steigen,
> Maar langsaam, by den schildpad, my te neigen.
> Myn laage lier onnut tot minnestof,
> Laat, van den luit, den luiden heldenlof
> Gewoon, uw deughd, en daaden oopenbaaren.

> But great Prince, O Prince of our land,
> O Sun, which burns of rays of wisdom,
> Who dares to light a match with sulphur powder,
> To give you a faint illumination?
> My wings, of softly cast wax,
> Remind me anxiously of the fall and crash of Icarus,
> And advise me not to ascend quickly,
> But to stay low along with the turtle.
> My lowly lyre is unsuitable for matters of love,
> Let the lute of someone else – who is
> Used to playing loud hymns to heroes –
> Reveal your virtues and deeds.

Six's poetic pen does not possess enough 'fire' to capture the 'sun' of Frederick Henry in poetry, he confesses; he manages only to light a 'match' to put a faint glare on the prince. His poetic tool is only a 'lowly lyre'. This opening is a show of humility – a common rhetorical gesture in Renaissance literature – but it is also more than that. It also fits Six's conscious self-portrayal as a down-to-earth druggist. One would expect the satirist to accept the consequences of his poetic reflections and to end the poem at the end of the introduction.[29] But he does not. What follows is a description of a hero's lute, adorned with gold and jasper, which Six, according to the text, himself does not have, and which is capable of 'revealing' Frederick Henry's virtues and deeds. Surprisingly enough, this segment makes up the main part of the poem (l. 22–96): The heroic lute brings the goddess Fama to life, we then read, so that she can blow her trumpet, which is adorned with a magnificent banner of the House of Orange and with images of great achievements accomplished under the guidance of Frederick Henry. Fama reminds us of 'staal, en 's Munniks blixemkooren' ('steel [of the sword] and the [accompanying] "choir" of the monk's thundering'), which were shot during large naval battles, and of valuables captured from hijacked Spanish ships: 'suiker, goud, tobak, en koetsjenilje [cochineal]' (l. 29–48).[30] Remembering the deeds of Frederick Henry gives the Dutch new strength, and fortifies them against the dangers to which they were exposed in the First Stadtholderless Period, such as the jealousy that neighbouring countries felt towards Dutch commercial wealth, and potential internal political conflicts (l. 49–96).

Once again, Six's poetry reveals strong contradictions and inconsistencies. This can be explained if we recall that Six's favourite poet was Horace, who also wrote deifying hymns about his political leader, Augustus. In fact, in some of these poems, Horace also operates with a distinction between high-flown and moderate poets – Horace speaks of himself as a poet inspired by wine and not by the water of the springs of the muses – and he also speaks of the necessity of a drunkenness when praising his emperor (see Ode III, 25). These poems have possibly formed a model for Six's *Vreughde-Zangen*. I will discuss these texts in the next chapter. Here, I want to concentrate on the poem with the most relevance for 'Hooghloffelijke gedachtenisse'. The *topos* of the fall of Icarus, which Six makes use of in the foregoing passage, is borrowed from Horace's Pindaric ode (Ode IV, 2).[31] In that poem, a young courtier in Rome asks the poet to write an ode in the style of the Greek poet Pindar, to the return of Augustus from his military campaigns in Spain and Germany, to Rome. The poem includes references to the imperial cult. It celebrates Augustus' return as

29 *Cf.* the abrupt end of Six's ironic praise poem to Queen Christina of Sweden: 'Duitschlands vreede, aan Kristina der Sweeden, Gotten, en Wenden kooninginne' ('Peace of Germany, to Christina, Queen of the Swedes, Goths, and Wends') (J361).

30 By 'monk', Six means Berthold Schwartz, the monk from Freiburg who is said to have invented gunpowder. See the preceding chapter.

31 For the *topos* of the falling Icarus in early modern Dutch literature, *cf.* also Stijn Bussels, 'Theories of the sublime in the Dutch Golden Age. Franciscus Junius, Joost van den Vondel and Petrus Wittewrongel', *History of European Ideas*, 2016, pp. 1–11.

a triumphal procession through the Sacred Hill up to the Capitol, and announces the advent of a Golden Age in the Roman Empire. Horace even outlines how he and the people will greet the emperor with an 'io Triumphe', 'Hail, Victor'. And it ends with the promise of the offering of incense and bulls to the Roman gods. However, Horace does not feel at ease with the request of the courtier. He himself advocates a poetry marked by sobriety and moderation. He therefore responds with a poem in which he argues that he would only fail at this. We read that, when he tries to follow Pindar's lofty verses, he falls, just as Icarus has done (Fig. 7.2). But through the rhetorical device of *praeteritio*, which, as we have seen, means that one says one is keeping mum about something even as one continues to talk about it, the poem shows itself to be a hymn to the divine Roman king: Horace's anti-Pindaric ode is in fact strikingly Pindaric in style and structure.

Six wants to distance himself from the baroque heroic language of the peace celebration, but at the same time he feels it is important to participate in a ceremony for the House of Orange at a time when the power of the Dutch States Party was growing. The basic tone of the other praise poems is not mocking, but sincerely respectful towards Frederick Henry. That said, in these texts, too, we find a number of relativising remarks about the use of glorifying language. In 'Op de komste der Vreegodinne in het Stadhuis' ('On the Arrival of the Goddess of Peace in the Town Hall') (J276), the Calvinist poet even depicts the Town Hall as a heavenly palace: Pax, the goddess of peace, who comes to earth to assist the peace negotiations between Spain and the Republic, was deeply impressed by the new Town Hall: 'ben ik noch by de Goôn?' ('am I still among the Gods?') (l. 4). As we have seen, Six solves the dilemma of the showcasing of the peace celebration in pagan terms by means of *praeteritio*. By describing in detail the 'hero's lute', which does not actually belong to his anti-aristocratic repertoire, Six manages to write a poem of praise for Frederick Henry without having to account for its non-Dutch idiom. He uses a similar strategy in the introduction to the poems of praise. After all, he tells the reader, he was 'drunk' with theriac when he wrote his Orange hymns. Therefore, he cannot be held responsible for the pagan-ecstatic content of the poems.

Deifying the king and queen of Spain

The Treaty of Münster is, at least indirectly, also the theme of another series of poems of praise that Six wrote in the same period: a series of poems to the king and queen of Spain. On 15 November 1649, while on a business trip in Spain, Six witnessed the Triumphal Entry into Madrid of Mariana of Austria, daughter of the German Emperor Ferdinand III. A month earlier, the young Mariana, from the German branch of the Habsburgs, had been married to King Philip IV, who belonged to the Spanish branch of

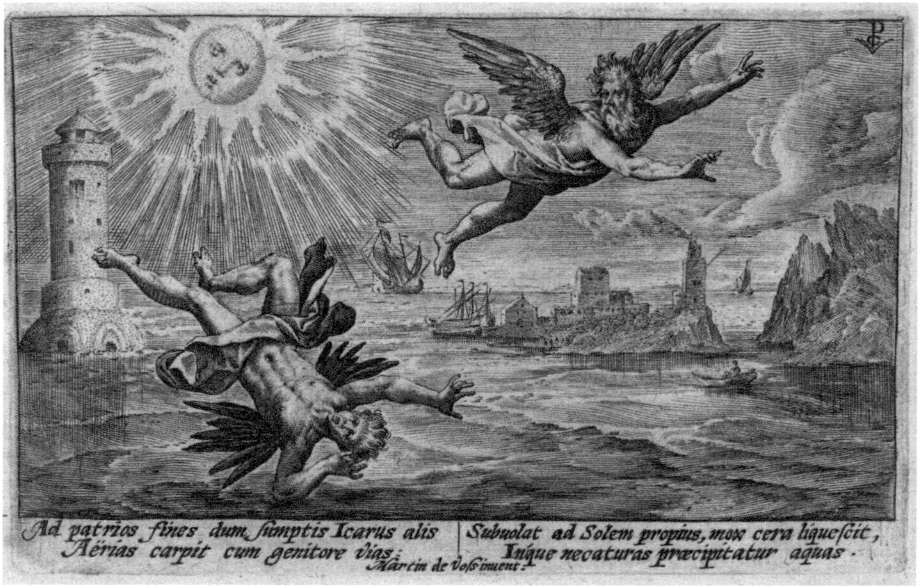
Ad patrios fines dum sumptis Icarus alis
Aërias carpit cum genitore vias.
Subuolat ad Solem propius, mox cera liquescit,
Inque necaturas praecipitatur aquas.
Martin de Vos inuent.

Fig. 7.2: Crispijn van de Passe (I), after Maerten de Vos, *The fall of Icarus*, c. 1602–1607. Engraving. (© Rijksmuseum, Amsterdam).

the family. Mariana was initially engaged to the crown prince of the Spanish Habsburg Empire, Balthasar Charles. When he died in 1646, his father, King Philip IV, took the place of his young son at the altar. Philip's first wife, Queen Isabella, had died two years earlier. The marriage between Philip IV and Mariana was not uncontroversial. Not only was Philip 30 years older than his Austrian bride – he was also her uncle. It was nevertheless carried through, as part of a geopolitical stratagem. The Spanish Empire was in an economic, political and royal crisis. The union of Mariana and Philip IV would increase the power and position of the Spanish and German Habsburgs. The grandeur of the arrival of the 14-year-old queen reflected these great expectations: this was the beginning of a new era for the Spanish Empire. At the same time, Six celebrates Philip IV as one of the architects of the Peace of Münster.

The festivities in Spain also took the form of a Royal Entry: they consisted of theatre spectacles, triumphal arches, and allegorical and mythological displays. The glorification of the royal couple ran like a connecting thread through the spectacle. The king and the queen were portrayed as two celestial bodies that were attracted to each other: Mariana as Aurora, the goddess of the dawn, who gets her light from Philip IV, who was portrayed as the sun god Apollo. The Royal Entry was also celebrated in literature: glorifying praise songs full of biblical and Catholic symbolism, printed in precious decorated books that were published in the same year. An example is *La segunda y esposa Triunfar Muriendo* by Pedro Calderón de la Barca. In this so-called *auto sacramental* (a Spanish allegorical drama genre of the mystery of faith), a spiritual reality is mixed with an earthly political reality: the glorification of the Roman Catholic Eucharist merges with the apotheosis of the royal wedding.[32]

Six's sequence of poems consists of seven texts that were published in *Poësy*. The texts were criticised in the Republic. Six's responses to this criticism were included in the same book. It is therefore possible that the series of poems had been disseminated among Dutch readers at an earlier stage, perhaps in manuscript form or as a pamphlet. I will discuss two poems in this group of texts: 'Blyde inkomste te [Joyous Entry into] Madrid, van Mariana van Oostenryk, kooninglyke bruid van Spanje' (J241) and 'Tempel, aan den kooningh van Spanje' (J246).[33] Other poems in the series, such as 'Vraage, van een Spanjaard, aan den Turkschen ambassadeur, en syne antwoorde' ('Question from a Spaniard to the Turkish Ambassador, and His Answer') (J245) and 'Op de schoonheit van de Kooninginne, aan de selve' ('On the Beauty of the Queen, to the Same Person') (J250), introduce beauty and hubris clearly as themes for the group of texts: the first poem thematises the contrast between the high costs of royal feasts and the high level of taxation in the kingdom, while the second places Mariana with Hera, Athena, and Aphrodite in the beauty contest that led to the Trojan War, thereby insinuating impending political catastrophe for the Spanish Empire. These texts give instructions on how to read the praise poems. The irony and the satirical tone here are more explicit than in the *Vreughde-Zangen*.

'Blyde inkomste te Madrid' brings us back to the Pindaric ode. This time Six himself imitates Pindar, the Greek Poet famous for his odes celebrating Olympic victories. Six could not have chosen a better lyrical form for the Royal Entry. This panegyric genre was reserved for sublime topics, and written for state occasions such as a ruler's accession, wedding, or funeral. In addition, the Greek ode was originally written to be performed by a chorus; the genre therefore has a triadic form: it consists of a strophe, followed by an anti-strophe and an epode. This was perfectly

32 For the Royal Entry of Mariana and Philip in Spain, C. Justi, *Diego Velazquez und sein Jahrhundert*, 1933, pp. 664–667, and especially Rina Walthaus, 'The Sun and Aurora: Philip IV of Spain and his Queen-Consort in Royal Festival and Spectacle', in: Martin Gosman, Alasdair MacDonald & Arno Vanderjagt (eds.), *Princes and Princely Culture 1450-1650*, part 2, 2005, pp. 277–308: Moreover, Walthaus, devotes space both to the *Noticia del recibimiento i entrada de la Reyne nvestra Señora*, the official report of the festivities, and to the aforementioned work of Calderón. 'No costs were spared to give evidence of [the] wealth and power that it [the Spanish kingdom] no longer possessed', says Walthaus, p. 307.

33 The other five poems written for the event and published in *Poësy*, are: 'Vraage, van een Spanjaard, aan den Turkschen ambassadeur, en syne antwoorde' ('Question, from a Spaniard, to the Turkish Ambassador, and His Answer') (J245), 'Opdracht van den tempel, aan den Kooningh van Spanje' ('Dedication of [my poem] "the Temple" to the King of Spain') (J247), 'Op d'aanstaande wandelinge van de kooninginne, na Casa del Campo, of het landhuis' ('On the Upcoming Walk of the Queen to Casa del Campo, or the Country House') (J248), 'Spanjes Heerschappye, afgebeeldt aan een der triumfboogen' ('The Reign of Spain, Depicted on one of the Triumphal Arches') (J249) and 'Op de schoonheit van de Kooninginne, aan de selve' ('On the Beauty of the Queen, to the Same Person') (J250).

suited to a state occasion in the form of a pagan procession. This choral structure is the basis of more than just 'Blyde inkomste te Madrid': Six also refers to choral performances in other texts in the series of poems. The theme of 'Blyde inkomste te Madrid' is how to approach a member of the royalty, or even a divine person, in this case the goddess of the dawn. Here Six offers the following instructions to the Spanish 'princes and princesses' present at the ceremony (l. 20–21): 'Versuim geen mirt, noch laaten roosenhoed, / Kroon Venus, strooi haar kruiden, onder voet' ('Do not leave out myrtle, or roses that are late for the season; crown Venus, and sprinkle spices at her feet'). At the same time, Six warns the earthly worshippers not to make direct eye contact with the 'Heemlsche Godin' (l. 9). His message here is that invoking a deity is possible only through a ritualised form of rapprochement.[34] The idea of enchanting eyes, the so-called 'fascie', is well known in the literature of the antiquity and the Renaissance. It was also part of the so-called imperial cult.[35]

Six includes himself among the characters in the poem: he steps forward among the worshippers. Through his words, the text appears as an altar, 'a middle wall', upon which the Dutch poet offers his own sacrifice to the sacred Mariana (l. 29–40):

Wat vordert al de sienelyke pracht,
Van u, zoo duur, en kostelyk betracht,
Misgunt het hart oprechtiger kleinooden?
Geen gulde glans, die Ofir geeft te vracht,
Noch mirr, noch rook van Arabiers gebracht,
Maar zielgom smaakt, op 't outer, aan de grooten.
Maar zoo de gloor, van uiterlyke gift,
Een teiken is van waarlike van binne,
Laat dat, als goud, van valsicheit geschift,
Klaar blinken, in myn kerkelyk gestift.

34 For an introduction of the Pindaric ode in Dutch Renaissance literature, see René Veenman, 'De Thebaensche Swaen. De receptie van Pindarus in de Nederlanden', *Voortgang. Jaarboek voor de Neerlandistiek XIII*, 1992, pp. 65–90: The Greek *encomium* (praise poem) was originally a choral song in honour of a hero or conqueror, which was performed during the round of honour at the end of the games or at the homecoming of a victorious player. This function is included in the odes of Pindar: see H. van Gorp, D. Delabastita and R. Ghesquiere: *Lexicon van literaire termen*, 2007, p. 14. For the Pindaric ode and the concept of poetic frenzy in Six's poetry, see also Chapter 8.

35 Compare the Roman historian Gaius Suetonius Tranquillus's description of the face of the Emperor Augustus in 'The Life of Augustus', 79, in: C. Suetonius Tranquillus, *The Lives of the Twelve Caesars*, 1913, p. 246. For the Roman imperial cult and its significance for the idea of divine kingship in the Renaissance, see Sergio Bertelli, *The King's Body: Sacred Rituals of Power in Medieval and Early Modern Europe*, 2001, pp. 10–34. *Cf.* the description of how the Spanish king is protected from the eyes of people, Ebben, 2005, p. 231. And *cf.* also 'Las Meninas' (1656) of Diego Velázquez, where the spectators do not look directly at the Spanish king and queen, but observe them through a mirror.

Aanbid aldaar uw Ryksgod, en Godinne,
Uw Kooningh, met syn groote Kooninginne.

What good is all this visible splendour
In your possession, so expensive and dearly pursued,
Does the heart reject more honest gems?
No shiny gold that Ofir brings to us,
Nor myrrh, nor incense from Arabians,
But the soul's gum pleases the great when laid on the altar.
But if the splendour of outward gifts
Is a sign of truthful inwardness,
Let it, like gold, purified of falsity,
Sparkle clearly in my church,
Worship there your Kingdom's God and Goddess,
Your King with his great Queen.

Six admits he could place 'gold from Ofir', myrrh and 'incense from Arabians', that is, frankincense, on his altar to the queen (l. 32–33): the three gifts that the three Magi from the East gave to the Infant Jesus, and the spiritual meaning that was attributed to them by the Church Fathers. Frankincense was a symbol of divine status. The apotheosis of Mariana would then become a foreshadowing of Christ. But in the following lines, he rejects the idea – gold and incense are but external, superficial sacrifices, the poet explains. He offers instead his odourless soul, his soul's 'gum resin' ('zielgom') as he calls it (l. 34).[36] Another modification follows: if outer beauty is a sign of selfless devotion, his sacrificial gifts may still shine on his literary altar to the Spanish goddess (l. 35–40).

What, then, is the significance of the poem? First, we note how Six contrasts inner and outward worship, which reassures the reader that he, as a Protestant, can take part in a quasi-religious event in a Catholic country without its infringing on his own faith – a line of argument that his Calvinist pastors back at home would hardly have accepted! Further, there is a curious material aspect to the poem: in offering his own luxury goods – incense and myrrh – to the queen, Six shows how taken he is with the spectacle. The exotic-spiritual vocabulary not only reflects Maria's exalted status – it is also part of the creation of this identity. The political and religious power of the princes is thus legitimised by the spiritual exotica in Six's apothecary. Six emerges as one of the Magi of the East contributing to a miracle – the apotheosis of a human being. The tone is, of course, ironic. It is only natural to read the poem as a satire on the Royal Entry.

36 'Gum' originally means odourless substances, *cf.* the fourth secondary meaning of 'gom' in the WNT.

Temple to King Philip IV

'Tempel, aan den kooningh van Spanje' (J246) follows the same structure – the poet includes himself among the characters of the poem: he takes the role of a poet-priest in a political-religious cult – this time in a temple devoted to King Philip IV. The poem to the Queen bride had the form of an *ekphrasis,* a vivid description of a scene or a work of art – in this case, a depiction of the altar to the Queen of Spain. This is even truer of Six's poem to the king; the poem is a description of a temple made for the king. But it is a literary temple: Six sees his poem as a contrast to the ephemeral ornaments of the spectacle, such as the triumphal arches raised for the Joyous Entry, and also as a contrast to the imperial cult of Ancient Rome, all of which are forgotten today. He says he will therefore 'een tempel van onsterflike gedichten, / Ter eer van Spanjes Vreegod stichten' ('found a temple of immortal poems, / in honour of Spain's God of Peace') (l. 65–66).

Nonetheless, Six incorporates elements from both the Joyous Entry and, especially, the Royal cult into the text: there are in fact more similarities between the cultic decorations of the Oranjezaal and this poem than in *Vreughde-Zangen*. Philip IV is 'een God' whose 'heiligh haar' ('sacred locks') outshine 'sonnestralen' ('the rays of the sun') (l. 15–18). He is thus the sun god Apollo. We are told that his virtues outweigh all the silver the Spaniards get from the silver mines in Peru (l. 23–28), in a comparison that we can only take ironically.[37] The Spanish monarch rides like a 'laurelled Augustus' (l. 37) into Madrid, Six writes. We then read about the four 'gold seegeboogen' ('golden triumphal arches') (l. 32) that were set up before the Royal Entry. Six is at pains to tell us that each one cost 38,000 reals (l. 64).[38] The fireworks that were set off during the Entry make Jupiter and Juno so enthusiastic that they even leave their 'gestarnte throonen' ('starry thrones') to take part in the party (l. 40–44): Here again, Six takes part in a ritual of worship in expressing the following wishes (l. 117–132):

Dat ik, als Priester, voor het outer, d'eerste reijen,
  Aan Eeuwigheit gewydt, mach leijen.
Dan zal ik, met de schaar van Kastals Sanggodinnen,
  Aldus een jaarliks lied beginnen.
Apollo groote God, en Vaader der gesangen,
  Door wiens genaa dit aangevangen,

37 Here Six could mean the so-called 'black legend' to which he refers more explicitly in another poem; see for example 'Op het koopergeld in Spanje' ('About the Copper Money in Spain') (J35). For the 'black legend', see Frijhoff & Spies, 2004, pp. 37–38.

38 Because of the high costs, the city of Madrid first planned to cut the number of triumphal arches to three: Walthaus, 2005, p. 300.

En uitgewrocht, ghy die gedichten geeft het leeven,
Wilt myn gedicht dat eeuwigh geeven.
Gun dat die Kooningin, naast haar onwinbren Kooningh,
Vereeuwe, met dees heilge wooningh.
Gun dat de Spaansche jeuchd, en jonglingen, en maagen,
Hier, alle jaaren, offer draagen.
Niet uit Faliskus wei, met witte, en gulde stieren,
Maar dat se, met myn lofsangh, vieren.
Uw heiligh outer zal ik, met een hals, berooken,
Die, onder 't juk, nooit heeft gedooken.

That I, as a Priest before the altar, may lead
The first choir songs, devoted to Eternity,
Then I shall, with the crowd of Castalian Muses,
Begin a secular hymn in this way:
Apollo, great God and Father of the songs,
By whose grace this song has begun
And been completed, you who give life to poems,
Would you give my poem that eternal life.
Grant that the Queen, with her invincible King,
May live forever in this sacred house.
Grant that the Spanish youth, and youngsters and virgins
Always come and offer sacrifices,
Not from Ager Falisus, white and golden oxen,
But grant that they add lustre to the ceremony with my hymn:
Your holy altar, I shall then incense
With a neck that never has bowed under the yoke.

The role that the druggist-poet assigns himself is far from modest. He presents himself as a high priest in his own temple, dedicated to Philip. He is also the cantor of the muses singing in a choir on Parnassus (the Muses of the Castalian Spring at Delphi), and of a choir of Spanish youngsters and virgins. And in that capacity he turns to Apollo, the god of poetry, and asks him to give eternal life to their 'secular hymn' and their 'hymns' about the royal couple. Then, this time as a priest offering a sacrifice, he consecrates the altar of his temple, not with a burnt offering of 'white, and gilded bulls', but with his 'neck' (thus his throat) – that is, with an offering in the form of a song: this hymn, which manifests itself as incense in the temple. But although he acts as the chief priest of this cult, Six emphasises that he has never been subject to Spanish rule. In conclusion, as a sign of divine legitimation, he reports that Apollo is pleased with the poem and that the other gods will find his literary temple worthy of entry (l. 137–138): 'My dunkt dat self Jupyn, en zoo veel Heemelgooden, / Sich eeven gunstigh laaten nooden' ('I think that even Jupiter, and also many Celestial Gods, would happily let themselves be invited [to the temple]').

'Tempel, aan den kooningh van Spanje' is a typically Sixian text, full of paradoxes and irony. The down-to-earth Dutch rhymester once again uses big words. Although Six's temple is a construction made only of words, the poet is not modest when it comes to its size and proportions. The similarities with the Roman imperial cult give further indications about the meaning of the text. First, Six's temple of peace evokes associations with the altar erected to Augustus in Rome, *Ara Pacis Augustae*, the monument to peace with Spain and Gaul mentioned at the beginning of this chapter. Second, as Jacobs notes, there is a remarkably high number of similarities between this poem and Horace's most important ode to Augustus, the *carmen saeculare* ('Hymn for a New Age').[39] For this glorification of the Roman Pantheon Horace was rewarded by his patron, the emperor, with the honorary title *poeta laureatus*. Six implies that he will receive the same title from the Spanish Augustus, Philip IV. While Horace, as the cantor of a chorus of Roman virgins and youngsters, sings of the deities of light, Apollo and Diana, and thanks the gods for peace and prosperity in the Roman Empire, Six leads a choir of Spanish 'youngsters and virgins', portrays Philip IV and Mariana as gods of light, and praises the peace and prosperity that obtain in the Spanish Empire.[40]

The problem of approaching a royal person is a theme in this poem, too. This is articulated already at the beginning (l. 1–6):

Och! dat die swaare straf, van 't al te trotse Babel,
    Myn tongh nu snoert, als met een kaabel,
En dat myn sanghgodin haar toegeneege luiten,
    Geensins op eedel Spaansch kan uiten.
Nochtans, o Klio, doe myn geest ten Heemel vaaren,
    Op luide Neederduitsche snaaren.

Oh, [how sad] that the heavy punishment of the all too proud [tower of] Babel,
Now twists my tongue, as with a cable,
And [how sad] that my muse
Cannot in any way utter her beloved lyre songs in noble Spanish.
Nevertheless, O Clio, let my spirit ascend to Heaven,
On loud Dutch strings.

39 Jacobs, 1991 II, p. 449.

40 *Cf.* also the poems Virgil (*Georgics*, 3.10–39) and Ovid (*Tristia* 4.2) wrote to imaginary Roman Triumphs. These poems also have some resemblance to the poem of Six.

Even though he feels as if his mouth is bound with rope, because of the fall of the Tower of Babel, he will try to write a poem in a 'noble Spanish manner', as he calls it. The reference to the 'overly proud Babel' not only indicates his disappointment at his lack of knowledge of Spanish and the need to use his own mother tongue. It also refers to a Babylonian hubris, thus making clear that his pagan temple to the Spanish king and queen violates Christian values such as modesty and sincerity.

How, then, can he make a poetic leap so that Clio, the muse of history, can make his 'spirit fly to heaven'? Six continues (l. 59–60): '[Ik] Wil eene kleine straal van varsche sucht doen blinken, / Die my d'olyfboom gaf te drinken' ('I will make a small spout of fresh juice glitter, which the olive tree gave me to drink').[41] Oil from an olive tree will give him divine inspiration and bring him into a state of *furor poeticus* – poetic frenzy. Six is probably referring to the ornaments of the spectacle: along the route, the royal newly-weds passed an artificial Parnassus, which was decorated with statues of the nine muses, Pegasus, and nine Spanish poets, and which was placed beneath an artificial olive tree, the *fuentes del olive*.[42] Six tells us, then, that his temple will contain 'een altaar van olistammen / Na 's Kooninghs vreedsaam hart gehouwen' ('an altar of olive trunks, carved into the shape of the peaceful heart of the King') (l. 89–90). Both the olive tree and the description of the king of Spain as Prince of Peace point to the Peace of Münster, which was agreed the year before the royal wedding, and which made it possible for Six to travel to Spain as a merchant, as Six emphasises in his poem (l. 57–58). Besides the olive tree as an iconographic symbol, Six addresses the materiality of the olive oil: he says he will drink directly from the peace symbol to get into a poetic rapture. This sounds strange to us today, but the cultural history of oil reveals that the liquid we now regard only as everyday cooking oil had a broader and more elevated set of uses in earlier times. Olive oil was used in oil lamps, as a sacrifice and as a raw material for perfumes. In the book of Exodus, God orders the high priest Aaron to include olive oil in a holy ointment for anointing the tabernacle and other sacred things. It was also widely used in early modern medicine.[43]

In 'Blyde inkomste te Madrid', Six spoke of gold, myrrh and incense, and here he speaks of oil – also an article that belonged to the pharmaceutical commodities of the early modern merchant-druggist. He introduces this product both as a

41 'Sucht' can also be translated with 'sigh', then as a metaphor the sound of dripping oil, or with 'desire', then pointing to the *furor poeticus* of the poet. I have translated 'sucht' with 'juice' as in 'watersucht', 'juice tapped from a tree', see 'watersucht, definition 4 in WNT.

42 For a description of this Parnassus, see 'Opdracht van den tempel' (J247).

43 Exodus 30:24. See also Rembertus Dodonaeus, *Cruydt-boeck*, 1644, pp. 1287–1289; and the English translation of Pierre Pomet, *Histoire générale des drogues* (1694): *A Compleat History of Druggs*, London 1737, pp. 156–157.

means of poetic inspiration and as a divine gift to the king. He portrays himself as a poet-priest who, by means of sacramental oil and incense, turns a civic festivity into an ecclesiastical ceremony, thereby endowing the new political leadership of Spain with a theological foundation.

The ironic tone is more pronounced here than it is in the poem to the Austrian bride. Six associates the turgid pretensions of the wedding celebration with the 'overly proud Babel'. In 'Tempel', more so than in 'Blyde inkomste te Madrid', he describes the wedding as a pagan ritual. We could simply read the poems as satires written by a Calvinist on the pathos of Catholic Spain, but things are in fact a bit more complex than that. As we have seen, Six is not only a satirist, but he presents himself as the supplier of materials for the pagan ceremony. He is even tempted to consume some of the luxury goods himself. An interesting question is whether Six, as a merchant in fragrances and oils himself, was involved in the city celebrations he describes in his poems.[44] Incense was a commodity that Dutch merchants bought in the Arabian Peninsula, brought to Europe, and sold to the Roman Catholic Church among others. We know that Six did at least travel to Spain to trade in olive oil. It was an important component in the production, in which Six was involved, of 'Spaense zeep' ('Spanish soap') in Amsterdam.[45] Six tells us, in 'Tempel, aan den kooningh van Spanje', that he was even among the first Dutch merchants to take advantage of the peace treaty between the Republic and Spain by seeking out the Spanish market (l. 57–58). These poems must surely have been relevant to the self-image of a merchant-druggist and importer of tempting exotic goods. I will come back to this presently.

'The goddess of France'

Six's 'Spanish eulogies' were the object of critical remarks by contemporary Dutch readers – none of whom are known to us today – but it is clear from his 'Verklaaringe teegen arghwaan, oover myn dicht ter eere van den kooningh van Spanje' ('Clarification [that Defends Me] against Mistrust of My Poem in Honour of the King of Spain') (J75) that his poems aroused suspicion in the Netherlands. The critic, or critics, blame him for bowing down to the Spanish monarchy. Six responds in

44 Spanish and Portuguese kings bought materials for their civil ceremonies and celebrations from Dutch merchants travelling in the Iberian Peninsula. See Tamar Cholcman, 'The Merchant Voice: International Interests and Strategies in Local *Joyeuses entrées*. The Case of Portuguese, English, and Flemish Merchants in Antwerp (1599) and Lisbon (1619)', *Dutch Crossing*, 2011, pp. 39–62.

45 When Six, in 'Brief aan myne Moeder' ('Letter to my Mother') (J454), talks about materials that a certain Nicolas Follin, has stolen from their company, he mentions, among other things, 'boomoli' (l. 28), *i.e.* olive oil.

'Verklaaringe teegen arghwaan' with a rhetorical question – why should his poetic quill not become 'geMadrilleest' (l. 7), that is 'Hispanicised', when Caspar Barlaeus comes across as 'Frans gezint', 'French-minded' (l. 8) in a series of panegyrics that he wrote to the French Queen Maria de' Medici?

Six is referring here to Caspar Barlaeus's *Medicea Hospes*, which celebrated the Royal Entry of the French Queen Maria de' Medici to Amsterdam in 1638. *Medicea Hospes* appeared in book form the following year, 1639 – thus almost 10 years before Six wrote his own poems.[46] His mention of Barlaeus's 'French' poem is no coincidence. In the literary criticism, *Medicea Hospes* is described as introducing a new artistic phenomenon to the Republic. This is D.P. Snoep's characterisation of the work:

> The book is considered the first official account of a Royal Entry held in the Netherlands. In this respect, the city took over a tradition from the south [the Spanish Netherlands], where city councils used to issue commissions for luxury editions of this kind in the mid-16th century.[47]

We are thus talking about the new mythological-allegorical style in the literature and art of the Dutch Republic: Royal Entries and the literary eulogies accompanying them – a phenomenon which had its origin in countries to the south of the Republic. Six says Barlaeus's work was Francophile.[48] The ideas for the Royal Entry in Amsterdam were the same as for that in Madrid. The link between political power, divinity and exotic materials is in fact also conspicuous in Barlaeus's text: during her visit to Amsterdam, the queen had been honoured as Cybele, the mother of the gods, and invited to the East India House for a banquet consisting of all kinds of exotica: drugs, spices, incense, dyes, and even saltpetre, the main ingredient in gunpowder (Fig. 7.3). In Vondel's translation, Barlaeus takes the view that these exotics were 'not only delicious for the tongue, but also fragrant, and pleasing to the eye':

> Here there was not such tastiness; but the fruits and plants of the Persians, Arabians, Moluccans, Japanese, and Chinese, served in large porcelain serving

46 Caspar Barlaeus's *Medicea Hospes* appeared in an exclusive, richly illustrated folio edition in which his New Latin original was printed along with French and Dutch translations (the latter was written by Vondel – *Blyde inkomst der allerdoorluchtighste koninginne, Maria de Medicis, t'Amsterdam*). Barlaeus received 1,000 guilders from the city authorities for his panegyric, see Snoep, 1975, pp. 39–76.

47 Snoep, 1975, pp. 41 and 42.

48 The Oranjezaal of Huis ten Bosch can also be called 'francophile', because Amalia of Solms-Braunfels was, when planning the ornaments, inspired by Rubens's decoration of the gallery of Luxembourg Palace, designed by Maria de' Medici. See Elmer Kolfin, 'Amalia's ambities. Een vorstenzaal voor de stadhouder', in: Magriet van Eikema Hommes & Elmer Kolfin, *De Oranjezaal in Huis Bosch. Een zaal uit louter liefde*, 2013, pp. 63–115.

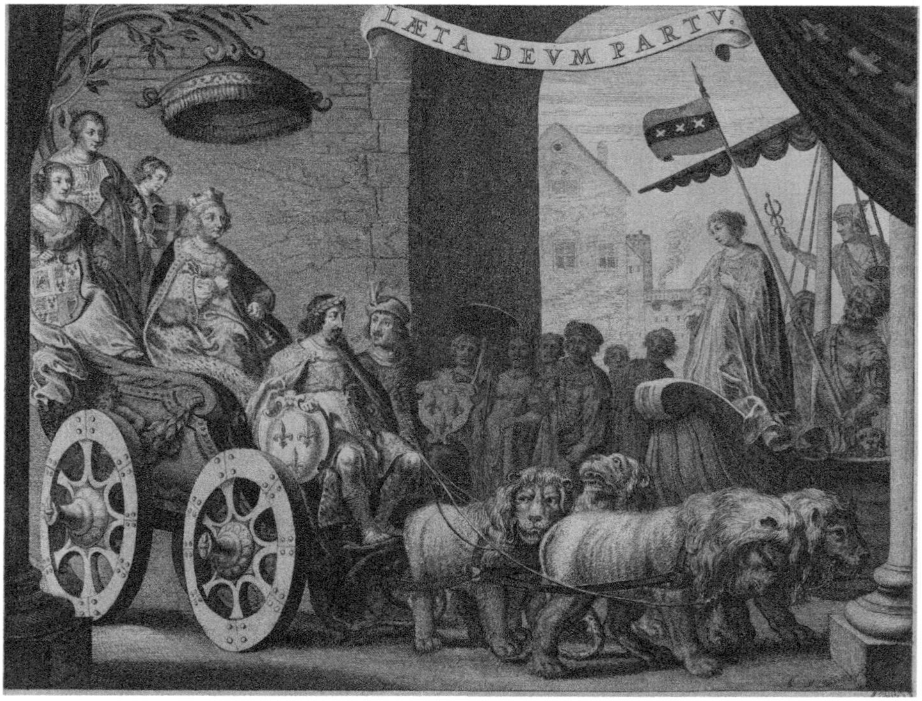

Fig. 7.3: Pieter Nolpe, after Claes Moeyaert, *Maria de' Medici as Cybele*, 1638. Engraving. (© Rijksmuseum, Amsterdam).

basins, arranged on a long table, the strangeness [vreemdigheid] of which delighted the Queen [...] The whiteness of the borax struck the eyes; the scent and smell of benzoin, the nose. Musk, styrax, sandalwood, indigo, and many other pigments lay in special saucers. This feast for the eyes also contained dragon's blood and cakes of mace resin, and gutta gamba as yellow as gold, which shone among the other dishes. Incense and myrrh from Saba, once used by pagans as sacrifices to their gods, served here as incense offerings to the Goddess of France. Cubeba, rhubarb, sugar, saltpetre, from which dreadful gunpowder is made, all lay in their places. She was even served lacquer, and wax that is made by bees, precious oils of macis, nutmegs, and candied and ordinary ginger.[49]

49 'Niet [alleen] tot leckerny voor de tong, maer oock welrieckende, en aengenaem in 't oog [...] Hier waren zulcke leckernyen niet; maer de vruchten en 't gewas van Persiaenen, Arabiers, Molucken, Iaponesen, en Chineesen, aengerecht in groote en ruime porceleine lampetschotels, die, op een lange tafel in orden gestelt, om haer vreemdigheid, de Koningin vermaeckten [...] De Borax bekoorde de oogen door haer wittigheid, en de Benzoin den neus door zijnen reuck en geur. Muskeliaet, Styrax, sandelhout, indigo, en meer andere verwen lagen in byzondere schotels. Oock was 'er, onder dit ooghbancket, Draeckenbloed, en koecxkens uit sap van foeli, en Gutta Gamba, zoo geel als goud, uitmuntende onder de andere gerechten. Het wieroock, en de Myrrhe van Saba, eertijds van de Heidenen den Goden geoffert, dienden hier voor reuckoffer aen de Godin van Vranckrijck. Cubeba, Rhabarber, suicker, en salpeter, waer van men het

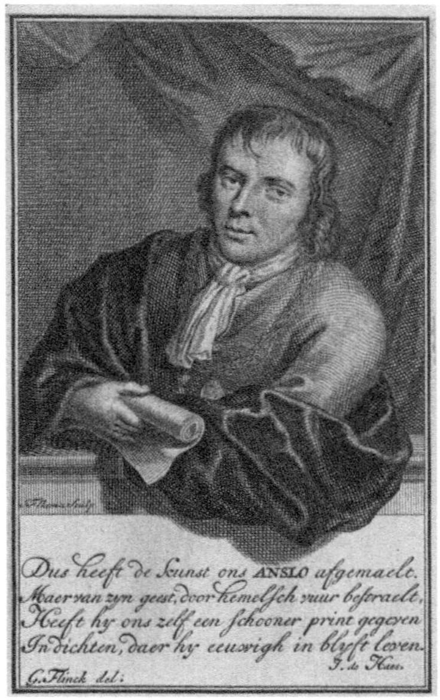
Dus heeft de kunst ons ANSLO afgemaelt.
Maer van zyn geest, door hemelsch vuur bestraelt,
Heeft hy ons zelf een schooner print gegeven
In dichten, daer hy eeuwigh in blyft leven.
G. Flinck del:

Fig. 7.4: Jacob Folkema, after Govert Flinck, *Portrait of Reyer Anslo*, 1713. Engraving. (© Rijksmuseum, Amsterdam).

The diversity of sensory impressions puts the queen into an ecstatic state. The text concludes with her imagining that she is a guest at a banquet in an exotic land. The exotica are thus a further sign of her divine status, and legitimise her political power. Obviously, Barlaeus recognised the moral problem entailed by the deification of a mortal person, because in the introduction to *Medicea Hospes*, he argues for using the concept of a royal cult, in part by pointing to the long traditions of divine kingship in European and other cultures: 'The knowledge of these things is deeply rooted in the minds of mankind.'[50]

That Six is ridiculing trends within the culture of the Republic becomes clear from texts by fellow poets of his who wrote in the Parnassian style. There are interesting similarities between Six's panegyric to the Spanish king and other Dutch praise poems addressed to royal persons. One poem that stands out in this regard is 'Zegetempel voor zyn Hoogheidt Fredrik Henrik, prince van Oranje. Toegewijdt den Heere P.C. Hooft' ('Temple of Victory, for his Highness Frederick Henry, Prince of Orange. Dedicated to the Lord P.C. Hooft' (1645) by Reyer Anslo, a literary disciple of

ysselijck bussekruid maeckt, lagen elck op hunne plaets. Oock diende men haer voor lack, en wasch dat van de byen komt, kostelijcken oly van macis, noten muscaten, en gekonfijte en ongekonfijte gengber', in: J.F.M. Sterck *et al.* (eds.), *De werken van Vondel*, vol. 3, 1929, pp. 629 and 630.

50 'De kennis van deze dingen zit diep in der menschen gemoeden', Caspar Barlaeus, *Blyde inkomst der allerdoorluchtighste koninginne, Maria de Medicis, t'Amsterdam*, 1639. 'Toe-eigeninge', un-paged.

Vondel (Fig. 7.4).[51] First, Anslo composes his poem as a literary temple. Anslo writes that this temple should be erected next to Muiderslot, the castle of P.C. Hooft, to whom the poem is dedicated. There, he says, the Dutch can worship the Prince of Orange as a god of peace and celebrate his heroic deeds, just as Anslo himself does in his poem. This temple was, of course, never built. It was a literary sanctuary. Second, such concepts as 'sacred altars', 'smell of incense' and 'sacrificial fire' occupy a central place in the text. They give the poem the necessary air of solemnity. The following lines, addressed to the god Mars, illustrate the tone of the praise poem:[52]

Ey gun, dat wy, eer Fredrik by den Goôn
Is in't gesternte onsterflijk opgevaren,
Oprechten, tot zijn eer, een Zegekerk;
En Koren van triumph, en dankaltaren,
En wierookreuk, en heilig offerwerk.

Oh, grant that we, before Frederick
Immortally ascends to the Gods among the stars,
May establish a Victory Church in his honour;
With Choirs of triumph, and altars of gratitude,
And the smell of incense and holy sacrifice.

The conclusion is clear: both of these 'Spanish hymns' show marked features of the language of the high Parnassus. In 'Verklaaringe teegen arghwaan', Six, picks up where earlier critics of Renaissance poetics, such as D.V. Coornhert, left off, and further develops the satirical function of his poems to the Spanish king and queen. We should read the series of poems, not just as satires on the spectacles in Madrid but, taken together, as a critical commentary on the exotic-ornamental language of poets such as Barlaeus, Vondel and Anslo. In Six's view, their poems represent what Coornhert had called a 'pronckelyc' ('flaunting') style incompatible with Dutch and Christian values.[53]

But my comparison also highlights differences that take us deeper into our analysis. Six uses this series of poems to portray himself as a druggist-poet. First, while Barlaeus and Anslo do not thematise their personae in their texts, Six not only explicitly portrays himself as a poet-priest in his poems – he also highlights his role as a druggist. Second, he stages the impact of the literary cosmetics on his own body. We saw the same techniques at work in *Vreughde-Zangen*, but in

51 M.A. Schenkeveld-van der Dussen (2007, pp. 59–60) has pointed to parallels between the poems.

52 R. Ansloo, *Poëzy*, 1713, pp. 175–181, quote on p. 176.

53 Coornhert, *Het roerspel en de comedies van Coornhert* (*The tragedy and the Comedies of Coornhert*), p. 156. For Coornhert's view on poetry, see the introduction.

Six's hymns to the Spanish king and queen, he dramatises to a greater extent his own role as an inspired poet at the ceremony. As we saw, his drinking of olive oil, the peace symbol of the Spanish king, brought Six into a state of frenzy. The change he experiences, however, is presented not as a divine transformation, but as a physical disturbance: his tongue twists when he sings in a Spanish manner. Six further describes the experience as psychologically delusional, paranoiac and megalomaniacal. He is, in a sense, diagnosing the Parnassian language.

According to the theory of humours, emotions were considered to be, not just psychological quantities, but also physical parts of the body, and, according to the concept of geohumoralism, emotional differences could be associated with different 'ethnic' identities. It therefore makes sense to consider the new baroque style in the Republic as both a social and a medical threat to Six's national identity. Barlaeus became 'French' by writing his eulogies to Maria de' Medici. Six argues that he would become 'Spanish' if his eulogies were meant seriously. This emphasis on an emotional-somatic basis for ethnic identities is confirmed if we look at other poems by Six where the physical reactions to an artistic style that he identifies as 'Spanish' are addressed. In the aforementioned 'Vraage, van een Spanjaard', Six points to 'dat eigen kittlende gemoed / Gebooren, in Kastiljes bloed' ('that self-caressing nature that inhabits Castilian blood') (l. 1–2). And there is actually one other poem in *Poësy* that addresses responses from Dutch readers to Six's 'Spanish hymns': 'Aan Pieter Klaaver' (J74). Here Six addresses what he sees as a rather different but equally misguided response to his ironic praise of Philip IV. In the poem, he rebukes a certain Pieter Klaaver for not only missing the irony in the poem, but actually praising its lofty tone. The exalted style of Six's poems to the Spanish king and queen are described as a physical disturbance. Six insists that his eulogies hurt his own 'needrige ooren' ('humble ears') (l. 11). 'Men kitt'le kitt'ligen, men pluimstryk Spaansche Gooden' ('One may caress the ones who like to be caressed, one may flatter Spanish Gods') (l. 12). Other poets may flatter those who like to be flattered. Six does indeed write about others, but he assures us that his humble Dutch ears make him immune to Spanish flattery. The attribution of exaggeration and paranoia to the Spanish was not an invention of Six's, but was quite common in Western European Protestant culture. According to early modern medical theories, paranoia and megalomania were widespread among Spaniards.[54]

54 For Dutch perceptions of Spaniards, see Marijke Meijer Drees, *Andere landen, andere mensen: De beeldvorming van Holland versus Spanje en Engeland omstreeks 1650*, 1997, pp. 79–99 and 106–114; Frijhoff & Spies, 2004, pp. 36–39: For an example, see the anonymous work *Wegh-wyser, ofte reysbeschryving* [...] *door de Konincrijcken van Spanjen en Portugael* [...] (1659): 'Van haer [the Spaniards] zijn de groote eer-namen, de manieren van pluymstrijcken, hooghdravende Ceremonien, en dierghelijcke rancken meer voortghekomen. al hun doen is maer op een uytterlijcke schijn en pracht ghestelt: hooren haer selfs gaerne prysen, en beelden sich ick weet niet wat voor grote dinghen, waer door sy in overmoedt Rodomantadas en opsnyery vervallen' ('From them [the Spanish] originate the grand titles, the way of toadyism, pompous

Although these sentiments are not explicitly expressed in the poems discussed in this chapter, it is natural to link them not only to the hot climate of Spain, but also to the use of drugs among Spaniards. From 'Uitroep om hoornafsetters', 'Op het blanketten van 't vrouwvolk in Spanje', and 'Afbeeldinge en wydinge van Roselle' (in which Six was also in Spain) – poems I discussed in earlier chapters – readers may recall the idea of drugs as contaminating cosmetics. In these texts, Six points specifically to the threat that the drugs referred to there represent to the human body. The same goes for the pharmaceutical ornaments in Six's poems to Philip IV and Mariana. The anti-cosmetic argument central to Farah Karim-Cooper's study is relevant here. Adam, the first man, was created in God's image; this 'beautiful panel' of God – as the human body is called in 'Afbeeldinge en wydinge van Roselle', VIII (J48) (l. 14) – is presented as sacred and inviolable. This argument is reflected in a well-known passage from the Bible in which the human body is also presented as a work of art and the *temple* of the Holy Spirit. Petrus Wittewrongel explained this passage as follows: 'Our Bodies, which are the Temples of the Holy Spirit (1. Cor. 6:19) may not be contaminated with it. We think particularly of that odious adornment through which people even try to improve the work of their God.'[55] In much the same way, Six's 'Spanish hymns' are based on a scepticism towards cosmetics as physically transformative, and on the idea of the druggist-poet as a creator of a perfect and divine world that is an offence to God's image. The choice between an inner and an outward sacrifice in 'Afbeeldinge en wydinge van Roselle' – the pure heart of the poet, as against luxury adornments – is analogous to Six's choice between the 'gum resin' of his soul and Arabic incense in 'Blyde inkomste te Madrid'. In both texts, Six chooses wrongly, thus making clear that he is aware of the sinful character of his act. And it is also possible that the temple Six erects to honour Philip IV and on which he

ceremonies, and suchlike affected manners. All their doing is aimed at outward appearance and splendour. They like to hear praise about themselves, and imagine themselves I do not know what for great things, through which they fall into the overconfidence of Rodomonte and bragging.'). Rodomantadas refers to Rodomonte, the arrogant and boastful king of the Saracens in Ariosto's *Orlando furioso.* Quotation from: Meijer Drees 1997, p. 108. It is important in this context, however, to underline that 'Spanish' also evoked positive connotations in the Dutch Republic, as the popularity of Lope de Vega's plays at the Amsterdam City Theatre has proven. See Lenor Álvarez Francés, 'Fascination for the "Madritsche Apoll": Lope de Vega in Golden Age Amsterdam', *Arte Nuevo: Revista de estudios áureos*, 2014, pp. 1–15: Six also wrote amiable, contemplative poems on the Spanish countryside during his travels through the land. See for example 'Op de ongelykmaaticheit der bruggen oover de rivieren van Sivilie en Madril' ('On the Distinction of the Bridges over the Rivers of Seville and Madrid') (J51), a poem that was probably inspired by the poetry of Luis de Góngora. See Jacobs, 1991 II, pp. 45–47. However, the connotations associated with 'Spanish' in the poems discussed here demonstrate that it was still was a term that aroused ambivalence in the Dutch Republic.

55 'Onse Lichamen, de welcke Tempelen des Heyligen Geestes zijn (1. Cor. 6:19) en mogen daer mede niet verontreynight worden. Wy sien insonderheyt / op die verfoeyelicke vercieringen, waer door de menschen / selfs het werck hares Godts, soecken te verbeteren', Wittewrongel, 1661, II, p. 1151.

places plenty of pagan incense and oil, contrasts with the concept of the human body as God's temple filled with the Holy Spirit.

Conclusion

Six's ironic eulogies to the newly-wed king and queen of Spain thus have several layers of meaning to them. At one level, these texts can be seen as satires on the pomp and ceremony of the Royal Entry to Madrid. The same goes for Six's responses to the critical comments he received from his compatriots on his series of eulogies, but here attention is directed towards his own compatriots. According to Six, the splendour of the Spanish court is no longer a purely Spanish phenomenon, but has spread to his own country. He points to new trends in the literature of his fellow writers, especially the 'Parnassian language', imbued as it is with references to incense, oil and other luxuries, an artistic style accompanying the early modern rebirth of the Roman Triumph: the Royal Entry. To fully understand these texts, we must also take into account the pharmaceutical and religious background of the poet, and read the poems as self-presentation, with self-scrutiny as a literary strategy. What strikes us first in this connection are the intellectual discussions that accompany Six's treatment of exotic goods. He draws his arguments from literary, medical and theological sources, and associates the consumption of exotics goods with moral, medical and social dangers. Second, Six's Northern European Protestant identity is important to any attempt to understand his writing strategies. Exotica are linked to various vices such as pride and hubris that Protestants associated with a South European, Catholic temperament. In the view of early modern moralists, the exchange of ethically reprehensible goods entailed the exchange of morally reprehensible sentiments. I have shown what this implies for Six's identity as a travelling merchant-druggist. He recognises the crucial role he plays when it comes to the transnational exchange of goods and ideas. In this respect, his quest for self-knowledge has a medical aspect: the importer of drugs is portrayed as a carrier of dangerous bodily desires.

But in this chapter, we have seen Six once again as a pragmatic poet. The artistic trends in Southern European court culture spread to the Republic in the 1640s, and became an important tool in the politics of the House of Orange. As an Orange supporter, Six participates in the apotheosis of Frederick Henry and other members of the Orange dynasty. Many of these poems, as we have seen, have an satirical tone, but it is not as obvious here as it is in his 'Spanish poems'. Through the use of exaggeration, irony and *praeteritio*, Six hits two birds with one stone: he succeeds in showing his respect for the House of Orange without being identified with the mythological-ornamental language through which princes are worshipped. Six wants to be seen by his readers as a sober, self-critical Dutchman above all – as someone who is aware of the pagan origins of his poetry and of his pharmacy, and who takes his distance from these.

8. Drugs as intoxicants

Abstract
In this chapter, I discuss the poetic inspiration that was associated in the Renaissance with such concepts as *furor poeticus* (poetic madness), ecstasy and *enthousiasmos*. I show how Joannes Six van Chandelier gives poetic madness a material foundation by linking it to exotic drugs such as cachou. I then show how Six, in a poem addressed to his doctor, Simon Dilman, and to the theologian Johannes Hoornbeeck, emphasises both the medical and the religious dangers of *furor poeticus*. Here Six presents himself as a weak and fragile rhymester, but in a positive sense, to distance himself from negative associations that poetic madness gave rise to, such as the thirst for divine knowledge and perfection. In other texts, some of which were addressed to the pastor Pieter Wittewrongel, we see how Six distinguishes between a Christian and a pagan ecstasy.

Keywords: Inspiration, enthusiasm, ecstasy, Calvinism, Johannes Hoornbeeck, Pieter Wittewrongel

Give me an ounce of civet, good apothecary,
to sweeten my imagination.
King Lear[1]

Poetic inspiration[2]

In one of his poems, 'Op de pinxterbloem der straatkinderen' ('On the Pentecostal Flowers of the Street Children') (J162), Joannes Six van Chandelier tells us how he would like to write. Children dressed up for Pentecost, he writes, travel around on St. Martin's Day, singing songs and asking for treats. He tells us how he – an adherent

1 Shakespeare, *King Lear*, Act 4, scene 6, l. 132–133.
2 A shorter version of this chapter has been published as 'Diagnosing the Poetic Inspiration: Medical Criticism of Enthusiasm in the Poetry of Jan Six van Chandelier (1620–1695)'; in: Jaap Grave, Rick Honings and Bettina Noak (eds.), *Illness and Literature in the Netherlands*, 2016, pp. 81–96.

Spaans, R., *Dangerous Drugs: The Self-Presentation of the Merchant-Poet Joannes Six van Chandelier (1620–1695)*. Taylor & Francis Group, 2020
DOI 10.5117/9789462983543_CH08

of a 'learned poetry on metrical feet' in 'a grand style' (l. 9–11) – is captivated by their unpretentious verses and how he himself would like to follow their style. He wonders who taught the children to rhyme like this (l. 25–36):

Het spoelde nooit, in Focidis dal,
Syn lipjes, met het henghste kristal.
Het sliep niet, op den dubblen Parnas,
Waar deur 't zoo draa een singertje was.
Het leerde niet, als 't extertje doet,
Uit honger, om het kostjen, een groet.
Wie onderwees dan singen, aan 't wicht?
Wie onderwees, na 't quam in het licht,
Het oeffnen van de reedlike tongh,
Met welke 't zoo natuurelyk songh?
Wie is er dan een rechte Poëet,
Die meest den dank syn moeder niet weet?

It [the child] never wet its lips in the Valley
Of Focis [where Mount Parnassus is located], with the crystal of the stallion.
It did not sleep on two-headed Parnassus,
Which immediately would make him a poet,
It never learned, as the magpie [in captivity] has,
To make a bow to get its food.
Who, then, taught the child to sing?
Who taught the child, when it was born,
To speak in a reasonable human language,
Through which it so naturally sang?
Who is then a true Poet,
But the one who can thank his mother for these skills?

The simple rhymes you learn from your mother, that's good poetry. Six borrowed both the light-footed, almost irregular metre and the opposition to Parnassian poetry from the classical poet Persius. In the prologue to his series of satires, Persius writes that he never drank from the holy springs of the Greek muses, and that he cannot remember dreaming on Mount Parnassus, for he is only a 'half-poet' – a *semipaganus*.[3] Persius' statement is meant as criticism of the high pretensions of the classical prophet-poets Ovid and Virgil. Although Six draws a contrast between the rhymes of the children and his own 'dignified tone', he uses Persius as a literary

3 *Juvenal and Persius*, 2004, pp. 43–45.

ideal in other texts. We have already seen many examples of this strategy earlier in this study.[4] In these texts, Six also portrays himself as a down-to-earth, abstinent druggist-poet – a self-image that is in line with the presentation of authorship in literary-historical research. The anti-idealistic Six does not need the inspiration of the pagan muses. His is a voice of dissent against poets such as P.C. Hooft and Joost van den Vondel.[5]

But it is not quite as simple as that. We have come to know Six as an ambivalent poet. Whereas Persius, in his satire on the high-flown poetics in antiquity, advocates a categorical abstention from divine inspiration, Six finds himself in a more difficult situation. The writings of the Renaissance scholar Julius Caesar Scaliger can help us get a better understanding of Six's position. Scaliger divides poets into two groups: one to which divine power comes from above – the so-called water-drinking poets, who drink water of the stream of the Muses – and another that is aroused 'by the fumes of unmixed wine, which draws out the instruments of the mind, the spirits themselves, from the material part of the body'. Scaliger regards Horace as belonging to the latter group.[6] As is clear from the poem I will discuss in this chapter, Six also places himself in this group with Horace, but as we shall see, that does not mean that Six's inspiration is of a purely earthly character. Six himself is, after all, a trader in materials that were associated with the mythological Parnassian language. And just as in the poems of Horace, we also find invocation of Apollo and his muses in Six's poetry (as a water-drinking poet), as invocations of Bacchus (as a wine-drinking poet). In the previous chapters, we saw that 'gods' is a frequent concept in Six's praise of high-ranking persons, along with references to pharmaceutical substances with transformative powers. We have also learned to know the playful way in which Six portrays himself as a down-to-earth poet. As we saw in his identification with drab species of birds (in Chapter 5), he did this rather coquettishly. We have a further example of this in the humorous 'Derde antwoord, aan den selven' ('Third answer, to the same person [Joan Radermacher]') (J442), in which Six writes that he identifies, not with 'high' animals such as the peacock, but rather with the sparrow, the squirrel, the lamb and the cod (!). This playful identification with birds is also a theme in the present chapter.

4 *Cf.* 'Afscheid aan myn rymen' (J120) (Chapter 2, p. 83) and 'Toewydinge aan de vreegodinne' (J218) (from the preceding chapter).

5 Jacobs, 1991 II, pp. 295–295; Schenkeveld-van der Dussen & De Vries, 2007, pp. 208–209.

6 Iulius Caeser Scaliger, *Poetices libri septem. Sieben Bücher über die Dichtkunst* (ed. by Luc Deitz), I, 1994, p. 83. For Horace's discussion on wine drinking poets, see his Epistle I, 19. The passage is ambiguous and it is possible that Horace waxes about wine as an inspiration, but that does not seem to effect Scaliger. The distinction between wine and water-drinking poet is a commonplace in classical writings, see J. Guépin, 'Het enthousiasme van dichters' in: *Bzzletin*, 1987, pp. 47–55.

In this chapter I focus on Six's own body. As just mentioned, invocations of the muses and the inspiration from the springs of Mount Parnassus are frequent *topoi* in his poetry: in 'Geluk op reis, aan Antoni Duivelaar' ('Have a Lucky Journey, to Antoni Duivelaar') (J302), Six speaks, for example, of the inspiration of 'Kastals geestigen fontein' ('the spiritual spring of Castalia') – that is, the spring in Delphi. In 'Ter eere van de fonteine Geronster' ('In Honour of the Spring at Géronstère') (J105), one of the poems Six wrote during his Spa cure, he compares the 'vloeijende metaal' ('liquid metal') (l. 21) of Spa with the water from the rock gorge of the Pythia (l. 7–30) – the crevice in Delphi from which rose the vapour that brought the Apollonian priestess to ecstasy. Six attributes the same transcendental effect to the goods he trades in. In a poem to one of his commercial contacts, 'Een stuk van een meloen, aan Manuel Spranger' ('A Piece of Melon, to Manuel Spranger') (J273) (Plate 6), Six describes the exotica as a 'goudvrucht van Parnas' ('golden fruit of Parnassus') (l. 1) and the beneficial effect of this exotic fruit on the human body (l. 5–10):

> Sie deese Haarlemer meloen
> Zal oogh, en neus, en tongh voldoen.
> Laat lyf, en ziel dat geele bloed
> Konfyten, van Apol gevoedt,
> En van syn lieve susters naam.
> Dit 's Gooden spys en drank te saam.
>
> See this melon from Haarlem,
> It shall please the eye, nose and tongue.
> Let that yellow blood candy
> Body and soul, [the blood] that is fed by Apollo,
> And that has its name from his beloved sister [the goddess Mellona].
> This is food and drink for the Gods.

The melon enchants the senses and pleases the body and soul of the one who eats it, in accordance with the concept of 'konfijten' we discussed earlier. But the literary representation of exotica as a source of inspiration is not always without problems. On the contrary, and as we have seen, the theriac and the olive oil in the previous chapters had a disruptive effect on the poet's body.

The question is therefore not what Six's position is with regard to pagan inspiration, but what strategies he uses to cast his identity as a druggist-poet in a favourable light. Six does not shrink from incorporating elements of his own identity in satirical verses. I will discuss four texts: the pair of texts 'Brief aan Hans Baard te Haarlem' ('Letter to Hans Baard in Haarlem') and 'Fooi' ('Farewell Drink') (J211, J212), 'Verrukkinge der sinnen, aan Joannes Hoorenbeek, dr., profr., en predikant t'Uitrecht: en Simon Dilman geneesheer' ('Rapture of the Senses, to the Preacher and Professor of Theology at the University of Utrecht, Johannes Hoornbeeck, and the Physician Simon Dilman') (J177), and 'Verrukkinge van sinnen' ('Rapture from the Senses') (J401). Drugs play a smaller role in this last two poems, but these texts teach us more about Six's perspective on the notion of *furor poeticus* and about who the intended audience of his poetry could be. The first three texts are a continuation of the poems discussed in the previous chapter: an ironising of the role of the poet-prophet in Royal Entries. The latter is of a more serious nature. Here he discusses the dangers that the concept of the mind-altering *furor poeticus* brings with it. At the end of the chapter, I will also discuss poems in which Six distinguishes between classical-pagan and Christian inspiration.

'The language of the Gods'

But before I turn to these poems, I would like to reflect on the early modern understanding of supernatural inspiration. In Renaissance literature, there is an important place for the concept of *furor poeticus*. This idea can be traced back to classical literature. A good starting point is the famous description of the poetic power of the Roman poet Ovid: 'There is a god in us; with him stirring us, we grow warm, it is his impulse that sows the seeds of inspiration'.[7] The concept of *inspiration* ('insufflation' in Latin) carries the sense that the poet is filled with a spiritual breath that comes from the outside. Full of this fervent enthusiasm, he begins to 'glow'. He becomes a *vates*, a prophet; his *genius* leads him to the supernatural and gives him access to heavenly ideas. In the Renaissance, this phenomenon is referred to by the term *furor poeticus*, 'poetic madness'. I will also use two other terms in my analysis of inspiration in Six's poetry: *enthousiasmos,* Greek for 'possession by a god', and ecstasy – *ék-stasis* in Greek, with the meaning 'to be outside oneself', a word that thus finds a parallel with the modern *altered state*.

The most important work in that respect, Plato's *Ion*, argues that poets are modern variants of the frenzied Bacchants of Greek mythology: 'when they are caught up in the music and the rhythm, they speak with Bacchic enthusiasm'.[8] In another work by Plato, *Phaedrus*, a distinction is made between the kind of possession that is divinely

7 'Est deus in nobis, agitante calescimus illo, impetus hic sacrae semina mentis habet'; *cf.* Vossius, 2010, II, pp. 1902–1903. See also Franciscus Junius, *De Schilder-konst der Oude*, 1641, p. 35.

8 Plato does not speak in the passage quoted; *Ion* presents Socrates' conversation with Ion. Plato himself attached less value to the irrational side of poetry than to the rational knowledge of philosophy. In the Renaissance, Plato's representation of the poet was seen as a person affected with madness, but in a positive sense. But the concept of the possessed poet goes farther back to a statement by Democritius about Homer. For more on this, see Vossius, 2010, II, pp. 1896–1915. See also Guépin, 1987. For Plato's ambivalent vision of poetry, see Johan Koppenol, 'Een tegendraadse poëtica. De literaire ideeën van Jan van Hout', in: K.J.S. Bostoen *et al.* (eds.), *Jan van Hout, Voorrede tot het gezelschap. Voorrede bij zijn vertaling van Buchanans Franciscanus*, 1993, p. 8, note 6.

inspired and that kind that must be regarded as an illness.[9] The work deals with four divine forms of madness (*furores*) that are considered to be positive: the prophetic (*e.g.* that of the Pythia in Delphi), the religious (*e.g.* that of priests in mystical rituals), the poetic (of poets), and the erotic: there is such a strong desire for sensual beauty that it turns into a longing for the contemplation of the idea of beauty. Each of these four forms of madness is linked to its own deity: Apollo, Bacchus, the Olympic muses, and Venus or Cupid. Other forms of madness, such as being in love, are seen as harmful.

Phaedrus also emphasises which genre the inspired poet-prophet uses, namely the dithyramb, the Ancient Greek hymn that was sung and danced during Bacchic processions, which I mentioned in the introduction to this study as a literary composition that Plato associated with intoxication and ecstasy.[10] In Plato's *Apology*, Socrates offers his views on the dithyrambic poets. Their verses, he believed, were not 'composed by wisdom': 'they were inspired, like prophets and givers of oracles, for they say many fine things, but know none of the things they say'.[11] The hymn was also known through Horace's Ode IV, 2, where it is linked to Pindar, the Ancient Greek poet who was regarded as the embodiment of the *furor poeticus*. As we have seen, Six imitated it on several occasions. Horace writes that Pindar's voice 'boils and surges' when 'he rolls down new words in his daring dithyrambs and is carried along in free, unregulated rhythms'.[12] But Horace not only waxes ironic over the dithyrambic poet. Ode III, 25, he presents himself as a poet chosen by the god of wine, and he – just as in Ode IV, 2 – tells that he has to have been in a Bacchic intoxication to be able to deify Augustus:

> Where are you hurrying me to, Bacchus, full as I am of you? Into what woods, what caves, am I being driven at such speed in a strange state of mind? In what grotto shall I be heard as I practise setting the eternal glory of peerless Caesar among the stars and in the council of Jove?[13]

For this reason, Dutch scholars in the Renaissance warned against the 'turgid and inflated style' of the dithyramb. In quoting Ancient writers, Gerardus Vossius says that 'the dithyrambic poet is excited and exhibits a great degree of frenzy by jumping

9 244a–245b, 249d–257b.

10 *Phaedrus*, 238D1–3. See Vossius, 2010, II, pp. 1124–1145.

11 *Apology*, 22B–C, in: Plato: *Euthyphro, Apology, Crito, Phaedo, Phaedrus*, translation by Harold North Fowler, 1982, p. 85.

12 'Seu per audaces nova dithyrambos / verba devolvit numerisque fertur / lege solutis', Ode IV, 2, l. 5–11, Horace, *Odes and Epodes*, translation by Niall Rudd, 2004, p. 223.

13 'Quo me, Bacche, rapis tui/ plenum? quae nemora aut quos agor in specus/ velox mente nova? quibus / antris egregii Caesaris audiar / aeternum meditans decus/ stellis inserere et consilio Iovis?', l. 1–6, Horace, *Odes and Epodes*, translation by Niall Rudd, 2004, pp. 200–203. For Horace, *furor poeticus*, and Dutch literature, see Piet Schrijvers, 'Een stralend nieuw lied. De Bacchus ode (3.25)', in: Piet Schrijvers, *Ik kan de Muzen niet haten*, 2004, pp. 75–98.

about and is made to rouse emotions, especially that suit the god [Bacchus]'.[14] When Vossius relates the exalted state of the dithyrambic poet to Bacchus, we have to remember that wine in early modern times was sometimes also mixed with drugs: As we have seen, Johan van Beverwijck spoke of wine blended with ambergris.

Theories about the etymology of the Greek term *dithyrambos* are interesting in the context of Six's poetry. Besides being an epithet of Bacchus, the word is linguistically linked to *triumphus*. In the previous chapter, Jupiter was presented as central to the Roman Triumph, but according to classical writers, in earlier versions of the triumph the religious ceremony was devoted to the god of wine: Pliny credited the invention of the triumph to Bacchus, and we find hints of a story of Bacchus's journey from the Far East in the opening of Euripides' *Bacchae*, a myth that had a formative influence on the military campaigns of Alexander the Great in India. The presence of an Asian element such as an elephant in the triumph, which is also depicted in the Oranjezaal in Huis ten Bosch, was seen as a Bacchic feature. 'The Triumph of Bacchus' was a popular motif in Renaissance art, and, as we shall see, Six used it himself in his poetry (Fig. 8.1).[15] Pindar is known, not just for his dithyrambs, but also for his victory odes. This type of poem has much in common with dithyrambs, and Six may not have distinguished between the two. Like many of the classical genres, the Pindaric ode was rediscovered in the Renaissance and became a popular model for Renaissance poets from Pierre de Ronsard to Joost van den Vondel, as René Veenman notes in his study of Pindar in Dutch literature. Here he points to Six's parodies of imitations of the Greek poet.[16] In this chapter too, I will discuss a parody by Six of Horace's Ode IV, 2, and I will also treat Six's imitation of other odes of Horace, wherein Horace presents himself as an inspired poet-priest with the power to deify Augustus, as Ode III, 25, and the so-called 'Roman Odes', III, 1–6.

Next to books that attributed poetry a divine origin, there were classical works that emphasise physiological concepts in explaining the nature of poetic inspiration. This is the case with *Problemata Physica*, a work that has long been attributed to Aristotle. Gerdardus Vossius describes this view as follows:

> He [Aristotle] was led to this opinion by the fact that from natural principles he could not acknowledge that there are gods. Therefore, he thought that this poetic frenzy did not originate with the Muses or with gods that poets invented, but from a black bile that he compares to wine.[17]

14 Vossius, 2010, I, pp. 1133, 1137.

15 Pliny, *NH*, VII, 191; VIII, 4; Mary Beard, *The Roman Triumph*, 2007, pp. 161, 315–318.

16 René Veenman, 'De Thebaensche Swaen. De receptie van Pindarus in de Nederlanden', *Voortgang. Jaarboek voor de Neerlandistiek*, 1992, pp. 65–67.

17 Vossius, 2010, II, pp. 1906–1907. 'In hanc eum sententiam impulit quod ex naturae principiis cognosci nequit esse daemones. Existimavit ignitur furorem hunc poeticum non esse Musis aut diis quos poetae

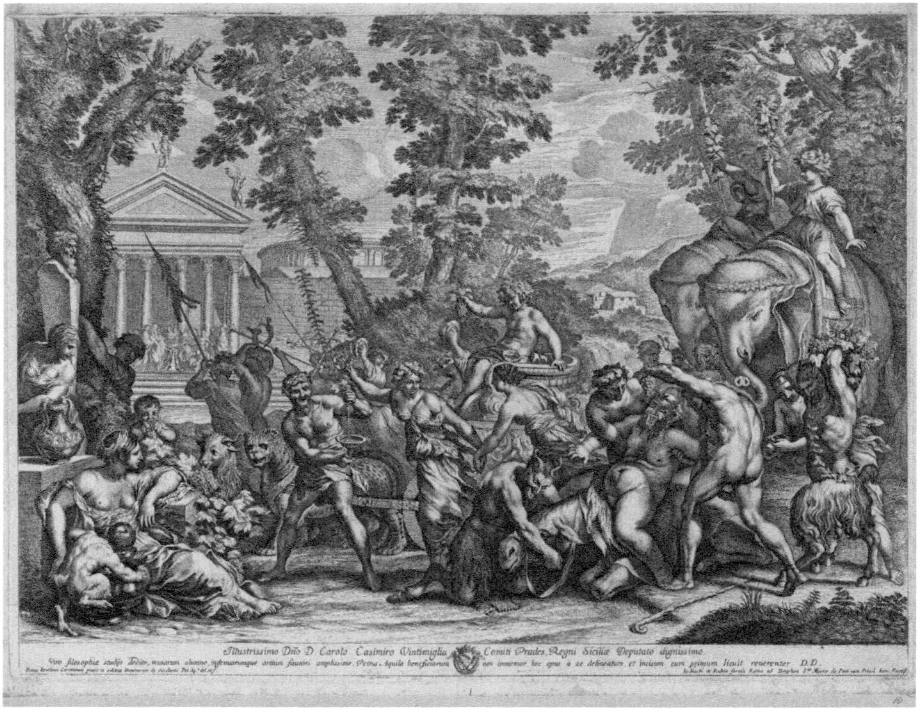

Fig. 8.1: Pietro Aquila, after Pietro da Cortona, *The Triumph of Bacchus*, c. 1660–1692. Etching. (© Rijksmuseum, Amsterdam).

The conclusion is that mad poets are people with a predominantly melancholic constitution, or who are under the influence of wine or strong emotions such as love and anger. The phenomenon must therefore be explained with medical theories – as a consequence of humoral-body processes and not as an effect of supernatural intervention. But this view did not exclude theories of inspiration where the physical was combined with the supernatural. In the Middle Ages, many doctors considered visions and delusions as symptoms of a melancholic syndrome, in line with the pseudo-Aristotelian explanation of poetic obsession, or even as the result of a devilish obsession. The Renaissance saw the remythologisation of *melancholia*; and *enthusiasm*, ecstasy and prophetic language were now seen in a positive light. The Italian humanist philosopher Marsilio Ficino, while not rejecting the physiological explanation of *furor poeticus*, argued that there was a positive, creative *melancholia* that could be distinguished from the negative variety. The

sint commenti, sed ab humore melancholico, quem vino similem facit'. (The English translation is by Jan Bloemendal, the compiler and translator of the new edition of Vossius's work.) And see Vossius, 2010, II, pp. 1908–1909.

positive kind, he argued, led to *furor poeticus* if the black bile did not prevail, but mixed well with blood. This balance of humoral body fluids depends on the state of the sensitive *spiritus* of the melancholic. When it glows, the poet is filled with an ingenious *imagination*. But if it merely burns, smoke rises to the poet's head, causing depression and hallucinations.[18]

The heavenly view of poetry is also reflected in the way poets were portrayed in other authoritative contemporary works. For example, we read in the Dutch translation of Cesare Ripa's famous *Iconologia* (1644): 'Following an old custom, pagans called poets Sacred Persons, a Heavenly family, Sons of Jupiter, interpreters of the Muses, and Priests of Apollo' (Fig. 8.2).[19] Ripa is probably referring to Horace, who calls himself 'a priest of the Muses' (Ode III, I, l. 3). In the aforementioned *Eglentiers poetens borst-weringh* by Theodore Rodenburgh – the Dutch adaptation of Philip Sidney's *An Apology for Poetry* – it is said that poetry creates a whole new reality, 'by the power of Celestial breath'. Behind this concept lies the Neoplatonic idea of a *spiritus mundi*, a 'world spirit' that lives in the universe.[20]

That Christian moralists should have warned against inspiration from the 'Priests of Apollo' can come as no surprise. The Christian Church also knows the concept of *enthusiasm*, namely in pneumatology, the teaching of the Holy Spirit. In a speech, Gisbertus Voetius warned against the appeal of poetry: 'Do not let Apollo – that is to say, your love of, and innate talent for, poetry – drive Christ from your heart'.[21] Six's interest in the Christian version of *enthousiasmos* is shown, among other things, in 'Op het boeck, Het Lof des Heilgen Geests, van Roelof Pieterse' ('On the book *The Praise of the Holy Spirit* by Roelof Pieterse') (J224). Six writes about the author of the book: 'Hoe saaligh is hy, o! wie schrijft in zulken sin? / Gods geest stuurt self de pen, en stort de stof der in' ('How blessed is he, oh, who writes in such a manner? It is the spirit of God that governs the pen, and pours substance into it')

18 Heyd, 1995, pp. 43–71, mainly pp. 51–52; Brinkkemper & Soepnel, 1989, pp. 172–184; D. Walker, *Spiritual and Demonic Magic: From Ficino to Campanella*, 1975, pp. 12–24.

19 'Poëten [werden] by de Heydenen, door een oude gewoonte, Heyligen genaemt, en een Hemels geslacht, Soonen van Iupiter, uytleggers van de Sangh-Goddinnen, en Priesters van Apollo' – see 'Furore Poetico. *Poëtische drift of geest*', in Cesare Ripa, *Iconologia*, 1644, p. 420.

20 'Door de kracht van de Hemelsche azem' (p. 9). See also the writings of Daniel Heinsius, an important ideologist in the development of the theory of Dutch Renaissance literature, especially with regard to his famous speech 'De Poetis et Eorum Interpretibus' (1603): J.H. Meter, *De literaire theorieën van Daniel Heinsius. Een onderzoek naar de klassieke en humanistische bronnen van De Tragoediae Constitutione en andere geschriften*, 1975. *Cf.* also P.C. Hooft's *Reden vande waerdicheit der poesi* (1614). And see Wouter Abrahamse, *Het toneel van Theodore Rodenburgh (1574–1644)*, 1997, pp. 33–36. According to Abrahamse, Rodenburgh tends towards Neoplatonic ideas, but without accepting all instances of them.

21 'Ne Apollo, hoc est genius et facultas poetica, Christum vobis de pectore excutiat', from Voetius's 1634 inaugural speech on the occasion of his appointment as professor at the Illustere School in Utrecht, *De pietate cum scientia contiungenda*. See Schenkeveld-van der Dussen, 1991, pp. 48–49; Els Stronks, *Negotiating Differences: Word, Image and Religion in the Dutch Republic*, 2011, pp. 129–135.

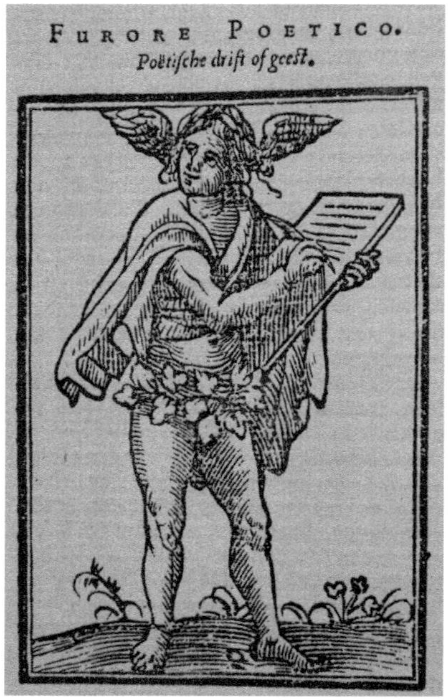

Fig. 8.2: Illustration of *Furor poeticus* in Cesare Ripa, *Iconologia*, 1644. (© Privately owned).

(l. 5–6). The Amsterdam preacher Roelof Pieterse is presented as a Christian *vates*, a mediator in higher wisdom: not he himself, but a spiritual force outside him has guided the pen for this book.[22]

If poetic inspiration is the theme, we should certainly not forget the Prince of Poets, Joost van den Vondel (Fig. 8.3). Vondel espouses Horatian ideals such as clarity and moderation, and in his poetic work *Aenleidinge ter Nederduitsche dichtkunste* (1650), he places more emphasis on systematic practice than on the language of ecstasy. Yet he, too, has an exalted vision of the origin and function of poetry. In *Aenleidinge,* he makes an important distinction between, on the one hand, the exercises of 'rijmers' ('rhymesters') who know their classics and, on the other, the 'hemelsche Poëzy' ('heavenly poetry') and 'de spraeck der Goden' ('the language

22 *'t Lof Des Heylighen Geestes: Dat Is: Korte Verklaringe Van Het Wesen, de Eygenschappen, ende Werckingen des H. Geestes: Over eenige bysondere Cier-namen, Ghelijckenissen, Afbeeldingen ende Cierlicke Beschrijvingen, die den H. Geest in het Oude ende Nieuwe Testament ghegeven worden* (1646). *Cf.* 2. Timothy 3:16. Roelof Pieterse (Rudolphus Petri) van Niedeck (1586–1649) is mentioned in two other texts by Six: 'Lykklaghte, oover Roelof Pieterse, Kerkenleeraar' ('Lamentation on the Dead Body of Roelof Pieterse, Parish Teacher') (J179), and 'Beklagh oover de dood van Jakob Holbeek, F. Kesseleer, en R. Pieterse, predikanten. Aan Katarina Jeheu' ('Lamentation of the Death of Jakob Holbeek, F. Kesseleer, and R. Pieterse, Ministers. To Katarina Jeheu') (J264).

of the Gods') used by poets who are filled with supernatural inspiration.[23] What is interesting is the social context to which Vondel relates the difference between good and bad poetry. As mentioned earlier in this study, Vondel makes a parallel between rhymesters and quacks peddling their jars of ointment (p. 44). And as we have seen, Vondel derived this medical-social hierarchy from the French poet Pierre de Ronsard: 'There is as much difference between a poet and a versifier, as between [...] a venerable prophet and a charlatan selling theriac'.[24] The *topos* of the quack selling theriac is also found in the art of the Dutch Republic. In 'The Quacksalver' by Gerrit Dou, which was possibly owned by the aforementioned chemist Franciscus Sylvius, the elixirs and oils on the quack's table are being contrasted with the domestically grown vegetables in the farmer's wheelbarrow to the left of the quack (Plate 11).[25]

I touched on aspects of Six's treatment of the concept of *furor poeticus* in previous chapters. The prevailing *mores* are not favourable for our druggist-poet. Not only is Six a merchant by profession and, as we saw, not only was his poetry associated with the empty screams of market vendors – *cf.* my discussion of 'Op quaade tongen' – but, as a druggist, he even traded in theriac too. 'Toewydinge aan de vreegodinne', discussed in the previous chapter, is thus also of relevance to this chapter, given its criticism of the socio-literary hierarchy and of the concept of *furor poeticus* – through Six's self-presentation as a rhymester intoxicated by theriac.[26]

23 Vondel [1650] (1977), pp. 44 and 55. *Cf.* also Porteman & Smits-Veldt, 2008, pp. 401–402; and Brinkkemper & Soepnel, 1989, pp. 172–184.

24 Pierre de Ronsard, *La Franciade*, 1983, p. 335; Vondel, 1977, p. 44. See also Schenkeveld-van der Dussen, 1983, p. 305. *Cf.* also how Andries Pels uses this topos: on the occasion of the spectacular performance of the plays by Jan Vos, Pels sarcastically asks himself 'whether there was "theriac for sale"': *Gebruik en misbruik des toneels* (1681), ed. M. Schenkeveld-van der Dussen, 1987, p. 67. The distinction probably goes back to a passage from Horace's *Ars Poetica*, the model for Vondel's *Aenleidinge*: 'Like the crier, who gathers a crowd to the auction of his wares, so the poet bids flatterers flock to the call of gain' ('Ut praeco, ad merces tubam qui cogit emendas, / adsentatores iubet ad lucrum ire poeta...') (l. 419–420): Horace, *Satires, Epistles and Ars Poetica*, transl. by H. Rushton Fairclough, 1991, p. 485.

25 Smith, 2004, pp. 203–204. This interpretation would correspond to the contrasting structure of the painting: Ronni Baer, *Gerrit Dou (1613–1675)*, 2000, pp. 101–103.

26 Since we have only literary sources to rely on, it is impossible to determine whether Six really wrote his poems of praise for Frederick Henry in a state of intoxication brought on by opium. In accordance with my analysis, the representation of inspiration by drugs in Six's texts has a rhetorical-polemical function. But even if he was not 'drunk' on opium when he wrote the poems, he may have relied on experiences with drugs from previous trials of commodities. *Cf.* Sijbrand Feitama's 'Op de vyf Zinnen', which I discussed in Chapter 4. I will come back to this question in the conclusion. The same goes for the state that *vates* poets were in when they wrote their poems. Some poets probably had faith in divine inspiration of some sort during the writing process: In 'Brief, aan R. Anslo, te Rome' (J468), Six mentions that Reyer Anslo covered his head with a cloth when he was writing (l. 87). Lambert Bidloo describes Anslo's custom: 'hy had zig een gereedschap doen maken, als een Zonne-Scherm, 't geen hy op en neêr kon schuyven, wanneer hy bezig was te Digten, en eenen goeden inval krygende, aanstonds

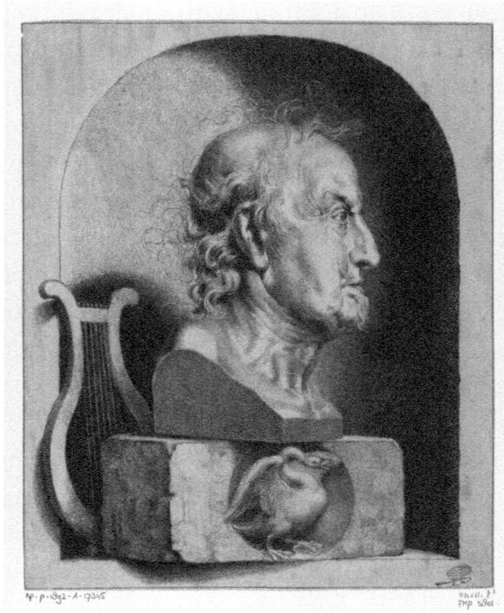

Fig. 8.3: Johannes Lutma, *Portrait Bust of Joost van den Vondel*, c. 1634–1689. Paper.
(© Rijksmuseum, Amsterdam).

In 'Oostkappele, aan Abraham Grenier den jongen' (J172), discussed in Chapter 5, Six thematises the process of poetic *imitatio* as a metempsychosis, which he rejects as an idolatrous act. He addresses this idea of a spiritual relocation explicitly in connection with the imitation of Horace's poetry in his satirical 'Horatius Liersangen, in Hollands vertaalt door J.v. Vondel. Aan den selven' ('The odes of Horace, translated into Dutch by Joost van den Vondel. To the same person') (J363). Here Six mocks the condition in which Vondel must have found himself when he made a prose translation of Horace's odes. When the spirit of Horace '[s]inloos, maar sinryk, Godlyk [Vondel] heeft beseeten' ('has divinely and senselessly possessed Vondel, yet full of understanding' (l. 11). Six concludes his poem ironically, telling us that an Italian translation of this work by the Vondel epigone Reyer Anslo will probably soon be published (l. 41–44). In these texts, Six comes across as a satirist. But he himself was a keen follower of Horace. This is evident from many of the poems that I will discuss in this chapter, and in which self-examination and self-criticism predominate.

ophaalen, en opstellen' ('he had made himself a tool like a sunshade, which he could slide up and down, when he was busy writing poems, and when getting a good bit of inspiration, he would immediately pick it up and set it up'), see Bidloo, *Panpoëticon Batavûm* (1720), p. 129. The reference is from Jacobs, 1991 II, p. 788.

Cachou

Just as in 'Toewydinge aan de vreegodinne', 'Brief aan Hans Baard te Haarlem' and 'Fooi' (J211, J212) present a particular medicine as a source of divine inspiration. However, this time it is not a classical remedy, but a novelty from the Far East: the plant extract cachou ('katsjoe'). The reason for writing the pair of texts can be found in the title to the second. The original meaning of 'fooi' is 'farewell drink' or 'farewell gift'. As the title shows, the gift is for a certain Hans Baert from Haarlem, a fellow merchant and a relative of Six's who shared his interest in foreign curiosities.[27] But Six also dedicates the poem to others who might accidentally get hold of it, namely a few literary stars of his time, such as Vondel and Jan Vos. This dedication means we can assume that the pair of texts served as a prologue to a cycle of poems.[28]

The first text, the prose prologue 'Letter to Hans Baard in Haarlem', addresses the difference between sincerity and pretending when it comes to praising someone. Six once again chooses pagan concepts that are linked to the panegyric as a theme. The poet stages the reception of a Bacchic inspiration (l. 2–6):

> Volgende myne somwyle gewoonte, maak ik u l. deelachtich een, of twee aalweelige luimen. Iuist zoodanige, gelyk se dan tuimelen, uit een ongebonden geest: die dikwils alleen door inbeeldinge van liefde, op Poësye, als dronkener is, dan wel de Bacchanten konnen zyn, van de lucht des Vaaders, van wien se hunnen Aadel beroemen.
>
> As I am wont to do on occasion, I am sending you, your kindness, one or two exuberant whimsies – just the kind that come tumbling out of an unbound mind, which often, solely by imagining love, writes Poetry, just as [the poet was] a drunk, as the Bacchantes could be, from the breath of the Father, to whom they owe their Nobility.

The poet must be in a trance to approach and glorify the one whose praises are being sung, as Horace wrote that he had to be in Ode III, 25. He must possess an 'unbound spirit', the *furor poeticus*. Our sober Calvinist allows that he himself also goes into ecstasy at times. At such moments he becomes a 'drunk' – inebriated by the 'breath' of Bacchus, or the Bacchic *spiritus*. The poets, he writes, are frenzied Bacchantes who owe their 'their nobility' to their god. Six returns in 'Fooi' to the exact nature and effect of his ecstasy. But, he then explains, if he were consistent in these great pretensions, he would not have sent these two prologue texts – possibly

27 See Chapter 3, note 22 and Appendix II.

28 Jacobs posits that it may be a lost pamphlet (1991 II, p. 363).

accompanied by a series of poems – to Baert just like that, but would have handed them over to him under cover of 'solemn ceremonies'. But Six emphasises that he distances himself from such corrupting poetry, which is, he tells us, merely a crude sacrifice to 'the false Goddess of flattery' (l. 6–13):

> Dit dicht, ik
> segh gerym, hadde immers behoort, en met braave ceremonien, u l. te werden toegewydt, gelyk de tweede voorsangh uitert: maar ik sende slechts een briefken. Aangesien myn gevoelen is, dat de meeste toewydingen niet beeters gelyken, dan een schetse beworpen, om de valsche Godinne der vleijerye wat cierlik te penceelen.
>
> This poem, I myself say rhyme, should actually be dedicated to you, your kindness, through solemn ceremonies, as the second strophe [of the poem] indicates: but I am sending you only a letter, since my feeling is that most dedications do not seem to be anything better than a sketch, intended to embellish the false Goddess of flattery.

Six therefore sends him a 'small letter' (this ironic prose prologue) instead of a heroic poem accompanied by a lot of ceremonial ado: here Six is referring to the next poem, 'Fooi'. The difference between 'ceremonies' and unpretentious 'rhymes' coincides with that between the poetry of the nightingales and that of the bastard birds from 'Toewydinge aan de vreegodinne'. The meaning of the text thus becomes clear. In an ironic prologue, Six expresses his dislike of the glorifying ode as a genre. The position of the *vates* serves to 'titillate' people in positions of power, so that the poet can make his social and literary career.[29]

If we shift our attention to 'Fooi' itself, we can see what Six means by 'unbound spirit'. As noted previously, the text is in the form of a Pindaric dithyramb. The farewell drink itself consists of an exclusive substance that is traded on the medical market. This is how Six describes the product in the first strophe of the ode, l. 1–10:

> 't OostIndisch huis bracht, uit Japon,
> Niet langh geleên, een groote ton,
> Met nieuwe waar. Een goet katsjou
> Genoemt. Dat ik gegraaven hou,
> Als Lemnosche aard. Schier rond van rand,
> Gelyk een bal, van korst verbrandt,

29 *Cf.* Vossius's discussion of a simulated poetic madness: 2010, II, p. 1899.

Van binnen malser, wit, en geel,
In 't eerste wringende de keel,
Van smaak zoo bitter niet, als roet,
Maar jongst, gelyk soethout, zoo soet.

The East-Indian House brought, from Japan,
Not long ago, a large cask
With a new commodity, a product called
Cachou, which I believe is dug out of the soil,
Like Lemnian bole. Almost round at the edges,
Like a ball, as burned crust,
Inside softer, white and yellow,
At first wringing the throat,
In taste not so bitter as soot,
But eventually as sweet as liquorice.

Once again, the professional pharmacist is holding forth. He meticulously describes the colour, taste and smell of the new product based on the impressions of his senses.[30] When he comes to talk about origin and classification, he bases himself on incorrect data: *terra japonica* means earth or clay, originating from Japan, while 'Lemnian bole' refers to medicinal *bole*, which was acquired on the Greek island of Lemnos – namely, *terra sigillata*, a remedy that was already known in classical times and that in the seventeenth century was very popular as a medicine, but also as a curiosity in the Wunderkammer. Cachou (or catechu) is actually a plant extract derived from tropical trees, mainly the acacia and betel palm from Southeast Asia, primarily Malaysia.[31] If we compare Six's characterisation of the product to the description of *terra japonica* in early modern medical reference works, we see there is nothing amiss. *Terra japonica* is a real *exoticum* – a novelty about which there was still a lot of uncertainty. Lemery says that 'we are not yet well informed on the nature of Cachou'. That said, Jan Huygen van Linschoten devotes a whole chapter to cachou and various types of betel nut: 'There is another sort which in the eating or chawing maketh men light in the heade, as they had drunk wine all

30 *Cf.* Lemery's description of cachou (or catechu): 1743, p. 163.

31 Pomet, 1737, pp. 415–416. *Terra sigillata* bore a special stamp and is therefore considered to be the first medicine to have a trademark. The medicine should not be confused with the fine red pottery that goes by the same name. See Arthur MacGregor, 'Medicinal *terra sigillata*: A historical, geographical and typological review', *Geological Society*, 2012. The seed of this tree, the betel nut, is chewed in the Far East together with other ingredients, and has a mild anaesthetic effect. Just as they are today, two types of cachou were distinguished in the early modern period: yellow (*uncaria gambir*) and brown (*acacia catechu*). Six is apparently talking about the former.

the day long.'[32] An English pamphlet from 1679 by a certain P. Brook explains why the new substance was popular: 'Japonick Earth', Brook tells us, helps against a range of conditions, including bad breath, toothaches and scurvy. Referring to Jan Huygen van Linschoten, Brook mentions that '[t]he King [...] and Lords of India, use Rolls made of Cattee, Aracca Camphir, Lignum Aloes, and Amber Greese, &c. which they continually eat mixt together'. It is no surprise, then, that this panacea is portrayed as a source of poetic inspiration.[33]

Did the narcotic effect of cachou, about which Huygen van Linschoten speaks, contribute to its representation as a Bacchic drink? In the next strophe, the 'antipode' to the Pindaric ode, Six discusses in more detail the kind of ecstasy that cachou causes (l. 11–20):

Ik haalde, van den dubblen top,
Een schaaltjen, met Kastaalisch sop,
Voor weinigh tyds, als in een droom.
My docht ik dronk die wyse stroom
En Naso gaf my strax een vorm,
Zoo dat ik spon, gelyk een worm
De syde spint. De draad scheen wreed,
En stram, maar naa se was gekneedt,
En wat gehaavent, vondt men ras,
Dat sy ook ergens quam te pas.

I fetched from the double peak,
A bowl of Castalian water,
In a short while, as in a dream,
I thought that I drank from the wise stream,
And Ovid gave me a shape,
So I spun like a worm
That spins silk. The thread seemed cruel

32 Lemery, 1743, p. 163; *Voyage of Jan Huyghen Linschoten, to the East-India*, vol. II, 1885 (the English translation was first published in 1598), p. 63. However, the question is whether Six associated *terra japonica* with Huygen van Linschoten's vegetable cachou. Huygen van Linschoten mentions in the same passage 'a cake or role made of certaine wood or tree called Kaate' (p. 63). This substance may have been conceived in Europe as a kind of earth. Although the yellow cachou (*uncaria gambir*) and the brown (*acacia catechu*) were often confused one with the other, *uncaria gambir* also has a stimulating effect and was chewed together with betel nut. See Hans H. Lauer, 'Zur Tradition exotischer Drogen: faufal (Areca Catechu L.) – die Betelnuß', *Sudhoffs Archiv. Zeitschrift für Wissenschaftsgeschichte*, 1966, pp. 179–204.

33 *A Brief Account, of the Nature, Vertues, Use, and Excellency of Indian Cattee*, 1679. And see Brian Cowan, *The Social Life of Coffee*, 2005, pp. 47–49.

And stiff but after it was kneaded
And battered, one quickly noticed
That it also was useful for something.

While eating the cachou, Six imagines for a moment that he is drinking from the Castalian Spring at Delphi, as if he were Ovid, the great *vates* of classical literature. The cachou causes in Six a creative and poetic urge: he 'spins' poetry.[34] But the great Bacchic ecstasy has yet to come. In an anticlimax, Six explains what poems his intoxication has brought him: poetry that is 'wry, hard and cruel'. Yet he emphasises that his poems will serve some purpose. The argument continues in the next strophe. Although this source of inspiration is hard on the outside and empty on the inside, some will find a 'ray of sunshine' in it, says Six (l. 21–28):

Zoo brengh ik weer papier in 't licht,
Op voeten, maate, en rym, gedicht:
Maar vies, en wrangh, en hard, en wreed,
Voor die ter loop het tast, of eet.
Maar wie het handelt als een dier,
Dat reeden heeft, zal daar een sier,
Of sonneveesjen goeds, of meer,
Sien in de keer, of weederkeer.

In this way, I bring poems into the light again,
On metrical feet, metre and rhyme:
But dirty, wry, hard and cruel,
For the ones who taste or eat it hastily,
But those who treat it as an animal
Possessed of reason [that is, a human being] will find a jewel
Or a little sunbeam of pleasure, or more,
In the strophe or the antistrophe of the poem.

So the intoxication from the cachou did not produce sweet-flowing Ovidian words, but 'slechte vaarsjes' ('poor verses') (l. 42). In the subsequent strophe (l. 31–40), Six turns once again to the recipient of the pair of texts, Hans Baert, but also welcomes others who may have become curious about his verses when they heard the printing

34 Six may have borrowed the image of the poet as a 'worm' (silkworm) spinning silk (making something precious or sublime) from another *vates* poet: in *Altaergeheimenissen*, 1645, first book, l. 18, Vondel identifies himself with a 'zyworm' that spins silk thread, in: J.F.M. Sterck *et al.* (eds.), *De werken van Vondel. 1640–1645*, vol. 4, 1930, p. 625.

press rattling. Who these people are, we find out in the next strophe (l. 41–50), where Six asks his 'bad verses' to greet the great 'Poets': Vondel, Jan Vos, Jan Six, Reyer Anslo and Geeraert Brandt. In closing (l. 51–60), Six expresses the hope that there is someone who will want to defend his honour when he is gone and slander is given free rein (l. 53–55): 'Zoo zal een dichter, goed van aard / Sien dat myn eere blyf bewaart, / Terwyl ik maanden ben van huis' ('In that way, a poet, friendly by nature, will ensure that my honour is preserved, while I am away from home for months on end').

The pair of texts raises many questions. Were they written for a particular occasion? In the last strophe Six announces that he has 'namaals' (l. 58) written to Baert, a term which A.E. Jacobs translates as 'after a dinner'. The poet also reports that he is about to leave for a business trip abroad. Six probably wrote these two texts in 1649, on the eve of his journey through Southern Europe (1649–1651).[35] If that is the case, Six's merchant colleague might have received these poems along with a specimen of *terra japonica*. We recognise the pattern from poems such as 'Dank, voor een gerookten salm, aan Pieter Loones' (J357) and 'Dankdicht aan Jakob Breine te Dantsich, voor een paar barnesteene hechten' (J165).

Given the references to 'solemn ceremonies', it is also relevant to read the pair of texts in the context of mythological poems in praise of Joyous Entries, such as the previously discussed 'Toewydinge aan de vreegodinne' to the Peace Treaty of Münster, which took place in the same period. If these two texts were written as a prologue to a cycle of poems, it is possible that the cycle included poems from Six's *Vreughde-Zangen*. A royal banquet such as that on the occasion of the visit of the French Queen Maria de' Medici to the East Indian House could also include exotica such as cachou. Since this dithyramb refers to an intoxicant from the Far East, there are also resonances with the Asian triumphs of Bacchus or Alexander the Great. Next to an imitation of Horace's Ode III, 25, that may have been a point of reference for Six while he was writing the text, even though he makes no explicit reference in the poem to any of these Far Eastern triumphs. But regardless of whether the series is aimed at a specific triumph, we understand Six's purpose in writing the poems: Six is waxing ironic over the concept of ceremonial use of poetry and drugs. Six honours Baets with divine poetry and exotics as if the Protestant merchant was a Roman Emperor. The contrast between the exalted use of language and the real situation, an informal dinner among merchant colleagues, would have made Hans Baert laugh. He would have appreciated Six's precious farewell gift and at the same time would have understood Six's relativisation of the religious connotations associated with foreign drugs. The commercial correspondence between Six and his business connections is, as we have seen, not devoid of quasi-religious

35 Jacobs, 1991 II, pp. 263, 366.

allusions, as the odiferous amber in 'Dankdicht aan Jakob Breine te Dantsich'. Six emphasises, however, that cachou does not offer divine insights. Here he is following the pseudo-Aristotelian explanation of poetic mania as a purely physical process. This time the physical effect of the substance is also not so drastic – after all, it is not an opium-containing drug, but rather a *soft drug*: cachou is 'eventually as sweet as liquorice', as Six writes.[36]

'Ecstasy of the Senses'

The mockery aimed at the elevated position of the poet-prophet reaches its zenith in 'Verrukkinge der sinnen, aan Joannes Hoorenbeek, dr., profr., en predikant t'Uitrecht: en Simon Dilman geneesheer' (J177), a text that in its form and content is in line with the texts in the prologue I discussed above. The first part of the title, 'Verrukkinge der Sinnen', means 'rapture of the senses' or, in modern English, 'ecstasy'. The rest of the title refers to the two people the text is addressed to: Johannes Hoornbeeck (1617–1666), a preacher and professor of theology at the University of Utrecht, and Simon Dilman, Six's physician, whom we met in Chapter 4. This poem too, is an imitation of Horace's Ode IV, 2, and we also find similarities with Ode III, 25, where Horace speaks of poetry as a 'sweet danger' (l. 18). And here again, Six's idea is to celebrate Frederick Henry as a Dutch Augustus. However, in the middle of the text, he changes his mind and, as the title makes clear, instead greets Hoornbeeck and Dilman. As we shall see, the reference to the Prince of Orange gives us reason to believe that the poem was written sometime after 1648, the year in which the Peace Treaty of Münster was concluded.

All of the elements of Parnassian poetry are present here, too: it is a Pindaric dithyramb with a triadic structure. The poet presents himself as a priest-prophet, possessed by a supernatural force, a sacred fervour, which provides him with the power to predict the future (l. 1–10):

Wat voel ik voor een seldsaam vier
Myn vadsich herssenslym ontsteeken?
Ik raak in brand, en schuimbek schier,
Als dolle lui, en weet met geen belul te spreeken.
De Poësy is soete raaserny.
De sienders, en Poeëten
Voorseggen, sonder toovery,

36 *Cf.* the taste of Six's verses/notes in 'Raad aan den Geenen, die myn rymen mishaagen' ('Advice to Those who Dislike My Rhymes') (J393).

Niet selden, sonder van voorsegginge te weeten,
Of wat het werden zal.
Hun Godheit straalt, en leert geen dingen by geval.

What a rare fire I feel,
Which ignites my indolent brain matter?
I catch fire, and almost foam at the mouth,
Like mad people, and do not speak with reason.
Poetry is sweet frenzy.
The seers, and Poets
Predict, without sorcery,
Not infrequently, without knowing that they are predicting,
Or knowing what is going to happen.
Their Divinity is radiant, and teaches us that nothing happens by chance.

What stands out here are the irony in the description of divine mania, and the attention Six pays to the physical reactions caused by the inspiration he feels. He feels the mystical union so strongly that he almost starts foaming at the mouth. Here, too, Six thus experiences ecstasy as a somatic disturbance. In summing up the contents of the poem, I will further analyse Six's description of this condition.

In the next two stanzas, Six discusses the relationship between Pindar and Horace when it comes to their different views on poetry. Anyone who tries to follow the high-flying style of Pindar will perish like Icarus, he tells us, referring to Horace's famous ode, in which, as we saw above, he was asked to sing, in the manner of Pindar, in praise of the Emperor Augustus' Roman triumph. He tells us he will never succeed in the task, comparing himself to the mythical hero who flew too close to the sun and fell back to earth. Horace turns down the request, telling us he lacks the talent for such a sacred task as singing the Emperor's praises. Nevertheless, Horace's ode is, as we know, remarkably Pindaric in both form and structure. Through the use of *praeteritio,* the ode does end up singing the praises of the Roman god-emperor. In his ode, Six explains Horace's apparent inconsistency. Horace could not help imitating Pindar, because he was blinded by the splendour of the Greek poet (l. 11–30).

Six tells us that Horace secretly stole feathers from Pindar's beautiful plumage, so that he becomes '[t]ienduisendmaalen schooner / De schoonste paradyser voogelen' ('ten thousand times more beautiful than the most beautiful birds of Paradise') (l. 23–34). Here Six welcomes a comparison to the early modern collections of naturalia: he refers to so-called birds of paradise – birds from the Far East with a particularly beautiful plumage (Fig. 8.4). Because they were brought to Europe without legs, European scientists thought they spent their whole lives flying. In descriptions of

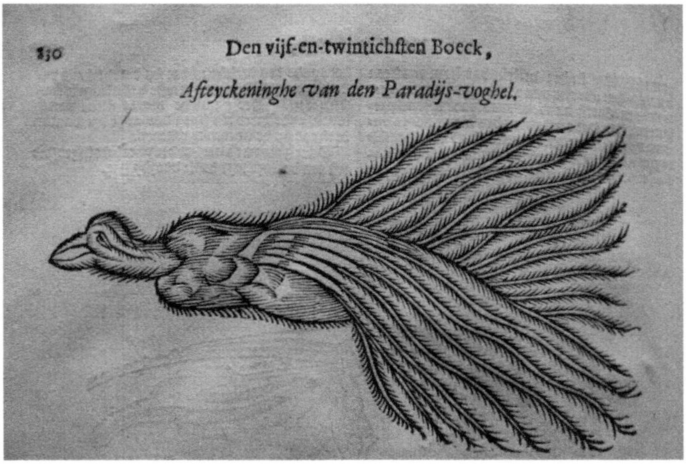

Fig. 8.4: Illustration of a Bird of Paradise in Ambroise Paré, *De chirurgie, ende alle de opera, ofte wercken*, 1636. (© Privately owned.)

the time, the bird is presented as an animal that has a special relationship with the sun, which fits in well with the myth of Icarus. According to Jan Huygen van Linschoten, the birds of paradise are 'Fowle of the Sunne' that 'flie, as it is said alwaies into the Sunne, and kéepe themselves continually in the ayre'. There was thus no bird more noble in Six's day. As a result, birds of paradise were very popular in curiosity cabinets.[37]

In the third stanza, Six tells us – once again with irony and hyperbole – that to '[o]ns Holland, parrel aan het oor / Des werldgodins' ('our Holland, a ring with a pearl in the ear of the goddess of the world') (l. 31–32) two Pindaric poets come flying in: Joost van den Vondel and P.C. Hooft (l. 38–40). Six parallels the opposition between Horace and Pindar and that between himself and the two stars of Dutch poetry. He tries to reach the artistic level of these 'bird kings' (l. 41), but admits that he will fall short (l. 51–56):

Maar of natuur, en dichtens kunste
  Gebaart, uit tyds, en oeffninghs schoot,
My weigerden haar Heemelgunste,
  Om gest te kneeden, in het brood,
  Van myn niet wel gereesen brein:
Zoo zal ik met myn riemen roeijen.

37 *Voyage of Jan Huyghen Linschoten, to the East-India*, vol. I, 1885, p. 118. See Jorink, 2010, pp. 274–276. Jacobs (1991 II, p. 321) has another explanation of 'birds of paradise': 'all birds ever created and living in paradise'.

But even if nature and the art of poetry,
Born of the womb of time and practice,
Denied me her Heavenly favour
To knead yeast in the bread
Of my not well risen brain:
Still I shall have to make do with what I have.

Although Six has inherited his talent from his mother, and masters poetic craftsmanship thanks to *exercitio*, he has been denied heavenly inspiration. He blames his own physical condition for this. He says he lacks an inner fire – the force required to achieve a high yeast, a ferment thus. 'Fermentatio' was a buzzword in the work of early modern chemists, for whom it was a form of 'natural transmutation' in which the character of substances was radically altered. They believed, among other things, that the life spirit resulted from a fermentation that took place in the heart. Six is probably poking fun at these ideas here.[38] But although Six does not achieve this transformation, as is apparent from the quote, he will have a go at it. In the next stanza (l. 61–70), he makes clear his intention in writing his ode. He asks Apollo to fill him with the power of the sun, so that – despite his lack of poetic imagination – he can compose a hymn to the marriage between Astrea, the goddess of justice, and the 'Oranjes vreedeprins' ('the Orange Prince of Peace'). The Prince of Orange thus emerges as Six's equivalent to Augustus as portrayed by Horace. If Apollo will give him inspiration, he says, he will be filled with divine power, so that 'vuur vloeije, uit een diamante pen, / Op dichtende papieren' ('fire may flow out of a diamond pen, onto poetic papers') (l. 65–66).

The lofty theme of the text, the planned celebration of the Prince of Peace, is, however, soon abandoned. It turns out that the poem is intended to be neither an apotheosis of a mighty person nor a celebration of a public event. With his Pindaric ode, Six has no higher intention than to greet two dear friends (l. 71–74):

Met sulken pen, o Haarlem, wil
Ik Hoorenbeek uw soon vereeren,
Die, met syn daagen in April,
Een vruchthoorn meededeilt, van goude soomerpeeren.

With such a pen, O Haarlem, I
Will honour your son, Hoornbeeck,
Who, with his [birth in these] days in April,
Presents a cornucopia of golden summer pears.

38 E.D. Baumann, *Francois dele Boë Sylvius*, 1949, pp. 67, 204; Elisabeth Berry Drago, *Printed Alchemists: Early Modern Artistry and Experiment in the Work of Thomas Wijck*, 2019, p. 220.

So much for the omniscient pretentions of the divine *vates*. The high poetic flight ends with an anti-climax: Six congratulates his friend Johannes Hoornbeeck on the birth of his son in April that year. The contents of the following and final stanza (l. 81–90) are equally prosaic: Six expresses his admiration for Simon Dilman's medical skills.

In 'Verrukkinge der Sinnen', Six argues that his innately humble nature is incompatible with the sublime style of poetry he intended to follow. The literary strategy he uses can be recognised from the texts discussed earlier. There is one text in particular that comes to mind: 'Hooghloffelijke gedachtenisse' ('Most Laudable Memory') (J215). Just as he does in that poem, Six tell us in 'Verrukkinge der Sinnen' that he cannot sing divinely because of a humoral lack of fire: 'my indolent brain matter' and 'my not well risen brain'. By emphasising his dry-cold condition, he means to prove his Dutchness: he is a Northerner with an innate sobriety that does not go hand in hand with the bombastic style of poetry of the Parnassian language imported from the South. His lack of fervour makes him – to continue with the medical terminology – *immune* to the inspiration of the muses.

But Six is not entirely blameless either when it comes to the high-flown style of Pindar. 'The Prince of Peace' whom Six mentions in the text is most likely Frederick Henry, the central figure in Six's own poems to the Peace Treaty of Münster.[39] As we have seen, the inconsistencies for which he reproaches Horace actually characterise his own poems of praise for the Peace in 1648. After all, the difference between Astraea, the goddess of justice, and Pax, the protagonist of 'Toewydinge aan de vreegodinne', who was also accompanied by a group of noble 'poet birds', is not that big. Ecstasy is therefore as much a hallmark of Six's authorship as it is of Hooft's and Vondel's. Six probably also wrote 'Verrukkinge der Sinnen' as a parody of his own *Vreughde-Zangen*.

This brings us to the recipients of the poem, Johannes Hoornbeeck, a minister, and Simon Dilman, a doctor. *Furor poeticus* is a concept that probably interested both of them: the doctor from a medical point of view, as a form of frenzy or drunkenness, and the theologian from a theological perspective, in connection with the notion of religious ecstasy, or *enthousiasmos*. Both were worried about Six's dangerous position, first as a follower of pagan-magical poetry, and second as a merchant-druggist, a trader in 'fiery' medicines. Both likely enjoyed reading Six's ridicule of the poetic madness of his fellow poets, but also understood that Six's 'medical

39 Jacobs (1991 II, p. 322) believe that 'Oranjes vreedeprins' (l. 70) is William II, but in my opinion Six is referring to Frederick Henry. In 'Het tweede Gezangh' ('The Second Song') (J609), which is not included in *Poësy*, the Astraea we referred to above in 'Verrukkinge der Sinnen' is also mentioned. Astraea, worshipped as the goddess of the Golden Age, is a popular figure within the early modern royal cult. *Cf.*, for example, the poems in praise of Elisabeth I: Frances Amelia Yates, *Astrea: The Imperial Theme in the Sixteenth Century* (1975).

confession' also related to his own body. Moreover, it is possible that laughter not only serves a rhetorical function here, but is also an end in itself. According to Johan van Beverwijck, laughter has medical properties: it dispels melancholy and invigorates the whole body.[40] Simon Dilman needs no further introduction here. He and his family would also have had a deeper interest in the subject of the poem. In 1654, one of his sons, Johannes, actually obtained his doctorate on the subject of frenzy. Six wrote a poem for the occasion: 'Welkomst, aan Joannes Dilman, van Leiden, naa hy geneesheer was gemaakt, alvooren hebbende beweert, wat raasernye was' (J381) ('Welcome to Johannes Dilman, from Leiden, after He Was Made Physician, Having Shown what Frenzy Is'). In his thesis, the young Dilman actually mentions characteristics of the disease along with methods of treatment that reflect medical discussions in Six's own texts. Dilman mentions hot food and drink as external causes of frenzy, characterises a 'trembling tongue' as a severe symptom, asks the patient to avoid strong feelings, especially anger, and recommends a diet consisting of greens such as endives and sorrel.[41] It could thus be that Six had discussions with the Dilman family on the 'sweet frenzy' of poetry and on possible medical explanations for the phenomenon. 'Ecstasy' can be seen as a medical self-diagnosis: Six shows that he is aware of the dangers of poetic excess. He demonstrates that his innate Dutch sobriety is incompatible with the presumptuous artistic style he was planning to follow. After all, he lacks the inner fire required to achieve the high 'ferment' of the prophet-poet.

Johannes Hoornbeeck

Let us now turn to Johannes Hoornbeeck. A surprisingly high number of the poems in *Poësy* are addressed to the theologian, who was a cousin of Six's and of Dilman's.[42] The texts discuss both personal and religious matters. Hoornbeeck sends him his theological works, for which Six expresses his gratitude in poems. Johannes Hoornbeeck, who was painted by Frans Hals, occupied an important position in the intellectual circles of the Dutch Republic (Plate 12). From 1644 to 1654 he was Professor of Theology at the University of Utrecht, and from 1654 he held the same position at the University of Leiden. Hoornbeeck, who knew thirteen languages and wrote a number of theological works before his untimely death, was one of the

40 Van Beverwijck, *Schat der gesontheyt*, p. 59. *Cf.* Anna Tummers, Elmer Kolfin, Jasper Hillegers (eds.), *The Art of Laughter: Humour in Dutch Paintings of the Golden Age*, 2017.

41 Johannes Dilman, *Disputatio Medica Inauguralis de Phrenitide*, 1654.

42 Johannes Hoornbeeck was the grandchild of Six's aunt, Susanne Six, and he was also related to Hans Baert, see Appendix II.

major figures of the so-called Further Reformation, a Dutch version of Puritanism.[43] Whereas Dilman serves as a medical supervisor for Six as he regains his health, Hoornbeeck seems to have the role of spiritual adviser to the merchant-poet in his search for salvation. At the beginning of his career, Hoornbeeck had been a pastor for four years at the Reformed Church 'under the Cross' in Mülheim am Rhein (now a district of Cologne). Because the reformed worship service was not permitted in Cologne, he focused mainly on the Protestant merchants in the city.[44] Hoornbeeck therefore had good qualifications to assist a reformed person travelling in Roman Catholic countries.[45] Considering the fact that Church history was Hoornbeeck's academic speciality, he was uniquely qualified to understand the obscure poetic language of Six, full of references to gods and religious practices of antiquity.[46]

But that does not mean that he categorically rejected all strange and new things from heathen countries. As revisionist research has recently underlined, the quality of global curiosity was not limited to radical thinkers in early modern Holland such as Spinoza, but was also present in apparently conservative Calvinists such as Hoornbeeck; his *De conversione Indorum et Gentilium* (1669), which was published posthumously and discusses the conversion of heathens to Christianity, is characterised by a surprising openness to, and curiosity about, ethnographic information.

43 T. Brienen, *Johannes Hoornbeeck (1617–1666): eminent geleerde en pastoraal theoloog*, 2008; Jan Pieter de Bie *et al.* (eds.), *Biografisch woordenboek van protestantsche godgeleerden in Nederland*, part 4, 1931, p. 277.

44 Ibid., p. 277.

45 *Cf.* 'Begroetenisse oover de eerstgeboorte van Joannes Hoorenbeek, doctr, professor, en predikant te Uitrecht' ('Greetings to the First-Born Child of Johannes Hoornbeeck, Doctor, Professor, and Pastor in Utrecht') (J284), in which Six, congratulates Hoornbeeck on the birth of his first-born by making fun of the Papal Jubilee year in 1650. Behind the humorous tone, however, lies a certain seriousness. The text was written in August 1651, after Six's return from his commercial trip through France, Spain and Italy (1649–1651). By distancing himself from the Roman Catholic Church, he showed that he had not been spoiled by his three years abroad.

46 See the presentation of the theologian in Johannes Hoornbeeck, *On the Conversion of Indians and Heathens. An Annotated Translation of De Conversione Indorum et Gentilium (1669)*, ed. by Ineke Loots & Joke Spaans, 2018, pp. 1–34. In this context, a recurring theme in the *oeuvre* of both Six and Hoornbeeck should be mentioned: criticism of the Jews. Many of Hoornbeeck's works, especially *Tshubbat Jehoedah* (1655), betray an aversion to Jewish culture. But Hoornbeeck's view of the Jews is not all negative. Although the theologian holds some common prejudices, such as the idea that Jews hate and deceive Christians, he opposed the much-heard accusation of ritual infanticide, which he describes as a product of collective fantasy. Hoornbeeck's main goal is to convert the Jewish people: Matthijs van Campen, *Gans Israël: Voetiaanse en coccejaans visies op de joden gedurende de zeventiende en achttiende eeuw*, 2006, p. 75. Things are no better in Six's case. The tone in some poems and text passages is stigmatising – see, for instance, 'Jooden kerkhof te Livorno' ('Jewish Churchyard in Livorno') (J253); 'Op de woorden: My dorst. Aan Jesus Kristus aan 't kruys' ('On the Words: I Thirst. To Jesus Christ on the Cross') (J323) (l. 4); ''s Amsterdammers winter' (J96) (l. 645–654). But his aversion is not based on the differences but on the similarities between himself and the Jews. As we have seen, many of Six's business connections were Jews.

This is also apparent from Hoornbeeck's friendship with the aforementioned physician Franciscus Sylvius, known in the Dutch Republic for his progressive medical ideas. The author of Hoornbeeck's biography in the posthumous edition of *De conversione Indorum et Gentilium* actually compliments Sylvius for not dismissing the ideas of antiquity in his search for new knowledge, and for entertaining instead a love for things both ancient and modern.[47] It is thus likely that Hoornbeeck shared Six's interest in exotic new products brought to Dutch ports by ships from the East and West Indies, but that he also called for caution in dealing with commodities from pagan countries, warning of the temptations that they might carry and that might bring him away from God.[48]

'Brief, neevens eenige rymen, aan Joannes Hoorenbeek, doctr, profr, en predikant te Uitrecht' ('Letter, in Addition to Some Rhymes, to Johannes Hoorenbeek, Preacher and Professor of Theology at the University of Utrecht') (J317) gives a further clue about how the exchange of writings between Six and Hoornbeeck worked. Given the title of this poem, it seems that Six would send Hoornbeeck not only verses specifically intended for him, but also other rhymes. The text is an expression of gratitude for the many theological works he has received from Hoornbeeck. Six describes these as injections of spiritual power. He also seems to see verses he sent to Hoornbeeck as a kind of penance. He continues to 'be indebted' ('schuldig staan') for the edifying books received (l. 10), he admits, and hopes that his 'rhymes' will be accepted as a form of 'payment' ('voldoeningh') (l. 11). So we should not take too literally the contempt Six displays for his own poems. Continual self-analysis and self-criticism were, after all, a characteristic of the Further Reformation.

Another 'epistolic poem' addressed to the theologian, 'Brief, aan Joannes Hoornbeek, te Uitrecht' ('Letter to Johannes Hoornbeeck, in Utrecht') (J236), supports my thesis here. In this text, Six brings up a moral dilemma: which of his literary examples, the psalms of David or the poems of Horace, does he value more? In the text, Six is faced with the choice between two types of poetic inspiration: ancient heathen and Christian. This test is worked into a story.[49] Six is on a business trip in France and, while he is crossing a rocky area in Anjou on horseback, his psalm book falls out of his pocket without his noticing. He has just been holding the other book he has taken along on his journey, by Horace, because, he says, he felt an enormous urge to read the pagan Roman: 'myn vaste Flakkus riep my, om syn

47 See 'Vita CI. Hoornbeek' (unpaginated), in: *De Conversione Indorum et Gentilium. Libri Duo*, 1669.

48 Jos Gommans & Ineke Loots, 'Arguing with the Heathens: The Further Reformation and the Ethnohistory of Johannes Hoornbeeck (1617–1666)', *Itinerario*, 2015, pp. 45–68.

49 For a more detailed analysis see: J.C. Arens, 'Studies over nawerkingen van Klassieken V: Six van Chandelier tussen Horatius en David', *TNTL*, 1961, pp. 114–130; Schenkeveld-van der Dussen & De Vries, 2007, p. 139.

disch te smaaken, / Vol ydelheits geschaft, om Davids niet te naaken' ('My regular companion Horace called on me, so that I could taste his fare, full of vanities, to keep me away from David') (l. 55–56). In the main part of the text, Six reflects on how he could have lost the psalm book. First he gives some possible, logical explanations: perhaps he forgot the book in the city he last visited, or perhaps it fell out of his pocket because he was riding on uneven terrain? But he chooses a deeper spiritual explanation: the devil – 'd'Onsichtbre Onkruidenier' ('the Invisible Poison Merchant') (l. 50) – was sitting behind him on the horse, and took the book out of his pocket and threw it away. 'Onkruidenier' is of course intended as a counterpart to an iconographic representation of Jesus that was popular in the early modern era: Christ as an apothecary.[50] The metaphor was not chosen by chance. It refers to Six's own identity as a merchant druggist.

The excessive desire for pagan, classical poetry that beset the poet was the work of the devil, he tells Hoornbeeck. When Six marks the contrast at the end of the text between the ambiguous predictions of Delos (the Pythia at the rock gorge) and the truth of the 'Priester van Apollon, / de Kriste Orakelgod, te Sion' ('Priest of Apollo, the Christian Oracle God of Sion') (l. 57–58), he shows all the same that he knows how to distinguish good Christian inspiration from the pagan variety. This reference would have been to the theologian's liking, for the Oracle at Delphi was one of his fields of research.[51] The next time he promises to write 'Kerkelyk, en aangenaamer' ('Religiously, and more pleasantly') (l. 64). Does he mean his plan to make his own rhyming translation of David's psalms?[52] In any case, 'Brief, aan Joannes Hoornbeek, te Uitrecht' supports my thesis that many texts in *Poësy* should be read as confessional literature. In this respect, it is not only the Christian theme of the poem that is interesting, but also its formal features. It could be that the story of the lost psalm book is based on an actual event, but for us the considerable value Six himself attaches to it is especially important. Six pushes the situation to the brink, so that the story acquires the character of a divine trial, but not, all the same, at the expense of Six's typical imagination, humour and irony. According to the Dutch humanist Gerardus Vossius, *ironia* is a device whereby what is said is the opposite of what is meant, but the rhetorical figure is also a way to show wit and engage in self-deprecation. This would have appealed to the humanistically learned Hoornbeeck, who was well read in ancient

50 *Cf.* the so-called *Christus medicus*. See also Chapter 4, p. 154.

51 *Cf.* the description of Ripa and Horace of the poet, mentioned in the beginning of this Chapter. See Johannes Hoornbeeck, *On the Conversion of Indians and Heathens. An Annotated Translation of De Conversione Indorum et Gentilium (1669)* (ed. by Ineke Loots & Joke Spaans), 2018, pp. 189–213.

52 *Cf.* Six's introduction to his psalm rhyming: he has been 'oover de twintig jaaren swanger' ('pregnant for more than 20 years') with the work, see Chapter 4, pp. 147–148. That means he started on it before 1654. According to Jacobs (1991 II, p. 417), 'Brief, aan Joannes Hoornbeek, te Uitrecht' dates from 1649.

heathens and those of his day; he would have had no difficulties getting Six's witty and subtle way of writing, such as his medical, moral and theological discussions of spiritual materials. He would also have understood the seriousness with which Six engaged in self-examination.[53]

The critique of *enthousiasmos*

What dangers does poetic madness actually bring with it? This is the subject of 'Verrukkinge van sinnen' (J401), a poem that has almost the same title as the text discussed above, but that uses a completely different literary strategy. The basic tone here is not relativising and humorous, but confrontational and serious. Six does not identify himself in the usual way with a humble bird species, but presents himself as a noble bird, a 'marvellous morning awakener' (l. 1–5):

Ik haat het onbesuist getier.
Den bek toe kraai, en kaauw, en exter.
Wat brein heeft luister naa myn lier,
Een wonderlyke morgenwekster,
In 't harte, aan brand van heiligh vier.

I hate the rash warbling.
Shut up, crow, and jackdaw, and magpie.
If you have brain, listen to my lyre,
A marvellous morning awakener,
In the heart, a sacred fire that burns.

The rooster (the 'morning awakener') as a metaphor refers to the omniscient prophet-poet.[54] Filled with heavenly inspiration, Six dares to ask some existential questions: what did God do before He created the universe and the earth, and why did He create the world (l. 6–10)? He then describes how he experiences a *metempsychosis*, a movement of the soul, and goes to a desert full of 'duursam goud / En schaaduwloose diamanten, / En onixen, en esmeroud' ('durable gold, shadeless diamonds, and onyx, and emeralds') (l. 16–18). But the ecstasy does not cause a Parnassian revelation this time either. A snow-white sheet with crimson letters comes down from heaven. The answer to Six's questions is on it: God has 'een roe

53 For Vossius's definitions of irony, see D. Knox, *Ironia. Medieval and Renaissance Ideas on Irony*, 1989.
54 See Vossius, 2010, II, pp. 1913–1914, where both the *topos* of the rooster and poetry as a Pythagorean movement of the soul are discussed.

van vuur [...] voor zulke goddeloose vraagen' ('a rod of fire [...] for such ungodly questions') (l. 27–28).[55] The high flight ends once again with an anti-climax. Scared to death, the poet falls back to earth.

The opening of the text is an *imitatio* of Horace's Ode III, I, in which the Roman poet asks the uninitiated mob to quieten down. For when he, the 'priest of the Muses', speaks, everyone must listen attentively.[56] If we think back to the poems discussed above, we can understand the meaning of the poem: once again the notion of the poet as a recipient of divine inspiration is criticised. Whereas Six explains the poetic inspiration in the texts we have looked at on the basis of medical theories, in this poem he approaches the *furor poeticus* with his thirst for omniscience from a theological perspective. In that sense, the text shows similarities to 'Brief, aan Joannes Hoornbeek, te Uitrecht'. Was the preacher perhaps also the intended reader of 'Verrukkinge van sinnen'? A glance at the writings of Hoornbeeck will help us understand the dangerous *curiositas* Six displays in the poem.

In Hoornbeeck's most important work, *Summa Controversiarum Religionis*, we find an interesting discussion that can shed more light on Six's poetry.[57] The sixth chapter, 'Enthusiastis et libertinis', is devoted to the concept of *enthousiasmos*. The theologian states that there is both a positive and a negative form of *enthousiasmos*. Each can be divided into two subcategories: ordinary and extraordinary. As for the good, extraordinary *enthusiasmos* – the direct divine inspiration of the prophets and the authors of the Bible – Hoornbeeck follows the strict Protestant point of view: miracles and prophecies no longer occur after the biblical era. The good, ordinary *enthousiasmos* is the power that emanates from the Holy Spirit and fills the community of true believers. The negative *enthousiasmos* is either imaginary or devilish in character, and is expressed in false revelations, visions and oracles.[58]

Hoornbeeck examines the concept mainly with regard to various religious sects and groups throughout the centuries: from the false prophets of the biblical era to the Rosicrucians of his own time. But as Michael Heyd emphasises, the reformed theologians do not always have a specific sect in mind. They refer to all kinds of groups that claim esoteric knowledge, such as prophecies and soothsaying, or whose psychological behaviours (ecstasies, convulsions, and so on) are associated with

55 The colour symbolism we recognize from 'Rariteiten te koop': on the one hand, red symbolises revolt and sin; on the other, divine anger and revenge – *cf.* Isaiah 1:18. I will return to the symbolic value of red in the last chapter.

56 Jacobs, 1991 II, p 698. For the description of ecstasy in 'Verrukkinge van sinnen', Six also borrowed elements from Acts 10:9–16. See also the definition of 'ecstasy' in comment 11 to Acts 10:10.

57 The first edition was published in 1653, but I use the augmented edition of 1658, which is also the starting point for Michael Heyd, *'Be Sober and Reasonable': The Critique of Enthusiasm in the Seventeenth and Early Eighteenth Centuries*, 1995.

58 Hoornbeeck, 1658, pp. 378–379.

enthousiasmos. This applies to the chapter 'Enthusiastis et libertinis' in Hoornbeeck's book in which the theories of the mystic Valentin Weigel are discussed. In this chapter it is not just Weigel who is treated: Hoornbeeck offers the reader a broader view of the *magica theologia* in the early modern era and thus also of the problem of how knowledge is acquired.[59] Although Hoornbeeck does not deal with the concept of *furor poeticus*, he does pay attention to a group of thinkers whose ideas are based on Neoplatonism, astrology and Pythagoreanism: Paracelsus and his supporters. Hoornbeeck warns against what came out of the 'hermetico-paracelsian ovens and flames'.[60] These Paracelsian scientists claimed that they had access to hidden knowledge. They regarded highly the works of the Florentine philosophers and their translations of mystical writings, such as Ficino's translation of the Hellenistic *Corpus Hermeticum*. Daniel Heinsius tells us that Homer was considered a universal sage, the father of all the sciences, and the voice of the Neoplatonists in the Republic. Could we then call the divinely inspired poet a kind of natural scientist, in possession of the so-called *prisca scientia* – secret knowledge about the origin of the world and the hidden meanings of natural phenomena – the knowledge Six seeks in 'Verrukkinge van sinnen'?[61] Hoornbeeck has his answer ready for such claims to omniscience: complete knowledge is impossible for humankind.

Both 'Verrukkinge van sinnen' and 'Brief, aan Joannes Hoornbeek, te Uitrecht' should, in my opinion, be interpreted against the background of this theological debate on *enthousiasmos*. The mystical experiences associated with poetic madness present our druggist-poet with epistemological dilemmas: how does a human being acquire knowledge? And how do they distinguish admissible from inadmissible forms of knowledge? In his poems, Six shows that he is aware of the dividing line between good and bad sources of knowledge. He does not want to be understood as a *poeta divinius*, whose hidden insights are acquired in a state of 'madness' or 'possession', such as the 'senseless' state in which Vondel found himself in 'Horatius Liersangen'. His opposition to the Parnassian poetics must be seen again in connection with his self-presentation as a sober merchant of drugs.

59 Heyd, 1995, p 22, Hoornbeeck, 1658, pp. 397–438: Six may have read Hoornbeeck's treatise on magic as early as 1646, because in that year he published *De Paradoxis et Heterodoxis Weigelianis Commentarius ubi et de Swencfeldo Aliisque Similis Indolis*. Brienen (2008, p. 22) tells us in this connection that 'he deals broadly with the basis and origin of all human knowledge and the eternity of the Holy Spirit'. See also J. W. Hofmeyr, *Johannes Hoornbeeck as polemikus*, 1975, pp. 118–130.

60 'Furnis & fumis Hermetico-Paracelsicis', Hoornbeek, 1658, p. 421. For the treatment of poetry as enthusiasm, see Méric Casaubon, *A Treatise Concerning Enthusiasme*, 1655, pp. 199–208.

61 *Cf.* Hoornbeeck's discussion on the mention of Homer in the Sibylline books, in: Johannes Hoornbeeck, *On the Conversion of Indians and Heathens*, 2018, p. 200. For the critique of 'philosophical enthusiasts', see Koen Vermeir, 'Imagination between Physick and Philosophy. On the Central Role of the Imagination in the Work of Henry More (1614-1687)', *Intellectual History Review* (2008), pp. 119–137. See also Peter Harrison, *The Fall of Man and the Foundations of Science*, 2007, pp. 125–138.

'Verrukkinge van sinnen' shows that Six's treatment of the notion of *enthousiasmos* is more complicated than it seemed up to this point. His approach cannot just be dismissed as the disturbance of the physical balance of a madman, as in the poems we discussed earlier. In this text, Six also adds demonic aspects to his representation of *furor poeticus*. Earlier we had clues about Six's spiritual worldview: in the texts just discussed, such as 'Brief, aan Joannes Hoornbeek, te Uitrecht', the poet links drugs to idolatry (*cf.* the depiction of the devil as a 'poison merchant'). 'Verrukkinge der Sinnen' can help us form a more nuanced picture of the issue. In that poem, the emphasis was on both the theological and the medical criticism of poetic madness. The text was, after all, addressed not only to Hoornbeeck, but also to Dilman, a doctor. Although Hoornbeeck discusses *enthousiasmos* in a theological context in *Summa Controversiarum Religionis*, the number of medical arguments in his discussion is striking. This is in line with the shift Michael Heyd points out in the views on *enthousiasmos* in the early modern period. Whereas sixteenth-century theologians identify it with demonic forces, theologians in the seventeenth and eighteenth centuries explain the phenomenon on the basis of medical theories. This in turn was based on the difference between so-called preternatural and supernatural wonders – the former refers to abnormalities and strange phenomena of various kinds that seemed to depart from the norms of nature. According to the Calvinist theologian Gisbertus Voetius, 'The devil cannot work against the direction nature takes [...]. Knowledge [...] of the miraculous, often toxic effects of all kinds of substances is important not only for theologians and philosophers, but also for physicians, because they must be able to distinguish between natural diseases, poisonings and demonic disorders'.[62] Andrew Keitt, who has studied enthusiasm in early modern Spain, writes that:

> The devil does not act as a medium, but is still present as a seducer. The devil, because of his former angelic status, was privy to secrets of nature inaccessible to the average man and could thus work wonders that surpassed common understanding, but it was commonly held that he was bound by the strict order of nature and that his seemingly miraculous effects were actually clever manipulations of purely natural causes.[63]

62 Heyd, 1995, pp. 55–57. For Voetius's vision, see M.J. van Lieburg, 'Voetius en de geneeskunde', in: J. van Oort *et al.* (eds.), *De onbekende Voetius: Voordrachten Wetenschappelijk Symposium*, 1989, pp. 175–176. The paraphrase is based on Voetius, *Selectae Disputationes*, 1648, I, pp. 1051–1059. For the difference between the preternatural and supernatural wonders, see Jorink, 2010, p. 8–10. And *cf.* Marcy Norton, *Sacred Gifts, Profane Pleasures: A History of Tobacco and Chocolate in the Atlantic World,* 2008, pp. 118–122.

63 Andrew Keitt, 'Religious Enthusiasm, the Spanish Inquisition, and the Disenchantment of the World', *Journal of the History of Ideas*, 2004, pp. 231–250.

I assume that the texts under discussion here are based on the same perspective. These principles are also reflected in the representation of precious exotica in these verses – in 'Verrukkinge van Sinnen' they are gems, for instance. They are not demonic in and of themselves, but they are illusory means that the devil uses to do his treacherous work, and it was thought that God often allows the devil to test His chosen ones. Their brilliance will enchant your senses, and tempt you to question Christian doctrines. Here again it is a matter of awareness of the moral dangers of stimulants and the passions they arouse – in this case, an un-Christian *curiositas*.

Christian versus pagan ecstasy

According to Hoornbeeck, genuine Christian *enthousiasmos* is inner and spiritual. Before concluding this chapter, I will discuss some examples in Six of what Hoornbeeck calls positive *enthousiasmos*. These texts give us more insights into the way Six handles the problem of inspiration.

'Pinxterfeest. Op de wyse van den 30 psalm' ('Pentecost. In the Manner of Psalm 30') (J203) has one of the most important stories from the New Testament as its theme: the outpouring of the Holy Spirit – an event that provided the Jewish Pentecost with a new Christian content and that is regarded as marking the beginning of a universal, Christian Church. After Christ's ascension, the apostles stayed behind alone, but Jesus promised them that the Holy Spirit would help them in his absence. Acts 2 in the Bible tells how the Holy Spirit descends upon the apostles and other believers present. Filled with a holy fire, speaking in foreign tongues and with prophetic eloquence – the gifts of the Holy Spirit – they go out into the streets to proclaim the gospel in their own language to the various nations gathered in Jerusalem at Pentecost. The listeners fall into wonderment and delight (see Acts 2:7 in the *Statenvertaling,* with comment 23) and ask whether the apostles are 'drunk' (comment 37). No, they are not. To explain their behaviour, Peter points to the words of Jesus, who had promised that the believers would be filled with divine gifts 'in the last days' (Acts 2:17).

The opening of the poem brings Six into a state of mind comparable to that experienced by the apostles whom Jesus has left, but in a Graeco-Latin context: 'Wat Godheit zal er in myn borst, / Die, om te spreeken, smacht van dorst, / Soet daalen, als den aavond daauw' ('What deity shall descend sweetly like evening dew in my bosom, which yearns for thirst, so that it will be able to speak') (l. 1–3). As a rhymester, he yearns for inspiration; as a 'thirsty druggist', he yearns for a liquid that will provide relief. Logically, the Renaissance poet goes to the poetic sources on Mount Parnassus. There, however, the reformed poet starts reflecting (l. 5–12):

Wat wonderrots zal my ontspringen?
Ik wil niet aardsch, maar Heemelsch, singen.
  Een singhsiek Kriste loop niet tot
  Der heidenen Orakelgod,
  Die door den helmond sprak, maar stom,
  Ter komst des Gods van 't Kristendom.
Die waare Apol leert liedren maaken,
Die God, en menschetongen smaaken.

From which marvellous rock shall a well spring out for me?
I want to sing, not in a worldly but a Heavenly way.
A Christian eager to sing does not go
To the pagan Oracle god,
That spoke through the mouth of Hell, but [fell] silent
At the arrival of the God of Christianity.
This true Apollo teaches us to make songs
That please the tongue of God and people.

Once again the text places Six in a situation where he must choose between Apollo and Christ.[64] True *mineralia* – to use chemical terms – do not come from 'the mouth of Hell', but as holy rain from above. Six refers to the mineral vapours from the rock crevice of Delphi, the sanctuary of Apollo.[65] In the following lines, the biblical Pentecostal story is outlined. Six finds the ideal solution to his own quest for inspiration. A drop of holy rain with fiery power (l. 17) descends upon the assembled apostles and other believers: the disciples '[v]erneemen Heemelsch windgedruis, / Dat hen vervult, en al het huis: / Hen hoofden geinsteren van tongen, / Die daar, als vlammen, booven hongen' ('sense a Heavenly sough of wind, which fills them and then the entire house: their heads flicker with tongues of fire, which hover above them') (l. 27–30): Six opposes the fire of the oracle of Delphi to that of the Holy Spirit. The Christian *mania* is brought about neither by a substance that has been ingested – the apostles are not 'vol wyn' ('full of wine') (l. 50) – nor by the inspiration of the Muses.[66]

64 Jacobs (1991 II, p. 352) reads 'wonderrots' ('marvellous rock') both as the boulder in Horeb that Moses struck and from which water came out (Exodus 17:6), and as a symbol for Christ (the 'spiritual rock': 1 Corinthians 10:4). But at the same time, in a classical reading of the poem, 'miraculous rock' refers to Mount Parnassus. The question is which of these 'marvellous rocks' is the right one.

65 *Cf.* my discussion of 'helmond'/'loogenmond' ('lying mouth') in 'Buskruids donder, en blixem, te Delft' (J396): Chapter 6, pp. 214–215.

66 *Cf.* the depiction of the Holy Spirit by Dutch poets in the fifteenth and sixteenth centuries – for whom it was also 'fire', 'water' and 'wind' – but from a Roman Catholic point of view: Moser Nelleke, *De strijd voor rhetorica. Poëtica en positie van rederijkers in Vlaanderen, Brabant, Zeeland en Holland tussen 1450 en 1620*, 2001.

A poem with a similar contrast between classical-pagan and Christian ecstasy as its theme, and in which the hand of the druggist is also recognisable, is 'Comfort to Sirikzee, oover 't verlies van Pieter Wittewrongel, kerkleeraar, hier beroepen' ('Comfort to Zierikzee over the Loss of Petrus Wittewrongel, Doctor of the Church, who Has Been Called to Come Here [Amsterdam]') (J123). The theme is the move by Wittewrongel, whom we know well from previous chapters, from Zierikzee, where he was a minister, to Amsterdam in 1638. Based on certain details in the text, however, A.E. Jacobs states that the poem was not written before 1644.[67] As in the case of Hoornbeeck, Six calls the reformed minister a 'Kristen Apolloon' ('Christian Apollo') (l. 70) and attributes physical properties to his edifying words; they have both an inspiring and a healing effect on the body of the listener or reader (l. 29–36):

Syn gulde mond ontsypt een Wrongel,
 Die puik van Nectargeur verkleint.
Syn heemeltongh smeert salf, en ongel,
 Om 't hart, in sondich bloed ontreint,
En van een scherpen pyl geschooten,
 Uit 's onderaardschen vyands ryk.
Ambroos, het brood der Godgenooten
 Heeft by dees seegen geen gelyk.

Out of his golden mouth flows a drop of Curd
Which surpasses the most delicious scented Nectar.
His Heavenly tongue smears ointment and tallow
Around the heart, which is contaminated by sinful blood
And hit by a sharp arrow
From the subterranean empire of the enemy.
Ambrosia, the bread of the Gods
Remains far behind this blessing.

Vondel's mocking pun on the name Wittewrongel is well known in Dutch literary history.[68] But this play with language in the quoted passage puts the preacher in a positive light: 'Curd' refers to a beneficial lactic fluid, while 'tallow' is a beneficial fat.[69] Nectar and ambrosia, the drink and the food of the pagan gods, fall well short of such 'native' nutrients. Wittewrongel's 'raasen' ('frenzy') (l. 59) is thus a

67 Jacobs, 1991 II, p. 228.
68 'Een zeeslang, wit van tong, zich wrong […]' ('a sea serpent, with a white tongue, twisted […]'), in: *Uitvaert van Apollo en Pan* (1654), l. 207. In: J.F.M. Sterck *et al.* (eds.), *De werken van Vondel. 1645–1656*, vol. 5, 1931, p. 799.
69 Jacobs, 1991 II, p. 229.

Christian variant of pagan poetic madness and evokes good passions in us.[70] The poet continues (l. 63–68):

Ghy raakt ons ingewand, zoo krachtigh,
  Dat wy schier Kristus neemen an.
Metaale tongh, doordringh uw spraaken,
  Uit saalicheits verborgen licht,
Wie voelt syn nierenvet niet blaaken?
  My parst ghe tot dit waare dicht.

You touch our intestines, so powerfully,
That we almost assume [the presence of] Christ.
Metal tongue permeates your speeches,
From the hidden light of salvation,
Who does not feel his kidney fat glow?
You press me to this truthful poem.

Wittewrongel's tongue is thus described as an exceptional specimen of *mineralia*. This 'Metal tongue' has a special purgative power: when Wittewrongel preaches, his listeners feel that their kidneys are glowing. According to early modern pathology, the kidneys boiled the blood to purify it and filter out the useless substances.[71] Wittewrongel's words also give Six true poetic inspiration.

Conclusion

In this chapter I have examined Six's approach to the question of supernatural madness or *enthousiasmos*. As we have seen, the concept of divine ecstasy in early modern times was not limited to the religious plane, but was expressed in several cultural areas – especially in the panegyric of Renaissance literature. In the pair

70 Acts 25. *Cf.* Wittewrongel's explanation of good and bad 'drunkenness': 1660 II, pp. 1094–1096 and 1105. *Cf.* also Stijn Bussels, 'Theories of the Sublime in the Dutch Golden Age: Franciscus Junius, Joost van den Vondel and Petrus Wittewrongel', *History of European Ideas*, 2016, pp. 1–11. Bussels shows how Wittewrongel ascend to a higher consciousness as long as it is Christian and driven by *humility*. Whereas I discuss this ascent in connection with the religious concept of *enthousiasmos*, Bussels is interested in a link between Wittewrongel's notion of a heavenly ascent and the concept of *sublimis* in the Greek writer Longinus.

71 Van Beverwijck, *Schat der ongesontheyt*, 1656, p. 148. *Cf.* the description of the physical effect of the tongues of Protestant preachers in early modern England: Jennifer Rae McDermott, '"The Melodie of Heaven": Sermonizing the Open Ear in Early Modern England', in: Wietse de Boer & Christine Göttler (eds.), *Religion and the Senses in Early Modern Europe*, 2013, pp. 177–197.

of texts 'Brief aan Hans Baard in Haarlem' and 'Fooi', Six gives madness a tangible foundation: he links it to the materials of his drugstore – we saw the same in 'Toewydinge aan de vreegodinne', which I discussed in the previous chapter. The druggist-poet describes the ecstasy aroused by these substances as a physiological process, and not as the result of divine revelation. In this way he offers a medical critique of the notion of *enthousiasmos* and the mystification of exotic drugs, and blurs the line between morbid and supernatural mania. This approach bears witness to the modern character of Six's ideas, which are dominated by the demystification of the world.

We could then conclude that, when Six defines poetic ecstasy as an illness, he is emptying the notion of its pre-modern, positive meanings.[72] We should stress, however, that the notion of illness is more complex than its appearance in Six's poetry might suggest. What is at stake in Six's criticism of *furor poeticus* is not so much a contrast between, on the one hand, rationality and health and, on the other, irrationality and illness, but rather an acceptance of one's humanity versus pretensions to divinity. In this context, pathological reactions are actually given a positive meaning. When Six emphasises, in 'Verrukkinge der sinnen', that he lacks an internal fire and is not capable of divine high flights, he is giving proof of his status as a fallible human being. Defectiveness is thus ascribed a positive value; the perfect and the divine, a negative one. Although the emphasis is more on pathologising than demonising *furor poeticus*, it is important to emphasise that Six also believes in the spiritual dimension: as 'Verrukkinge van sinnen' shows, the devil can use *enthousiasmos* to lead a person away from God. The last poems discussed show a positive variation of *enthousiasmos*, namely the power of the Holy Spirit. In contrast to the pagan classical inspiration associated with the food of the gods, the Christian *enthousiasmos* is presented as an immaterial force – a 'Heavenly sough of wind'. This immateriality implies that this force has no seductive taste, colour or odour. It looks more like indigenous, wholesome milk products than the fragrant substances of some exotic origin. Although Six puts emphasis on the immateriality of this force, it has a striking physical effect on the human body. Our druggist-poet describes these wholesome goods in medical terms.

Another paradoxical point that deserves a deeper explanation is the significance of the Further Reformation for Six's self-presentation. Continual self-analysis, penance and repentance are characteristics of the Further Reformation.[73] What is

72 For intoxication as a positive artistic force, see Marty Roth, *Drunk the Night Before: An Anatomy of Intoxication*, 2005.

73 *Cf.* Strengholt, 'Tekenen van de Nadere Reformatie in de poëzie van Revius, Cats en Huygens?', *Documentatieblad Nadere Reformatie*, 1987, pp. 109–125. The themes of self-examination, penance and repentance are actually not specifically pietistic. They can be traced back to a broader, Catholic tradition of devotion, see Terence Cave, *Devotional Poetry in France*, 1969, p. 104.

particularly interesting is the use of the idea of 'noble pagans' in combination with moral self-criticism in the literature of the Further Reformation. The behaviour of sophisticated Chinese intellectuals such as Confucius makes Europeans blush with shame, writes Hoornbeeck.[74] Turning the hierarchy of civilised and barbaric peoples on its head lies at the root of the 'European exotica' in 'Rariteiten te koop': It is not the heathens, but rebellious Europeans, who are the real cannibals. I will return to this point in Chapter 9. More problematic, however, is the literary style of *Poësy*. Six's poems are characterised, not by puritan austerity and edifying content, but by baroque poetic language. *Poësy* is not a collection of religious verses, but for the most part contains texts on profane matters. In addition, when later in his life Six was working on his own rhyming translation of David's psalms, he stayed in touch with Johannes Coccejus, a self-declared opponent of the Orthodox Calvinists. It is also worth mentioning that one of the writers of the laudatory comments in Six's translation, Frans Burman – whom I mentioned in Chapter 4 – promoted the ideas of Descartes.[75] But as Jos Gommans and Ineke Loots emphasise in their study of Johannes Hoornbeeck, the term Further Reformation dates from later on: it originates from the beginning of the nineteenth century. Research on the movement should therefore be done with a more open mind than has been the case so far by many researchers.[76] This relativising view of the Further Reformation concerns not only Six, but also theologians who were linked to the movement. We must take into account a certain affinity for literary references and devices among theologians who have a humanist education and who are well read in the great names of classical antiquity. The relativising view also goes for the language of the preachers of the Further Reformation. As Herman Roodenburg has stressed, the 'grand style' was also used among Protestant pastors. At the same time as Protestant theologians dismissed all 'sophist' preaching – an ornamental rhetoric with the purpose of shining and sparkling – they advocated a style marked by vividness, drama and expressivity, with the goal of moving believers' hearts. Hoornbeeck himself wrote in his preaching manual that a sermon should be 'emotive, moving

74 Gommans & Loots, 2015, pp. 45–68 and 50. *Cf.* also Bettina Noak: 'Foreign Wisdom: Ethnological Knowledge in the Work of Franciscus Ridderus', *Journal of Dutch Literature*, 2012, pp. 47–64.

75 Schenkeveld-van der Dussen & De Vries, 2007, pp. 244–246. For Frans Burman (Franciscus Burmannus), see Doede Nauta and Johannes van den Berg (eds.), *Biografisch lexicon voor de geschiedenis van het Nederlands protestantisme*, vol. 2, 1983, pp. 111–113.

76 Enny de Bruijn's words about the poet and preacher Jacob Revius are useful in this connection. She takes the view that 'Revius is a fine illustration of the fact that the usual frameworks and contradictions do not always suffice, and that the theological world of the seventeenth century is more complex and confused than is suggested by concepts such as "confessionalisation", "Voetian versus Coccejusian", "further reformation", "pietism" or "biblicism"'. Enny de Bruijn, *Eerst de waarheid, dan de vrede. Jacob Revius 1586–1658*, 2012, p. 511.

and penetrating'.[77] Hoornbeeck is also known for his scholastic style of writing – a technique of argumentation where arguments *pro* and *contra* play a central role. In several poems we have looked at in this study, we have seen a similar rhetorical method, where various moral dilemmas connected to drugs, cosmetics and ornamental language are systematically scrutinised. However, Six includes his moral trials in both serious and playful narratives, and his use of irony and *praeteritio* means that Six does not always give a clear answer of these ethical questions. Rather, he leaves it up to the reader to come up with answers themselves.[78]

In this context it is also worth mentioning that Hoornbeeck took courses in literature from Daniel Heinsius when he was a student at Leiden.[79] The pastor would, as we have seen, appreciate the humour and exaggerations Six used. The same goes for the performative style of the texts I have discussed in this chapter, such as 'Verrukkinge der sinnen' and 'Brief, aan Joannes Hoornbeek, te Uitrecht'. This theatrical template is the basis for poems to which I have devoted a great deal of attention in this book, and which I consider to be highlights in Six's *oeuvre*: 'Gierigheits woninge en gestaltenisse' (J99), 'Uitroep om hoornafsetters' (J244), 'Afbeeldinge en wydinge van Roselle, en haare bestraffinge' (J59–64). It is possible that Six had Hoornbeeck in mind when he wrote these 'rhymes'.

77 Herman Roodenburg, 'The body in the Reformation', in: Ulinka Rublack (ed.), *The Oxford Handbook of the Protestant Reformations*, 2017, pp. 643–666. On Hoornbeeck, see p. 657. In his commentary on a Christian grand style, Roodenburg refers to Debora K. Shuger, *Sacred Rhetoric: The Christian Grand Style in the English Renaissance*, 1988. *Cf.* also Freya Sierhuis' mention of a positive pathos with other Dutch poets and ministers: Freya Sierhuis, 'The Passions in the Literature of the Dutch Golden Age', *Tijdschrift voor Nederlandsche taal- en letterkunde*, 132 (2016), pp. 333–365.

78 For Hoornbeeck's scholasticism, see J.W. Hofmeyr, *Johannes Hoornbeeck as polemikus*, 1975. *Cf.* these poems of Six: 'Afbeeldinge en wydinge van Roselle, en haare bestraffinge. I–V' (J59-64), 'Op het blanketten van 't vrouwvolk in Spanje' (J41–50), 'Bruiloftsangh, aan Joannes Abeels getrouwt met Anna de Bra' (J171), 'Oostkappele, aan Abraham Grenier den jongen' (J172), and 'Lykbalsem' (J405), and 'Damspel, om geld teegen ooverblyfselen van heiligen, van kapucynen, met den scheepskoopman, op zee tusschen Alikante en Genua' (J256) in the following Chapter. For the technic of the scholastic disputation on literature and art, see Spies, Marijke, '"Op de Questye...": Over de structuur van 16e-eeuwse zinnespelen', *De nieuwe taalgids*, 1990, pp. 139–150; Koenraad Jonckheere, 'An Allegory of Artistic Choice in Times of Trouble: Pieter Bruegel's Tower of Babel', *Nederlands Kunsthistorisch Jaarboek*, 2014, pp. 151–177. *Cf.* also Schenkeveld-van der Dussen's (2007, pp. 250, 273) comments on Six's discussing style.

79 Gibertius Voetius, for instance, valued satire positively, provided it was not written to satisfy personal vengefulness. See C.A. de Niet, 'Voetius and Literature', in *Nadere Reformatie en literatuur. Speciaalnummer van Documentatieblad Nadere Reformatie*, 1995, p. 35. Hoornbeeck as a student in Leiden, see. J. W. Hofmeyr, 'Johannes Hoornbeeck, a Monumental 17th century Dutch Theologian: Continuities in His Thinking on Doctrine and Life', *Acta Theologica*, 2016, pp. 19–48.

Part III

Divine Blood for Sale

9. The human body as a drug

Abstract
In Chapter 9, I discuss poems by Joannes Six van Chandelier where three types of 'human' drugs play a role: *mumia* (ground Egyptian mummies), Catholic relics, and human blood, more specifically the blood of the executed king of England, Charles I. The blood of the king is praised as a divine drug in 'Rariteiten te koop'. I argue that the praise is ironic and that the lust for the blood must be understood as a 'cannibalistic lust for power' – a disease that forms a threat to the 'body' of the Dutch Republic. I argue that this and other poems serve a medical function in purging the Dutch nation of that illness. In this Chapter, I also show how Six gives a new interpretation to the name of his profession: 'druggist' as a 'thirsting' person, in the sense of longing for the blood of Christ.

Keywords: Charles I of England, human blood, mummy, relics, body politic, blood of Christ

And cynnamone, and odours, and ointments, and frankincense,
and wine, and oile, and fine floure, and wheat, and beasts,
and sheepe, and horses, and chariots, and slaues, and souls of men.
Revelation 18:13[1]

Medical cannibalism

In this chapter, we will return to 'Rariteiten te koop'. In many ways, the poem is a culmination of themes, motifs and exotic medicines that are present in Six's poetry. It is therefore also a culmination of topics and drugs that we have looked at in this book. Six discusses drugs as food, as material and linguistic ornaments, as gifts – even his Roselle receives blood as a gift in the poem – as a religious and royal attribute, and as a means of poetic inspiration. Drugs from all 'the three

1 *King James Bible*, 1611: kingjamesbibleonline.org/1611-Bible/ (consulted 17 May 2019).

Spaans, R., *Dangerous Drugs: The Self-Presentation of the Merchant-Poet Joannes Six van Chandelier (1620–1695)*. Taylor & Francis Group, 2020
DOI 10.5117/9789462983543_CH09

natural kingdoms' are treated: plants, minerals and animals. As regards this last category, the drug at the centre of 'Rariteiten te koop' – originating from 'the animal endowed with reason', the human being – is a product from none other than a king: fresh blood from, a 'cut in the King's carotid' (l. 48), following the beheading of the King of England, a grotesque product that surely no one would want to consume. But in fact, yes, they would. In the early modern period, Europeans were indeed hungry for human blood, especially that of a king.

In this chapter I will discuss three poems in which Six deals specifically with 'human drugs': 'Lykbalsem' ('Corpse Balm') (J405), on *mumia* as medicines; 'Damspel, om geld teegen ooverblyfselen van heiligen, van kapucynen, met den scheepskoopman, op zee tusschen Alikante en Genua' ('Draughts, for Money against Relics of Saints, [Played] by Capuchin Monks with the Ship's Merchant, on the Sea between Alicante and Genoa') (J256), about Catholic relics, before I come back to 'Rariteiten te koop' (J158), on the blood of King Charles I of England. 'Rariteiten te koop' is a complex poem, not only because of its rich intertextuality, but also because of the references it makes to the so-called cult of Charles the Martyr, a concept replete with theological and political connotations. Other texts about the cult, both English and Dutch, should therefore be included in the analysis. The same goes for the large number of poems that Six wrote during the First Anglo-Dutch War (1652–1654), where he expresses his concern about the broken relationship between the Dutch and the English, two kindred Protestant peoples. In some of these texts, the English republicans are portrayed as people filled by a 'cannibalistic lust for power' – a lust that Six describes as a disease that is dangerous for the bodies of both England and the Netherlands. This time he does not relate the illness to his own body, but to the body of his country, the so-called 'body politic'. In this section I argue that 'Rariteiten te koop' serves a medical function in purging the Dutch nation of this illness. Before concluding the chapter, I will also look at three short poems that Six wrote about the blood of another 'Martyr King', Christ. In these texts, Six introduces a form of human cannibalism that is permitted: consumption of the body and blood of Christ.

But first I will explore the early modern appetite for the human body. The human body not only took in medicines. In the early modern period, it was thought that it was the other way around, too – that the body also had medicinal powers. Body parts, secretions and faeces were available not only from shady characters in medical markets such as quacks and charlatans, but also from qualified doctors and pharmacists. They were included in the official pharmacopoeias as *simplicia* or as components of *composita*. In Lemery's reference work on drugs, we find the following anthropophagous substances, among others: skull (*cranium humanum*), brain (*cerebrum humanum*), blood (*sanguis humanus*) and a speciality from the gallows field: a fungus growing on skulls (*usnea humana*).[2] There was also medicinal *mumia*, embalmed human beings in powdered form, to which I will return presently.[3] We may be shocked to read about items of this kind, but the pharmacist or chemist who dealt with them on a daily basis used the same criteria as for other medicines. Here, too, purity and authenticity were the usual quality-control requirements, and forgeries had to be guarded against. For example, Lemery – when basing himself on the doctrine of signatures, which states that herbs and drugs resembling various parts of the body can be used to treat ailments of those parts – advises his readers to select the best type of *cranium humanum* – a substance that was good for brain disorders such as falling sickness and strokes:[4]

> The skull must be procured from a young, vigorous, but recently killed and as yet unburied man. The skull should then be grated and pulverized, but not calcined, like the ancients did because the sal volatile, where its main strength lies, evaporates through calcination.

Why were human substances actually used as medicines? Lemery does realise that many readers will censure him for including 'man in a inventory of drugs', but he defends this medical cannibalism. The argument for this can be found in his definition of a human being: 'the most wonderful being of all creation. It is the animal provided with reason and judgment'.[5] The implication, then, is that a creature created in the image of God was an appealing ingredient for medicines.

The use of human substances as medicines cannot be attributed to a single cultural sphere of influence. The literary historian Louise Noble places 'Hippocratic

2 Lemery (1743, p. 761) describes the latter productas follows: 'Een kleen groenachtig Mosch twee of drie lynen hoog, zonder reuk, een weinig ziltig van smaek, groeijende op de bekkeneelen der lyken van mannen en vrouwen, die langen tyd aen de lucht zyn blootgestelt geweest' ('A small greenish Moss, two or three lines high, without smell, a little salty of taste, growing on human skulls, both men and women, which have been exposed to air for a long time'). Its use is no less repulsive: 'Het is zeer 't zamentrekkende, goed om de neusbloeding te stuiten, als het in de neusgaten gestoken word' ('It is very astringent, and good at stopping a nosebleed when inserted into the nostrils').

3 Other human substances that are discussed are hair from scalps, breast milk, nails, earwax, saliva, urine, and stones from bladder and kidneys – 'human bezoar stones', according to Lemery (1743, pp. 129 and 340).

4 'Men moet 't Bekeneel van een' jong mensch van eene goede gesteltheit, die aen eenen geweldigen dood gestorven en niet begraven is geweest, verkiezen, en zich vergenoegen van 't te raspen, en 't tot poeder te brengen zonder het te verkalken, gelykals de Ouden [mensen in de oudheid] wilden, dewyls men door de verkalking het vlug zout, waer in zyne voornaemste kracht bestaet, laet vervliegen', Lemery, 1743, p. 224. For the doctrine of signatures, see H.A. Bosma-Jelgersma, *Poeders, Pillen en Patiënten*, 1983, p. 103.

5 'Den mensch in eene Beschryvinge der Droogeryen [...] 't heerlykste van alle levende schepselen, of de dier begaaft met verstand en reden', Lemery, 1743, pp. 339–340.

dirt therapy and the drug corpse-food' in a 'cross-cultural and intra-Greek pharmacological continuum'. Medical cannibalism was practised in all ancient European civilisations, although the view of this macabre medicine varied from culture to culture. Galen, for example, found the habit of drinking sweat, urine and menstrual blood 'scandalous and disgusting', but at the same time recommended animal faeces as a remedy.[6] As far as the early modern use of human medicines is concerned, we must look at the tradition of Paracelsus, whose followers thought that the beneficial properties of plant, mineral and animal substances were to be found in their 'life spirit'. And they also thought this was true of 'the animal with reason', the human being. For the Paracelsians it was important, as we saw from the above quote from the iatrochemist Lemery, that the human material for the preparation of drugs came from healthy people who had died in a violent way, because their spirits were, they believed, still present in their bodies. Richard Sugg explains the origin of the use of human medicines as follows:[7]

> To fully understand the logic and attraction of corpse medicine, we need to realise, first, how densely and precisely the Christian soul pervaded the human body. That will allow us to grasp one of the more startling aspects of European corpse medicine: certain Christian practitioners seem to have believed that it was possible to consume the powers a human possessed. Secondly, we need to look at how an increasingly scientific medicine sought to make use of the force of the soul, alchemically processing and transforming the raw material of the body. Thirdly, we will find that, for much of Northern Europe, medicinal cannibalism was not only a deeply religious practice, but a quite emphatically Protestant one.

Just like the exotic drugs discussed in this book, the medical use of human medicines was linked to magical ideas. This also made human medicines popular for other, non-pharmaceutical purposes, even cosmetic and ornamental use. In Six's poetry we find examples of the use of human medicines. Many of the skaters that Six portrays in ''s Amsterdammers winter' (J96) wear colourful clothes, and one of them shows off 'met / Een haairkuif van een doode slet, / Of galgebrok' ('with a wig made from the hair of a dead slut or a gallows bird') (l. 625–626). But the dismissive attitude expressed in the poem – other skaters who notice the headdress make fun of it – makes it clear how Six thinks about these kinds of drugs.

In another of Six's poems in which human substances are presented as magical ornaments, 'Lesse aan het mesje van Roselle' ('Lesson to Roselle's knife') (J155), the

6 Louise Noble, *Medicinal Cannibalism in Early Modern English Literature and Culture*, 2011, p. 19.

7 Richard Sugg, *Mummies, Cannibals and Vampires: The History of Corpse Medicine from the Renaissance to the Victorians*, 2011, p. 173.

druggist-poet does not seem to show such loathing. In this Petrarchan love poem, Six refers to a knife of Roselle's that he has stolen, but which he now gives back as 'love medicine'. Six admits that he had the knife in his mouth while he was eating, that he even kissed it, and that he used it to cut the ribbon that wrapped this poem. Six urges the knife to be careful with Roselle when it goes back to her, so she will not cut her finger. M.A. Schenkeveld-van der Dussen interprets the underlying meaning of this passage as follows: the penetrating action of the knife suggests an erotic invitation, and losing blood stands for losing virginity. In other words, this would then be an intimate, playful love poem that plays a daring game with Petrarchan conventions.[8] But from line 74 onwards the poem takes a remarkable turn. Attention shifts from Petrarchanism to pharmacy: Six advises Roselle to use this poem, which is attached to the knife, as a plaster on 'het wond' ('the wound'), so that her 'eedle bloedkoraalen' ('noble blood corals') are not lost. Where the knife causes the wound, the attached poem will stop the bleeding and collect her blood drops, for they are (l. 81–90):

Kraalen, en robyne vonken,
Schooner, dan uit zeespelonken,
En uit Indiaansche bergen,
Die Europes gronden tergen,
Met hun prachtige juweelen,
Ciersels van de kroonprieelen.
Kom ik dan dit blad t'aanschouwen,
'k Zal er konstigh van gaan vouwen
Vermiljoene braseletten,
En myn erm daar mee besetten.

Beads and sparkling rubies
More beautiful than the ones from sea caves
And from Indian mountains,
Which make European grounds jealous,
With their brilliant jewels,
Ornaments of the royal pleasure gardens.
If I then catch sight of this [drenched] sheet,
I will artistically fold it
Into a vermilion bracelet,
And use it as decoration on my arm.

8 Schenkeveld-van der Dussen, 2007, pp. 40–41.

Six values blood from the body of his beloved more highly than pearls and gems from exotic countries. We read that, if he can see this paper again, he will fold it to make a vermilion bracelet and wear it himself.[9] In the last lines of the verse, Six tells us he is confident that people will find this a more beautiful decoration than a bracelet belonging to Venus herself. The different services involved in this sexual exchange are interesting: if the 'knife' that Six is giving back is allowed to 'cut' her, Six will honour Roselle by elevating her virgin blood to a *mirabilium*.[10] The druggist-poet wants to show it off as the most precious commodity he has ever acquired and as the most beautiful poem he has ever written. The blood will thus serve as a literary adornment and as a miraculous ink.[11]

Were there no ethical objections to the use of human substances as medicines? According to Christianity, a person's mortal remains are sacred and destined for eternal rest until Judgment Day. In this chapter I want to show that human substances were an important part of the early modern drugstore trade, and that it was therefore a moral problem for Six's self-portrait as a down-to-earth, responsible druggist. One text that highlights ethical concerns regarding the trade in human body is 'Lykbalsem'.

Mumia – a 'divine spice'

'Lykbalsem' ('Corpse balm') (J405) is about the most remarkable human medicine in the seventeenth century: *mumia*. The fact that there was great interest in this article in scientific circles may not come as a surprise – mummies were the showpieces in early modern curiosity cabinets. But it is more difficult to understand that there was also a demand for it among those who were sick. *Mumia* was among the most expensive substances on the list of exotic medicines, and miraculous therapeutic properties were ascribed to it (Fig. 9.1).[12]

9 For vermilion, see Chapter 5, note 32.

10 *Cf.* other 'gift poems': 'Aan Arnoud van Someren' (J336), 'Dankdicht aan Jakob Breine te Dantsich, voor een paar barnesteene hechten' (J165) and 'Dank, aan Bonavontura Koegelen van Dortmond, Geneesheer, voor het geneesen mynes hands' (J444). Like the knives and forks in these poems, the knife from 'Lesse aan het mesje van Roselle' is decorated with exclusive *naturalia*, which make it an appealing object for curiosity cabinets.

11 Compare 'Aan Elisabet van Baarle, &c.' by Jan Vos, where tears from the eyes of the person mentioned in the title is presented as an exclusively 'human drug' with a wide range of applications; Geerdink, 2012, pp. 35–36, 140–141, 250–253.

12 The aforementioned *exoticotamia* of the druggist Joan Breyne contained, for example, 'twee voeten en een hant van Mumia' ('two feet and a hand of Mumia'), *Catalogus van een groote partij extraordinaire curieuse Rariteyten* [...] (*Catalogue of a Large Batch of Extraordinarily Curious Rariteyten* [...]) (1693), p. 17. For more than two centuries, Amsterdam was an important import port for *mumia*: J. Smits, *De Verenigde*

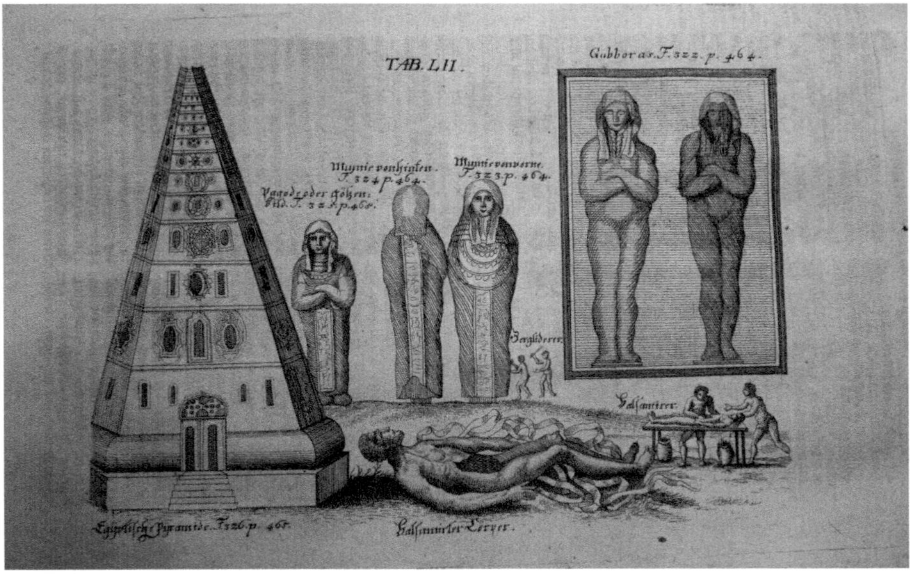

Fig. 9.1: Illustration of *Mumia*, in: Pierre Pomet, *Der aufrichtige Materialist und Specereÿ-Händler* [...], 1717. (© University Library of Oslo).

The text opens with an attack on the phenomenon that was considered the great religious *hybris* of antiquity: the Egyptian custom of burying pharaohs 'in een naald / Van hardsteen, toorenwys verheeven / Als het prachtigh graf van Cheopes' ('in a pyramid of freestones, rising tower high, as the magnificent grave of Cheops') (l. 4–6), and mummified with precious spices, 'mirre, en aloës' ('myrrh, and aloe') (l. 8). In contrast to this vain pride, Six sets the actual process of decomposition that every person, regardless of their social origin, undergoes when they die. Death 'keurt, ten einde van de daagen, / Geen onderscheid, in knecht, en heer' ('makes, at the end of days, no distinction between servant and lord') (l. 19–20).[13] In the rest of the text, the focus shifts to *mumia* as a medicine and a commodity. Six wants to show that the hubris of the ancient Egyptians also relates to his own time and to his own professional reality. Unlike the imaginary 'horn' of the 'Uitroep om hoornafsetters', which I discussed in Chapter 4, *mumia* and embalming were real phenomena in early modern medicine.

Nederlanden op zoek naar het oude Egypte (1580–1780), 1988, pp. 165–167. In the same passage, Smits discusses the price level of *mumia*: at the Amsterdam fair in 1631, 400 guilders was paid for a counterfeit mummy from the 'sea of sand'. See also the interest in *mumia* with regard to the *prisca scientia*, the lost knowledge of nature from before the Flood and Babel: Jorink, 2010, 278–289. The physician Otto Heurnius (1577–1652) called Egypt 'the ancient tutor in every branch of science' and praised the medicinal powers of *mumia*. Quoted from Jorink, 2010, p. 285.

13 *Cf.* 'Myn uiterste wil' ('My last will') (J606).

Six leaves no doubt about what he thinks of drugs of this kind. A Christian may not turn man into a commodity or a medicine. Six provides several arguments for this view. First, the forged *mumia* on the market come, not from the divine bodies of 'Egiptens kooningen' ('Egyptian kings') (l. 23), the so-called *mumia vera aegyptiaca*, but from the corpses of criminals who have recently been hanged: 'galgelyken / Gereeuwt, gebracht, en valsch verkocht' ('gallow corpses, smashed, transported, and sold under false pretences') (l. 33–34) – Six is at pains to say that it is Jewish merchants who carry on this kind of trade.[14] As we saw, Van Beverwijck warned against trading with unbelievers, who he believed had no qualms about deceiving Christians.[15]

Six then wonders what ethical consequences this might or might not have had for consumers of *mumia* themselves: 'Wat scheelt dit van de menscheneeters? / Vier stuivers 't pond van menschevleesch. / Weet nu een Kristemensch niet beeters, / Dan dat men mensch, met mensch, genees?' ('What separates them from cannibals? Four stivers for a pound of human flesh. Is a Christian not wiser than to believe that one can cure man with man?') (l. 37–40). Reduced to a commodity, the individual loses his human value. That is why Six chooses the low price of four *stivers*. In reality, *mumia* was a much more expensive product.[16] At the same time, the consumer is guilty of the most primitive of all lusts: cannibalism. Stirring *mumia powder* through your drink (l. 36) is therefore actually double self-deception. First, there is a false belief that a human being can be medicine. Second, there is the illusion that one is taking royal substances when in reality these are the remains of corrupted people: criminals and murderers.

The theme is noticeably a sensitive one for Six. The specialised description of the preparation process reveals a professional familiarity with *mumia* and the spices

14 *Cf.* the negative discussion of *mumia* by the French doctor Ambroise Paré. In his collected works, he describes a conversation between a fellow-doctor and a Jew in Alexandria, who had 'een geheel packhuys vol mommye' ('a whole warehouse full of *mumia*'), and 'verwonderd was / dat de Christenen soo lecker waren / ende so gheerne doode lichamen aten' ('marvelled greatly that Christians were so eager to eat the bodies of the dead'), *De chirurgie, ende alle de opera, ofte wercken*, 1636, p. 368. See also Lemery, 1743, p. 469: 'Men moet niet gelooven, dat de gemeene Mumië, die men ons brengt, de oprechte Mumië van Egypten zy, die uit de graven der oude Egyptenaren gehaelt is; deze is te zeldzaam, en indien men 'er iets van heeft, bewaert men 't in kabinetten als een groote rariteit. Die men by de Droogisten vind, komt van de lyken van verscheide menschen, die de Joden of zelfs de Christenen [...] balsemen' ('We should not believe that the common mummies that are brought to us are the true mummies from Egypt, obtained from the graves of Ancient Egyptians; these are too rare, and if one has examples of these, one keeps them as rarities in cabinets. The ones you find by at druggists are from corpses of different people, which Jews, and even Christians [...], embalm.')

15 Many of the arguments used in this poem against the medical uses of *mumia* can also be found in Van Beverwijck, *Heelkonste* ('Surgery'), 1656, p. 16. For the views of other Dutch contemporaries of Six, see Smits, 1988, pp. 167–168.

16 *Cf.* the low price of royal blood in 'Rariteiten te koop' – see Appendix 1 – and of incense in 'Afbeeldinge en wydinge van Roselle', Chapter 5.

used in embalming. In addition to the aromatic substances myrrh and aloe, which we have seen above, Six mentions 'Griekse pek' ('Greek pitch') (l. 32) and a substance with the strange name 'Sodoms teer' ('Sodom's tar') (l. 33). Consulting early modern pharmaceutical reference works gives us some clarity about these raw materials. 'Greek pitch' (*pix græca*) is boiled pitch (that is, resin) from pine trees – a kind of turpentine.[17] By 'Sodom's tar', Six means *bitumen judaicum*, 'Jews' pitch', a bitumen or asphalt that in earlier times served as a preservative, medicine and dye. Bitumen was a raw material that was crucial to the mummification process. The Arabic word for it is *mumiya* (from which *mumia* and 'mummy' also come). This brings us to the original reason for the trade in mummies: the interest in Egyptian mummies initially did not concern the human content at all, but the *mineralia* that were used.[18] In the sixteenth and seventeenth centuries, however, there was still a lot of uncertainty about the significance of both bitumen and *mumia*. Some doctors thought that the therapeutic effect of *mumia* came from the substances used in embalming. For example, the famous French surgeon Ambroise Paré – a name to which Six refers in *Poësy* – is at pains to say that the falsified *mumia* in which he says Jews trade, comes from 'the corpses of common people, which are embalmed only with common asphalt gum', while the real thing – *mumia vera aegyptiaca* – was embalmed with precious asphalt from the Dead Sea and spices such as myrrh and aloe.[19]

'Sodom's tar' is a term with strong ethical connotations. The description Lemery gives of the origin of the substance and of the health hazards associated with its collection explains its strange name:

> It is found swimming upon the Surface of the Lake, or Asphaltite Sea, otherwise call'd the Dead Sea, where stood some Time ago the Cities of Sodom and Gomorrah. This Bitumen is cast up from Time in the Nature of liquid Pitch, from the Earth that lies under these seas [...] The Birds that fly a-cross it fall down dead, and it is call'd the Dead Sea, because of the stench, Bitterness, and excessive Saltness of it, so that neither Fish or any other Creature can live upon it.[20]

17 See Lemery, 1743, p. 204; Kooijmans, 2007, pp. 105–107.

18 Lemery, 1743, pp. 104-105. Later on, in the writings of medieval Arabic doctors, the whole mummy was given the status of a medicine, and 'mummification' came to mean 'embalming': K. Dannenfeldt, 'Egyptian Mumia: The Sixteenth Century Experience and Debate', *Sixteenth Century Journal*, 1985, pp. 163–180. Today, asphalt refers first and foremost to the black material used as surfacing for roads. But the history of the material's use is long: Asphalt, or bitumen, is a mineral resin produced by slow oxidation of oil. It was mainly collected on and near lakes where it had floated as a liquid resin. The most precious asphalt came from the Dead Sea.

19 'Ghemeyne volcken / die alleene met ghemeyne gomme Asphaltum ghebalsemt waren', Paré, 1636, pp. 375–380, quote on p. 378. *Cf.* Sugg, 2011, pp. 15–16, especially note 47; Noble, 2011, pp. 131–132.

20 Pierre Pomet, *A Compleat History of Drugs*, with additional comments from Nicolas Lemery, 1737, p. 388.

But there are still further explanations of the name 'Sodom's tar', says Lemery. Because of a confusion between 'bitumen' and 'pitch' – thus *vegetabilia* instead of *mineralia* – the substance was associated with the burning 'clods of pitch' under which Sodom from the Old Testament was buried, according to the apocryphal books of Ezra.[21] The city was buried under its own luxury product, according to Lemery's interpretation of Ezra. Bitumen is a flammable substance. Why Six calls 'Jews' pitch' 'Sodom's tar' is not hard to understand in view of this explanation.

Emphasising that 'lyksalf', 'corpse ointment' (l. 41) contains decadent ingredients thus has a deeper meaning. The sinful nature of this luxury symbolises for Six the physical and moral dangers that his own body and his hometown, Amsterdam, run. Six has every reason to warn the buyer of the pathogenic consequences of *mumia*. The conclusion reads as follows (l. 45–52):

Al wat men, laaci, meint te schuimen,
Uit kooksels van gebalsemt bloed,
Dat loost de beurs, in sieker fluimen,
En ongemerkt, in schoorsteenroet.
O menschen, wilt ghy u besorgen,
Van balsem, en een piramyd?
Versorgh uw zielen alle morgen,
Met goude deughd, die nimmer slyt.

All that they – how regrettable – claim to skim
From the stew of embalmed blood,
[that] empties the purse [of the sick], causing sicker fluids.
O man, do you want to provide yourself
With balm and a pyramid?
Equip your soul each new day
With golden virtue that never wears out.

However, there is still more to discuss in the poem. Lemery compares the mummification process in ancient Egypt with that in his own time. Ancient Egyptian mummies, he writes, keep for four thousand years, while those from the seventeenth century last only three hundred years.[22] He refers in this context to the renewed interest among pharmacists and doctors of his time in the art of conservation. Interest in the composition of Egyptian mummies seems to have been particularly

21 'Pek' versus 'aardpek', and 'peck-schollen', see the Dutch translation of Lemery, 1743, p. 105, and see 2. Esdras 2:9.

22 Lemery, 1743, pp. 468–469.

strong in the Netherlands. In the early modern period, the Republic was a centre for medical experiments and medical research. As we have seen, Ancient Egyptian civilisation, home to Hermes, had considerable influence on the science and culture of the Renaissance.[23] According to classical doctrine, besides maintaining health and curing illnesses, prolonging life was the third task of medicine.[24] The process of preserving corpses was about removing the fluid from the body so it would not decompose. Drying was therefore equivalent to preserving, as illustrated by certain 'natural mummies': bodies that were naturally preserved because of the heat and drought in the North African desert.[25] But the way in which ancient Egyptian mummies were preserved – which had remained wonderfully lifelike thanks to a lost technique – exerted a strong fascination in the early modern period. It was thought that in ancient Egypt the divine insights from before the flood of Noah – knowledge from Adam's time – had been preserved, and that the Egyptian mummification technique could stop and preserve the exhalation of the spirit of life, which normally leaves the body at death. As Harold Cook writes, 'In the seventeenth century, then, methods to preserve the bodies of living things seemed almost miraculous.'[26]

Thus in Cook's view it was not surprising that a lot of time and money were spent on experiments with mummification. The legitimacy for this renewed revival of a pagan custom was found in the Bible, which describes how King David is embalmed.[27] According to an English surgeon, a contemporary and compatriot of Six's, Louis de Bils (1624–1669) was 'the greatest Master of Ambalming in our Time'.[28] His experiments with the conservation of human bodies garnered attention. Not only did he develop a 'bloodless' dissection technique in which not a drop of blood or other fluid was lost from the deceased, as he demonstrated in

23 For the meaning of *mumia* in connection with the fascination for ancient Egypt, see Karl H. Dannenfeldt, 'Egypt and Egyptian Antiquities in the Renaissance', *Studies in the Renaissance*, 1959, pp. 7–27. For the interest among Dutch physicians and scholars in ancient Eastern cultures, see Jorink, 2010, pp. 285–289; Smits, 1988; Cis van Heertum, 2012. On the art of embalming, see Smits, 1988, pp. 161–164; Harold J. Cook, 'Time's Bodies', in: Pamela Smith & Paula Findlen (eds.), *Merchants and Marvels: Commerce, Science, and Art in Early Modern Europe*, 2002, pp. 233–247; Kooijmans, 2004, pp. 44–48.

24 Both Francis Bacon and René Descartes believed that this could be achieved during their lifetimes (Cook, 2002, pp. 228–229).

25 See Lemery (1743, p. 469) on forged *mumia*: 'Men vind somtyds op de kusten van Lybië doode mensenlichamen, die al daer door de baren van de zee geworpen zynde van 't zand doordrongen en gedroogt' ('Off the coast of Libya one sometimes finds bodies that have been carried there by the waves of the sea, and permeated and dried by the salt').

26 Cook, 2002, pp. 228–230. *Cf.* also attempts by Dutch chemists to make *mumia*, as a fifth element: Ibid., p. 231, note 28.

27 Genesis 50:2.

28 Cook, 2002; Kooijmans, 2004, pp. 20–24.

anatomical presentations he organised and gave to important people and famous scientists such as Robert Boyle. His embalmed human beings also looked 'freshly dead'.[29]

This brings me to a point that is relevant to my analysis of 'Lykbalsem'. When De Bils's sensational technique became known, people began to write wills in which they stipulated that their bodies were to be mummified after they died.[30] The opening of 'Lykbalsem', in which people who want to be embalmed are directly addressed, should therefore not only be understood in the light of the historical mummification process the Egyptians used. It was actually directed to the poet's contemporaries. Six means, not necessarily De Bils's experiments, but the great confidence his contemporaries had in the miraculous power of medicine. So it is with people who harbour such vain desires (l. 21–29):

Wie specerye, en trotse wooningen
  Besorgen dart, voor syne dood,
Die werd, gelyk Egiptens kooningen,
  Gesteurt, en van het graf ontbloot.
Verscheept, geveilt, gekrookt, gebryselt,
  Uit dommigheit, van Artseny,
En, in d'apteek, tot stof, gevyselt,
  Gemenght, in drankjes, voor mumy,
Ter heilinge van halve dooden.

He who dares to provide himself
With spices and proud houses,
Will, like kings of Egypt,
Be disturbed and robbed from the grave,
Shipped, sold, broken and mashed,
Because of foolish medical theories,
And ground to powder in the apothecary,
Mixed in drinks as *mumia*,
As medicine for people who are already half-dead.

'Lykbalsem' thus relates *mumia* (in the sense of both medicine and preservative) to a series of negative phenomena: superstition, blasphemy, hubris, cannibalism and disease.

29 Ibid., pp. 274–275.

30 De Bils asked for 6,000 guilders to embalm a certain Count Hautreppe in 1663 (Jan Reinier Jansma, *Louis de Bils and the Anatomy of His Time*, 1919, p. 76). According to other sources, he also received similar requests when he lived and worked in Amsterdam, see Smith, 2004, p. 294.

And as usual, the poet is not just criticising others, but also engaging in self-reflection. Six himself is, after all, practising the art of conservation and the prolonging of life, not only as a druggist, but also as a poet. As we have seen, his verses are full of references to methods of preservation, such as 'confijten', and immortalising incense and spices. *Poësy* also contains examples of literary imagery featuring mummification. In 'Sucht oover de dood, van Jakob Breine den Ouden, te Dantisch' ('A Sigh at the Death of Jacob Breyne the Elder, at Danzig') (J365), Six uses *mumia* as a metaphor to recall a dear friend and business associate – Jacob Breyne the Elder who had died of the plague in 1655. When he re-reads the last letters he received from his friend, his tears 'bewenen' ('bewail') the paper, and he wishes that the letter 'strek myn geheugh, gelyk mumy, / Beweent gesalft, ten schildery' ('may serve my memory as a portrait – like a mummy, embalmed with my tears') (l. 49–50): His 'embalming' tears mummify the letter into an immortal work of art.[31] *Mumia* – the 'godlik kruid' ('divine spice'), as Six calls it in 'Lykbalsem' (l. 42) – will therefore have held a certain attraction for Six himself.

Relics

Embalming and perfuming corpses with aromatic spices are not only hallmarks of Egyptian funeral rites. This practice was also followed throughout the Middle Ages and in the early modern period. The remains of dignitaries were embalmed and then kept in richly decorated tombs. The cult of relics is also relevant here. The Roman Catholic Church was interested in the art of embalming. Unspoilt, fragrant corpses were considered a miracle to which beneficial properties were ascribed. In the seventeenth century, a large number of 'human medicines' were thus to be found as relics in churches and monasteries. And since the crusades of the Middle Ages, there had been a lively trade in the remains of saints.[32] The question is how a Protestant merchant managed to distinguish between the trade in human medicines and the trade in relics. Once again, drugs seemed to evoke unwanted associations with Catholicism – a fact that Six was concerned about. Indications of this can be found in 'Damspel, om geld teegen ooverblyfselen van heiligen, van kapucynen, met den scheepskoopman, op zee tusschen Alikante en Genua' (J256) – a long, narrative poem about the relic trade that I will discuss here.[33]

31 For *mumia* as a literary symbol of immortalisation, see Philip Schwyzer, *Archaeologies of English Renaissance Literature*, 2007, pp. 164–165.

32 See for example Joan C. Cruz, *Relics*, 1984; Susanne Evans, 'The Scent of a Martyr', *NUMEN*, 2002, pp. 193–211; and Patrick Geary, 'Sacred Commodities: The Circulation of Medieval Relics', in: A. Appadurai (ed.), *The Social Life of Things: Commodities in Cultural Perspective*, 1986, pp. 169–191.

33 For Six's discussion of Catholic saints and relics, see also 'Om geneesinge myner miltsiekte, aan de spafonteinen' ('To Cure My Spleen Disease, to the Spa Springs') (J102, l. 36), 'Op het heiligh graf' ('On the

The title already suggests that a double morality is one of the themes of the text. What takes place in the poem was apparently based on actual events. At the start of 1650, Six travelled by ship from Spain to Italy.[34] During this trip, he witnessed a strange scene: to kill time, Catholic monks were playing dice with the ship's merchant, with relics brought along as collateral. Six reacts to this and is not sparing in his anti-papist criticism. Many of the arguments on which his reasoning is based also apply to a true Roman Catholic: gambling is a sin according to general Christian morality. When monks gamble, they also break with their holy vows (l. 1–22): Capuchins or Friars Minor are begging monks who have taken a vow of poverty. And the slew of sins just keeps on growing: by playing and gambling with the relics of saints – who, according to Catholic doctrine are 'followers of Christ' – the monks are in fact guilty of once again tormenting the body of Jesus, and therefore of blasphemy (l. 23–50). That does not bother the Capuchins. Even a critical remark about the possibility that their relics are fake prompts no repentance or remorse. On the contrary, they dismiss this criticism as irrelevant. It is not so much a matter of the essence of faith, they argue. The most important thing is to earn money for the Catholic Church and to convert people. Perhaps, they say, the ship's merchant will be convinced to switch to Catholicism (l. 71–92). With these remarks they are guilty of more sins: lying, swindling and hypocrisy. If we win, we will have money for our passage, and for those who gave us money we will say a thank-you prayer during the Catholic mass, they conclude at the end of the poem (l. 93–106). Here Six puts his finger on the sin that is actually at the heart of 'Damspel': simony, the buying and selling of spiritual goods or services (l. 12).[35]

The list of sins committed by the monks is unrealistically long. The text reads more as an anti-Papist diatribe than as the account of real events it presents itself as. The choice of Capuchin monks, for instance, is no coincidence: they played almost as important a part as that of the Jesuits in the Counter-Reformation in converting people to the Catholic faith. We recognise the pattern from other poems of Six's: the poem is just as much about Six himself as it is about Catholic monks. Although the story may be rooted in a real event, that reality has been manipulated in such a way that Six is able to convey his message: he wants to rid himself of the undesirable associations that the trade in drugs could evoke. This is made clear by a closer examination of a passage from the text (l. 51–70):

Holy Grave') (J226) and 'Geusemirakel' ('Geuzen Miracle') (J426).

34 Jacobs, 1991 II, p. 256.

35 See 'simony' in Acts 8:18–19. See also another source referred to in connection with the Protestant critique of the cult of, and trade in, relics: John 19:23–24, which tells the story of the Roman soldiers who cast lots to see who would win Jesus' undergarment. Six refers to this in l. 27–31.

Maar Vaaders, fyne religieusen,
Wy loopen, met geen houte neusen,
Als reukeloose Tempelgooden,
Vergeefs den wierook aangebooden:
Wy ruiken wel, die brokkelingen
Niet bleeven, van geheilghde dingen,
Of schoon een nette greine kasse,
Voor elk een laadjen had van passe,
Voor oogen weigerigh, met deurtjes,
En syde strikjes, van veel kleurtjes,
Waar in, beschreeve ceeltjes laagen,
Met antwoord van den naam, op vraagen.
Die beentjes sommige uitgebranden,
Van kruinen, ribben, schenkels, tanden
Gelyken alzoo wel van stieren,
En bokken, als bereende dieren:
Gelyken alzoo wel van fielen,
Of ongesaaligde, als gesaalgde zielen.
Ghy braght se, seght ghe, mee van Romen,
Se konden ook, van Tunis koomen.

But Fathers, you fine religious persons,
We do not walk around with wooden noses,
As Temple Gods without a sense of smell,
[To whom] the incense is offered in vain:
We smell very well that these [earthly] remains
Do not come from holy things,
Even though the pinewood chasse
Had a drawer shaped for each of the relics,
[Which was] hidden from sight with small doors
And silk bows in many colours,
Where pieces of paper are found
With answers to questions about the name of the relevant saint.
These bones, some of them charred,
Of skulls, ribs, shanks and teeth,
Are quite similar to those of bulls,
And goats, as those reasonable animals [human beings]:
Are quite similar to those of crooks,
Or unblessed, to those of blessed souls.
You brought them, you say, from Rome,
They could also come from Tunisia.

'Temple Gods' and 'incense' – these have become familiar motifs for us in Six's poetry. Six asserts that we are not consecrated images of saints (*cf.* 'Afbeeldinge en wydinge van Roselle'), but people made of flesh and blood, with real senses. The poem is not just about religious discord. Six also shows here that he has experience checking goods: even though the monks' substances are so seductively packaged, a well-trained druggist's nose can tell that they do not come from saints, but from animal carcasses, or from corpses from the gallows field. They do not come at all from the holy city of Rome, but from North Africa, where, in the desert sand, completely desiccated corpses are sometimes found – the 'natural mummies' I mentioned earlier.

Whether the story is actually based on a real event is therefore less important than the confessional content of the poem. Relics have the same exotic origin, can be transported just as easily, and have the same supposedly transformative powers as early modern drugs. They are thus closely related. Like the trade in exotic oils and fragrances, the trade in human substances was an international business that had originally arisen from religious needs. The 'ship's merchant' of the title is interesting in this respect, because he is the one the monks are trying to persuade in the poem. But his position remains unclear: he is not introduced any further and we do not get to know his reactions to the monks' behaviour. Or is Six himself behind the 'we' used in the poem, and does he stand, as it were, for merchants as a whole, among whom the poet also counts himself? This is one plausible explanation. Six shows us that, as a merchant, he understands the immoral commercial practices of the monks.

As for the portability of, and the transformative powers ascribed to, relics, sacred objects played a role in the most diverse parts of early modern society. Thus the remains of saints were used as gifts and means of exchange, and even – as was also the case in 'Damspel' – as means of payment.[36] Religious goods of this kind were also in circulation in Protestant countries. In the scientific collections of members of the Dutch Reformed Church, there were all kinds of *devotionalia* from religions from all corners of the world. One section of Bernardus Paludanus's famous naturalist collection was entitled *reliquiae,* and included a reliquary containing the bones of fourteen martyrs. Although placed in a more or less profane context, the relics still had the character of *mirabilia*. They illustrated biblical and Christian history, and were widely seen as a highlight of the collection. How did the Protestant collectors get their hands on these 'holy curiosities'? Among other things, they got them from Dutchmen who had been on trips in Southern Europe – travelling merchants such as Six.[37]

36 *Cf.* Geary 1986.

37 For Paludanus's cabinet of curiosities, see Jorink, 2010, pp. 269–278. See also Jorink's discussion of the relics and biblical *naturalia* in the collections of Andreas Colvius, a pastor from Dordrecht (pp. 293–296) and

A Protestant blood relic

I will now return to the blood of King Charles I of England, the miraculous product from 'Rariteiten te koop' (J158). According to my initial discussion of the poem at the beginning of this study, what is involved is the marketing of the blood of Charles I as a 'rariteit', a *curiosity* or *mirabilium*. The text, which comprises 162 lines, is a panegyric to a new, and until then unknown, commodity that has appeared on the market. It is, of course, an ironic panegyric. In terms of content, three parts can be distinguished in the poem: the introduction (l. 1–36), the conclusion (l. 151–162) and in between them the main part, a comparison between the new commodity and already existing exotic substances on the Dutch market (l. 37–150).

At the beginning of the text, a 'merchant' (l. 3) speaks to us. That the role of this trader is important for the understanding of 'Rariteiten te koop' is shown by the fact that 'merchant' is capitalised (l. 1–3), 'Alle stoffe heeft een maakler, / Andersins een vryen kaakler, / Die des Koopmans wille peilt' ('All commodities have a broker, or an independent hawker, who represents the interests of the Merchant'). In the business world, there is a dealer for every kind of substance. Nothing escapes the commercialising hands of the merchant – not even a king's blood. This dealer – given the context, he is likely an importer or wholesaler – is looking for a 'broker' or a 'hawker' (l. 1–2) – a middleman or a street vendor – who is prepared to offer the blood to Dutch consumers. Whoever dares to act as a broker, however, falls into a trap: he is going to get his hands dirty with blood money (l. 31–34):

Wie zal 't maakelampt bekleeden?
Die volght nu geen Judas schreeden:
  Want dit bloedgeld dient de wraak,
Om wat houts, en touw te koopen,
Om syn moorders op te knoopen [...]

Who shall be the agent for this commodity?
He does not follow in the footsteps of Judas:
Because this blood money should be used
To buy timber and rope for revenge:
To hang the murderers of the King [...]

Nicolaes Witsen (p. 326–333). Jorink writes about the latter's relics: 'In the *Catalogue*, after the description of these relics, we read something almost apologetic: 'Zynde deze dingen door diverse Reizigers mede gebracht' ('things that are brought to me by various travellers').

Any potential broker is compared to Judas, who sold Jesus. The comparison with the story of Christ's passion is no coincidence: the English king was presented by royalists as an *Imitatio Christi*. I will come back to this presently. But Six emphasises the distinction between the two royal histories of suffering. Rather than a return of the 'thirty pieces of silver' (Matthew 27:3–10), this blood money must be used to get revenge.

The blood not only serves as an image for the sinful temptation of merchants who are looking for profit, but also for that of Dutch consumers, keen to have what is the latest and most chic item on the market. This shift in focus marks the transition from the introduction to the main body of the text, which contains a list of all kinds of luxury goods on the Dutch market. All these precious drugs are compared to the English novelty, but none of them surpasses the blood in lustre and radiance. This section can be divided into five subsections, based on five main categories that Six already mentioned in the introduction to the text (l. 25–30): The first subpart deals with dyes (l. 37–66), the next part is about stones and gems (l. 67–102); the third part (l. 103–108) lists fragrant exotic woods. In the fourth subpart (l. 109–126), Six devotes attention to the category of flowers, although only one type of flower is mentioned: roses. The last part treats blood as ink, and therefore also as a source of inspiration (l. 127–150): As I mentioned at the beginning of this study, the poem includes a total of 25 different expensive exotic drugs. In Appendix I, I give a detailed overview of all goods. These are expensive and rare commodities, such as cochineal, blood coral, jasper and red sandalwood. It is possible that red dyes belonged to the assortment in 'De Vergulde Eenhoorn'. An indication of this is the fact that one of Six's most important trading contacts, Jacob Breyne, had so-called Polish cochineal as his main trading product.[38]

They consist for the most part of drugs that existed in early modern times. But the pigment I discussed earlier in this study, the purple of the purple snail, and to which Six pays a lot of attention in the text, was a mythical substance in his day, although some rarity collectors in Amsterdam claimed to have specimens of the purple snails in their cabinets of curiosities. The recipe for the purple dye was lost in the fall of Constantinople in 1453. This brings the fictitious character of the text to the fore. It is about drugs that appeal to the imagination and dreams of people in the early modern period. That is evident from an oil sketch that Rubens made of the myth of the discovery of the material. Red was, as we know, an important colour in Rubens's paintings (Plate 13).[39] The same goes for the rose of the fourth

38 The son of Jacob Breyne the Younger, Johann Philipp Breyne, even wrote a treatise on Polish cochineal, see Fleischer, 2019, pp. 107–135.

39 See Aneta Georgievska-Shine and Larry Silver, *Rubens, Velázquez, and the King of Spain*, 2017, pp. 107–108. For the purple snail in Dutch cabinet of curiosity, see the notes to the poem in Appendix I.

part: If someone in this season – Charles I was executed in winter – wants to have roses to braid wreaths of flowers with, they must be in England, according to the text. There were already painted roses on the coat of arms of the Stuart royal family, but now these roses are *alive*: they bloom 'to Charles's fame' (l. 111–114): in a macabre allegory, in which the double meaning of 'bloeien' ('blooming' and 'bleeding') is played out, the blood flowing from the king's body is presented as an eternal, miraculous, blooming rose. The metaphysical motif is continued in the lines that follow (l. 119–123):

> Stuart is een roos herbooren,
> En van Jesus hoogh bemint.
> O! hoe voel ik 't hart opluiken,
> By dees vroege lentparruiken,
> Van dat duursaam martelbloed?

> Stuart is reborn as a rose
> Which is highly loved by Jesus.
> Oh! How I feel my heart open
> At the sight of the bouquet of early flowers
> From that precious martyr's blood?

The rose of Stuart, the text continues with a reference to Christian mysticism, is similar to the bride in the Song of Songs, 'the rose of Saron'. In the biblical exegesis, this bride is referred to as Christ.[40] The text passage points to a religious subtext in the poem that has already been felt in the comparison between the seller and Judas: an allegorical comparison between the death of Charles I and that of Jesus Christ. There are more allusions to Christian traditions in the text. In l. 64–66, a passage on dyes, Six characterises Charles's blood as the 'bloed van Santen / Opgesopt, met neusdoek kanten' ('blood of saints soaked up in a handkerchief'). Red as a symbol of pain also refers to a sacred, divine pain: the suffering of saints and martyrs. The blood emerges as a Protestant blood relic. If we follow this Catholic path, we will also understand that the identification of the blood with luxury drugs is based on more than just an outward comparison: Six speaks of direct metamorphoses: 'that miraculous blood' that turns into ink, paint, roses, wood and stone (see l. 25–28 and 153–155). The idea of the royal blood that is subject to transformation is in keeping with the core concept of the Roman Catholic Church: the sacrament of the Eucharist, in which transubstantiation takes place – the transformation of bread

40 Lemery, 1743, pp. 343 and 483; Jacobs, 1991 II, p. 288, and comment 2 to Song of Songs 2:1 in the *Statenvertaling*.

and wine into the body and blood of Christ. The description of the miraculous effect of the blood and the ecstatic reactions the Dutch have to it should be understood in this light. The idea of the transmutation of base products into a miraculous red substance is also in accordance with concepts within alchemy. The final stage of gold making, the 'red stage', also called *rubedo*, involved the production of the red philosopher's stone, which was thought to have power to produce gold and cure all diseases.[41] Although this link to alchemy is not as clear as the link to Catholic theology, it is likely that Six, who was well versed in chemical symbolism, is also alluding to gold-making in mentioning the blood.

Six himself is one of those who reacts excitedly to the blood. As always, he does not describe the incident remotely, but puts himself in the shoes of consumers who are keen on the miraculous blood. Six presents himself in the poem as a merchant, a poet and a young man in love. The blood would be a beautiful 'roosenhoed' ('rose garland') for his Roselle. In the form of ink, it could do wonders for his career as a poet, giving life force to his 'rhymes' (l. 124–141): However, he acknowledges – if ironically – that he is not the only rhymester on the Dutch Mount Parnassus who desperately needs inspiration. In the following lines, he advises his 'peers' to follow his example (l. 144–146): 'Wat beleeft deese eeuw Poeëten! / Die men dan alzoo zou heeten' ('Oh, what Poets does this century experience! / Then they [the rhymesters] will be called by that name'). By using miraculous human blood as ink, Dutch rhymesters could fulfil the ideal of a Golden Age. Only then could Six and his fellow rhymesters call themselves poets. The red ink probably alludes in this context to the sacred books of the Delphi oracle, since Six mentions in another poem that Sibyl's prophecies were written in golden letters.[42]

The hope that the most secret dreams will come true also concerns other consumers. The blood produces an ecstasy, a collective daze, among consumers in the Dutch marketplace for exotica. By wearing clothes dyed with this blood – 'kooninglyke drachten' ('kingly costumes') as splendid as those of the biblical Solomon – one grows in stature (l. 37–51). Wine that is mixed with this blood tastes like the 'blood of saints' (l. 61–66). The use of this blood as an adornment on the new Town Hall of Amsterdam makes this 'eighth wonder of the world' surpass the temple of Jupiter on

41 Lawrence M. Principe, *The Secrets of Alchemy*, 2012, pp. 124. According to the English philosopher Roger Bacon human blood was more important than all other ingredients in making gold, see Sven Dupré, Dedo von Kerssenbrock-Krosigk & Beat Wismer (eds.), *Art and Alchemy. The Mystery of Transformation*, 2014, p. 56.

42 'Koddenaartje' ('Chaffinch') (J232), l. 29–32. 'Purple', 'gold' and 'red' are, strictly speaking, different colours. Six probably took as his starting point the Latin meanings of the words. For example, the meaning of purple was wider than ours: the colour includes a whole range of shades, 'from very dark violet to fairly bright red', according to Nicolaas Vels Heijn, *Kleurnamen en kleurbegrippen bij de Romeinen: The Names and Concepts of Colours among the Romans*, 1951, p. 28.

the antique Capitol in splendour (l. 79–96). And by painting their interiors with this blood, middle-class Dutch women can realise aristocratic Italian ideals (l. 97–102).

However, as we have seen, the poem ends with an anti-climax. Six lets his rhymester friends know what to do about their poems if no one recognises their genius (l. 147–150). Royally gilded poetry is worth no more than 'gilded' toilet paper:

> Werden wy zoo niet gehult,
> Vrienden, wat 's er aan geleegen?
> Die wat heimliks moeten veegen,
> Maaken al ons rym verguldt.

> But if we are not praised,
> Friends, what does it matter?
> The ones who need to wipe their buttocks
> Gild all our rhymes

This renunciation of gold-making with a reference to 'wiping someone's bottom' is a *topos* both within the poetry of Six and images of the alchemist in Dutch art.[43] The anticlimax also concerns other Dutchmen hungry for this blood. In the end, the miraculous blood is worth no more than Judas's pieces of silver (l. 159–162):

> 'k Wensche, dat ik maar ontfongh
> Dertigh stuivers, sonder dingen,
> Vry wat min, dan silverlingen,
> Waar sich Judas om verhongh.

> I wished I had just received
> Thirty stivers, without bargaining,
> A good deal less than the pieces of silver,
> For which Judas hanged himself.

The social metamorphosis that the consumers of the divine blood hoped to undergo has not taken place.

What is the message of 'Rariteiten te koop'? From a pharmaceutical point of view, the similarities to the *mumia* and relics discussed above are significant: this blood is not only a substance originating in the human body, 'the most glorious of all living creatures', in the words of Lemery. It is a substance from the body of a holy

43 *Cf.* 'Raad aan den Geenen, die myn rymen mishaagen' ('Advice to Those Who Dislike My Rhymes') (J393), 'The Quack' by Gerrit Dou; see also Drago, 2019, pp. 172–173.

person, a king. Also, the human medicine in 'Rariteiten te koop' is characterised by both ambiguity and ambivalence, like other tempting drugs discussed in this study. But the text also evokes a larger reality. The execution of the English king was a shocking political event throughout Europe, and it is this that gives this 'drug' the greatest symbolic value in Six's poetry.

Charles the Martyr

In order to really understand 'Rariteiten te koop', we will therefore have to focus our attention on the large body of royalist texts published in the wake of the execution of the English king, which also includes 'Rariteiten te koop'. What resemblances are there between 'Rariteiten te koop' and other royalist poems? Helmer Helmers has pointed to the special position of 'Rariteiten te koop' within the Dutch reception of the English regicide. Like Helmers, who speaks of a shared Anglo-Dutch public sphere, I also include English literature. Six bought and sold goods from and to England, and had good connections there, so it is also likely that he read English texts. According to Nigel Smith, the so-called Cavalier poets in England, poets who supported King Charles I during the English Civil War, were even inspired by continental poets such as Six.[44] I will then take a look at other texts in Six's *Poësy* that devote attention to the execution of Charles.

One of the most important royalist propaganda texts was the autobiography *Eikon Basilike – The Pourtrature of His Sacred Majesty in His Solitudes and Sufferings* (1649), which was published just after the execution and which gained enormous popularity: just a few short months after the beheading, twenty different editions of it were in circulation.[45] In it, the king staged the story of his suffering and death as an *imitatio* of the story Christ's passion. The apotheosis of King Charles I, the so-called cult of Charles the Martyr, forms the basis for the large number of royalist texts that would follow *Eikon Basilike*. Some of them can shed light on 'Rariteiten te koop'. Of particular interest is the group of texts on the cult that deal with the healing powers of the royal body. The most famous example of this is the anonymous pamphlet, published in the same year, *A Miracle of Miracles: / Wrought by the Blood of King Charles the First, / Of Happy Memory, / upon a Mayd at* Detford, *foure miles from* London, */ who by the violence of the Disease called the* Kings Evill *was blinde*

44 See Helmer J. Helmers, *The Royalist Republic. Literature, Politics and Religion in the Anglo-Dutch Public Sphere, 1639–1660*, 2015, pp. 137–139. *Cf.* the long list of English books owned by Abraham Grenier, Six's friend and travelling companion in England, in Leneth Witte, *The English Book in the Dutch Golden Age*, 2018, pp. 15–16. And see Nigel Smith, 'Cross-channel cavaliers', *The Seventeenth Century*, 2017, pp. 433–453.

45 For *Eikon Basilike* and other royalist works, see Lois Potter, *Secret Rites and Secret Writing: Royalist Literature 1641–1660*, 1989. For the cult of Charles I, see Andrew Lacey, *The Cult of King Charles the Martyr*, 2003.

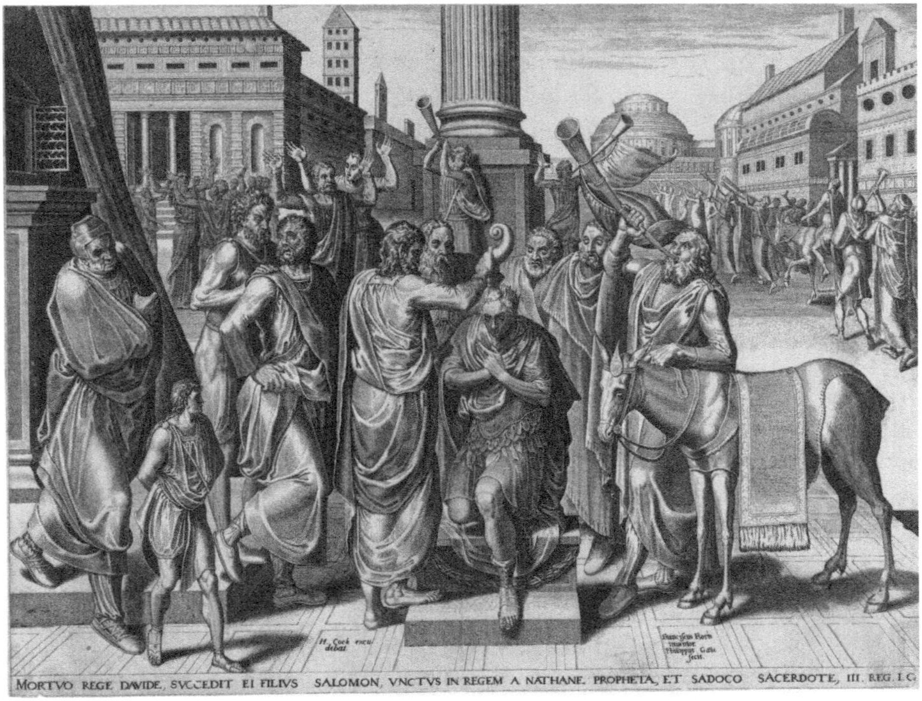
H. Cock excudebat
MORTVO REGE DAVIDE, SVCCEDIT EI FILIVS SALOMON, VNCTVS IN REGEM A NATHANE PROPHETA, ET SADOCO SACERDOTE, III. REG. I. C

Fig. 9.2: Philips Galle, after Frans Floris (I), *The Anointing of King Solomon*, c. 1557–1570. Engraving. (© Rijksmuseum, Amsterdam).

one whole yeere; / but by making use of a piece of Handkircher [handkerchief] *dipped in the Kings blood is recovered of her sight. / To the comfort of the Kings friends, and astonishment of his Enemies. The truth hereof many thousands can testifie.*[46] The text needs no further description. The long title tells us exactly what it is about.

The pamphlet is based on the tradition of the *royal touch* – the ceremony of the royal laying on of hands, a practice that went back to the idea of the king as a holy person: the concept of the 'divine right of kings'. This notion was in turn traced to the biblical story of the anointing of Solomon and David as kings of Israel (Fig. 9.2). Since the Middle Ages, anointing was also seen as an important part of the coronation of a Christian king. A highlight of the ceremony, which had the character of a mass, was the application of 'holy oil' to the king's forehead, chest and hands. In early modern Europe, a king's authority was thus based, not on a worldly, but on a divine right. The king was 'the Lord's Anointed'.[47] In line with the concept of the king as a beatifier or

46 For the complete text, see http://anglicanhistory.org/charles/miracle.html.

47 See Sergio Bertelli, *The King's Body: Sacred Rituals of Power in Medieval and Early Modern Europe*, 2001; and Roy Strong, *Coronation: a History of Kingship and the British Monarchy*, 2005, pp. 9–12 and 243–267.

saviour who brought peace to earth, the anointed king was also seen as a healer. The body of the king, having been anointed, became an ointment itself. Several times a year, those suffering from the so-called 'King's Evil' (scrofula) came to their king to be healed by the laying on of hands. Especially early modern English and French monarchs did this to confirm their *droit divin*, their divine right to rule. This is apparently an issue that occupied Six's attention. In one poem, 'Op de Reedenstryd, oover de kooninghlyke siekte, te Leiden gehouden, door Geeraard Worst, voor syn Geneesheerschap' ('On the Disputation on the King's Evil, Held at Leiden by Geeraard Worst, for His Doctorate in Medicine') (J423), he describes the ritual of the royal touch, and distances himself from this kind of superstition (l. 31–36 and 40–42).

> De kooninghs siekte wierd wel eer
> Geneesen, van een Hongersch heer,
> Of Kooningh, door verborgen kracht:
> Gelyk het kooninghlyk geslacht,
> In Vrankryk, erfelik aan't regeeren,
> Met raaken heilt de gorgelseeren
> [...]
> Maar wie nu bygeloovigh was,
> En siek, tot artsen, niet wou keeren,
> Zou syn gesondigheit ontbeeren.

> The King's Evil was earlier
> Healed by a Hungarian lord,
> Or King, through a hidden force,
> In France, [a king who had] inherited the crown,
> [Could], through touch, cure people of an ailment of the throat.
> [...]
> But he who is superstitious,
> And ill, but does not turn to a doctor,
> Will have to manage without recovering.

The fact that Six is contemplating 'King's Evil' and the royal touch is in the context not so strange, as he himself is a trader in 'royal' substances.[48] We also then

48 About Charles I as a practitioner of the royal touch, see Marc Bloch, *The Royal Touch, Sacred Monarchy and Scrofula in England and France*, 1989, p. 210. Geeraard Worst does not himself mention royal touch in his disputation: *Disputatio medica inaugaralis de Morbo regio*, 1655. The pastor-poet Joannes Vollenhove tells in the diary he wrote during his stay in England in 1674 that even Dutchmen travelled to England to be healed by Charles II, see Joannes Vollenhove, *Het dagboek van Joannes Vollenhove, Engeland, 17 mei–30 oktober 1674*, 2001, pp. 103–105.

understand the message of *A Miracle of Miracles*; the text serves as a royalist proof that the royal touch is still present in the remains of the king: a sign that Charles was a rightfully anointed king.

This brings us to another event that underlies *A Miracle of Miracles*: after the beheading of Charles I, and as was the custom at public executions in the early modern period, spectators flocked to the scaffold to dip their handkerchiefs in his blood. This is depicted in the painting 'The Execution of Charles I' (Plate 14a and 14b).[49] Not all blood was used as a medicine. As we now know early modern multifunctional drugs, they could also be used as status symbols, exhibition pieces, and political markers. Some of the blood was also used as ink and dye for royalist propaganda literature. Perhaps the most remarkable contribution to the cult of Charles the Martyr is the panegyric 'Upon the Kings-Book bound up in a Cover coloured with His Blood' by the poet and deacon Abraham Wright. By 'Kings-Book' Wright means a copy of *Eikon Basilike*. The appearance of such a 'strange piece' – such a rarity – puts the poet into a state of religious ecstasy: 'This sacred blood doth Rome a Relique show / Richer then all her shrines, and then all those / More hallowed far, far more miraculous'.[50] Is the representation of the royal blood in these English propaganda texts comparable to that in 'Rariteiten te koop'? The glorifying character of the English poems of praise is at least reminiscent of Six's ironic hymns to royals, especially 'Blyde inkomste te Madrid' and 'Tempel, aan den kooningh van Spanje'. Can 'Rariteiten te koop' also be regarded as a satire – in this case in the quasi-religious tone of royalist propaganda? If so, Six could be compared to the English Puritan John Milton. In his *Eikonoklastes* (1649) – the most important response by the parliamentary Puritans to *Eikon Basilike* – Milton warns of the dangers of the monarchy by emphasising the seductive splendour of royalist rituals. 'For Milton, the true worship of God was entirely inward and did not need or depend on any external rite', notes Andrew Lacey in his discussion of the work.[51] But this comparison is problematic. Although at the beginning of the English Civil War there was a certain sympathy for the Puritans, almost the whole of the Netherlands reacted with horror to the beheading of Charles – Orthodox Calvinists as well as Remonstrants and Catholics.[52] This is also evident from the other poems Six wrote about the beheading. Royalist sympathies apparently outweighed any objections

49 Lacey, 2003, p. 62. My thanks to Helmer Helmers for the referral.

50 The text is printed in *Parnassus Biceps. Or Severall Choice Pieces of Poetry, Composed by the best Wits that were in both the Universities before their Dissolution*, 1656, pp. 54–55. The book *The Bloody Court, or the Fatall Tribunal* is also worth mentioning in this context. Just like 'Rariteiten te koop', it is printed in red ink (Potter, 1989, pp. 175 and 188). However, if the dating is correct, this book did not appear until 1660.

51 Lacey, 2003, p. 88. *Cf.*, too, Richard F. Hardin, *Civil Idolatry: Desacralizing and Monarchy in Spenser, Shakespeare, and Milton*, 2007.

52 See Helmers, 2015.

to the religious form of the royalist propaganda. And as Helmer Helmers shows in his study of how the execution of Charles I was regarded in the Netherlands, the concept of *droit divin* was, moreover, not exclusively regarded as a right of royalty: regents in the Dutch Republic also invoked a divine right to rule. Tyranny was therefore a trap into which not only the monarch or emperor could fall, but also the republican head of state.[53]

Taking into account the high degree of self-reflection and self-criticism Six engaged in, the question arises whether 'Rariteiten te koop' might be an exception within the group of pro-Stuart texts in *Poësy*. Six's support for the House of Orange is not in question, but we now know how uncomfortable he feels in the role of 'priest-poet' engaging in the quasi-religious worship of the Princes of Orange. Can the ironic panegyric also be read as a way of coming to terms with his own role in the apotheosis of Charles I? The possibility cannot be ruled out.[54] 'Six was one of the very few Dutch authors who expressed his scepticism in print', we read in the conclusion to Helmers's analysis of the poem.[55] But in my opinion this interpretation is not sufficient: the complex layers of meaning in 'Rariteiten te koop' also leave room for other interpretations.

New Market-Fayre

The differences between 'Rariteiten te koop' and royalist literature are as striking as the similarities. The action in the text takes place on the worldly stage of the market square. The blood of the English martyr king is presented not only as a relic – as was the case in the royalist texts discussed above – but also as a commodity. This

53 Ibid., p. 132. This view is at the root of Six's ironic verses in 'De Waarom, van myne vrymoedige reise, naa Engeland' ('The Reason for My Self-Assured Journey to England') (J404): The text describes a – probably fictitious – encounter between Six and Cromwell. 'Ik had syn handen niet gekust: / Noch staarelinghs geooght, op oogen, / Voor welkers sterke son de mijne eerbiedigh boogen' ('I would not have kissed his hands; nor fixed my eyes on his eyes, for whose strong sun my eyes bow respectfully') (l. 18–20), Six writes ironically.

54 Six was a supporter of the monarchy as a form of state, as can be seen from 'De koninghlyke regeeringe, met de byen, vergeleeken' ('The Royal Government Compared to the Bees') (J356). In the Netherlands, the struggle between supporters of the State and Orange supporters was intertwined with religious disputes. Six's own support for the Princes of Orange was of a piece with his background as a Calvinist. But to what extent Six identified himself with the faith of Charles I is more difficult to answer. Both during his life and after his death, the Anglican king represented non-protestant ideas. The Stuart kings advocated the use of more ceremonies in the Anglican church. In 'Kooninghlyk schavot te Londen, in plaat gesneeden, door Krispyn van de Pas' ('Royal Scaffold in London, in an Engraving Made by Crispijn van de Passe') (J169, l. 21), Six calls him, a bit optimistically, 'een steun van Gods hervormde woord' ('a supporter of God's reformed word'). *Cf.*, too, K. Exalto's discussion of Cornelis van Niels's remarkably positive appreciation of the Stuart kings: K. Exalto, 'Cornelis van Niel en zijn "Welrieckende balsem", 1683', in: K. Exalto, *Beleefd geloof. Acht schetsen van gereformeerde theologen uit de 17^e eeuw*, 1974, pp. 107–108.

55 Helmers, 2015, p. 138.

indicates other uses of royal blood. According to an observation by Sir Robert Manley, not only sick people, but also people more generally, were eager to profit from the king's blood:[56] 'They were inhumanly barbarous to his dead corpse. His hair and his blood were sold by parcels [...] which were greedily bought up, but for different ends [...]'. 'From a demi-god to commodity in a bare few seconds', is how Richard Sugg describes this extreme metamorphosis.[57] This story can serve as a starting point for a text within another category of royalist texts, the satirical poems on Cromwell: the pamphlet *A Tragi-Comedy called / New Market-Fayre, / or a / Parliament / Out-Cry: / of / State-Commodities / set to sale* (1649), written by John Crouch (signed with his usual pseudonym, 'Man on the Moon'). The text shows interesting similarities to 'Rariteiten te koop' and thus helps us to get a better understanding of Six's poem.[58]

The theme of the text is the auction of the king's possessions, which had been confiscated by parliament. This sale actually took place: not long after the execution, many of the assets of the royal family – the regalia and other valuables – were auctioned off to raise money for the English Commonwealth (the republican government).[59] But the text is more theatrical in nature; Crouch also refers to the king's blood: 'Here be cloaks, hats and gloves, Rings and Bracelets of His Dear Loves; Here be boots and spurres, and bloody handkerchers [...] Here you may all things buy that belong to Monarchy' (p. 4), says the 'Cryer', who speaks in the pamphlet. Although the auction was organised on the initiative of the English Commonwealth, Crouch not only has the new republican rulers act as sellers – he also casts Cromwell and Fairfax as the most fanatical bidders. The tragicomedy ends with as much intensity as it began. Royalist troops hunt down republican soldiers – and at the same time the people themselves turn against the republicans. One aspect of *New Market-Fayre* is particularly interesting in connection with 'Rariteiten te koop' and deserves our further attention. In both texts, transformative power is attributed to the royal objects. The luxury goods enchant both the buyer's and the seller's senses. 'O yes, O yes, O yes', the 'Cryer' shouts excitedly as he praises the beauty of his goods: 'Here be Jewells of wondrous price, they will dazzle both your eyes' (p. 3). In 'Rariteiten te koop' we read that the blood 'd'Oogen scheemren doen, van vier' ('dazzles the eyes, like fire') (l. 138). Just like the blood in the royalist texts discussed above, the royal goods are depicted as physically altering agents. But whereas, for

56 Quoted from Robert Partridge, *'O Horrable Murder': the Trial, Execution and Burial of King Charles I*, 1998, p. 97.

57 Sugg, 2011, p. 86.

58 For analyses of the text, see Laura Lunger Knoppers, *Constructing Cromwell: Ceremony, Portrait, and Print 1645–1661*, 2000, pp. 27–30; Potter, 1989, pp. 111–112.

59 Knoppers, 2000, p. 27. Six mentions this sale in his poetry, and accuses Dutch politicians of taking part in it. See 'Neetelen' ('Nettles') (J332).

royalists, the blood is like a ritual drink that has healing powers and offers hope and comfort in anticipation of the wicked times to come, the 'consumption' of these royal substances is tantamount to endangering the republican body. 'Here 'tis Sir; try it on: So, now 'tis sure / And makes you look more like a King *then Brewer*' (p. 4), the auctioneer promises when he has placed Charles's 'Golden Crowne' (p. 3) on Cromwell's head.[60] The social metamorphosis that the consumers of the divine blood hoped to undergo, has not taken place. This is because of an incompatibility between the social origins of the republicans – Crouch emphasises that Cromwell comes from a family of brewers – and the elevated status of the royal regalia. The dazzling power of the royal objects has the opposite effect: it creates a divide between the republican allies Cromwell and Fairfax.

New Market-Fayre occupies a special position in royalist literature. The text is unique in the sense that the blood of Charles and the other royal *devotionalia* do not emerge as symbols of royalist loyalty, but as 'objects of lust'. This is of course because of the satirical nature of the text: Crouch's theme here is not the relationship between the blood and its 'royalist worshippers', but the appeal it has for the enemies of Charles I, the power-loving republicans. The republican uprising and the assassination of the kings led to the collapse of English society, and *New Market-Fayre* describes the consequences this had: 'the monarchy' has become a tradable commodity available to everyone, regardless of social status. See also the painting 'Allegory of Charles I of England and Henrietta of France in a Vanitas' (c. 1650–1655). The painting has the same message as *New Market-Fayre*: the king has, like luxury goods such as red corals, become an item that is no longer elevated and immortal, but vulnerable and transient (Plate 15). That is the most important point of similarity with Six's satire. The poem confirms that the ironic tone of 'Rariteiten te koop' does not necessarily mean that Six is distancing himself from the royalist cause. Just as Crouch does, our merchant-poet describes the effect of the blood on people who want to get their hands on it, not because of any loyalty to the king, but out of self-interest: as a means to realise their personal ambitions.

'Rariteiten te koop' does have much in common with *New Market-Fayre*, but it also contains elements that are absent from the English text. It is precisely these elements that make 'Rariteiten te koop' a more meaningful and interesting text. On the one hand, Six plays on both the classical and Christian moral symbols associated with the colours red and purple. Horace is ambiguous in his portrayal of these colours: in his poems of praise to Augustus, he writes that 'Augustus will drink nectar with purple lips', and he sings of 'the blood of gods', but he also

60 This is a commonplace in royalist literature. The *Mercurius Elencticus* newspaper, for example, emphasises the plain origins of the insurgents, who are 'Brewers and Bakers, Coblers, Peddlers and Tinkers' (quoted in Knoppers, 2000, p. 27). *Cf.* Helmers, 2015, p. 217.

warns against 'purple-clad tyrants'.[61] And we know, of course, the most prominent reference to purple in Western culture: the embodiment of the city of the antichrist, the whore of Babylon. The comments in the Statenvertaling attribute both a 'royal splendour' and a 'bloodthirstiness' to the colour.[62] On the other hand, the royal blood is integrated into the process of self-examination – this we know from other poems of Six's. It is not so much the English or Dutch anti-royalists, eager to get their hands on royal substances, who are being mocked, but all kinds of people from Dutch society. And Six scrutinises his role, not just as a royalist, but as a poet, a merchant, and a druggist. Blood is thus integrated into the discourse on the dangers of exotic drugs. Taking as a starting point Crouch's argument about blood as a physically altering agent, Six expands this perspective by including alchemical ideas, according to which processes that took place in the body were analogous to those that took place in the laboratory. In 'Rariteiten te koop', Six portrays royal blood as a tincture, a golden essence that, if dissolved in the human body, has the power to transform it physically (thus making the individual healthy and perfect), cognitively (giving them divine knowledge), and socially (turning them into a king).

'English frenzy'

A final puzzle piece of my analysis of 'Rariteiten te koop' can be found in other texts of Six's about the execution of Charles I. Six wrote a number of poems about the execution. I will confine myself to those texts that shed light on 'Rariteiten te koop' and on Six's discussion on the corrupting effect of drugs.

The title of 'Engelsche raasernye' ('English frenzy') (J157) brings us back to concepts I have discussed in previous chapters. The druggist-poet diagnoses the uprising as an intoxication in accordance with the concept of 'frenzy' or 'drunkenness' – and which can also be associated with *ira,* one of the seven deadly sins.[63] Here Six describes Cromwell and his supporters as people being 'drunk' on the 'Koonings aard' ('nature of the King') (l. 82): they are intoxicated by the nature of the King. At other points in *Poësy,* these *mania* are described more precisely as 'staatsucht', a word that translates both as 'thirst for power' and 'desire for higher status'.[64] The description in another poem, 'Kooninghlyk schavot te Londen, in

61 'Augustus recumbens/ purpureo bibet ore nectar' (Ode III, 3. l. 11–12), 'deorum sanguinem' (Ode IV, 2, l. 13–14), 'purpurei metuunt tyranni' (Ode I, 35, l. 12).

62 Reinhold, 1970, pp. 20–24 and 42–57; Rev. 17:3–4, comment 11: 'Conincklicke pracht', 'blood-dorsticheydt'.

63 Johan van Beverwijck, *Schat der gesontheyt*, 1656, pp. 87–114.

64 *Cf.* 'Engelsche staatsucht' (J164) and the meaning of 'staatsucht' in WNT: 'Sucht' meant 'pathological hunger', while the first part of the word, 'staat', was originally understood in a broader sense than 'state power'; it meant 'status', 'high position', and 'material wealth'. 'Ambitious of honour' is the translation

plaat gesneeden, by Krispyn van de Pas' (J169) ('The Scaffold in London, Carved in Engraving by Crispijn van de Passe'), of the beheading of Charles I explores this *mania* further. The building where the execution took place (l. 28–33).

> Dat Withal heet, de plaats van 't kruis,
> Bequaamer, voor een rooden hal,
> Gescholden, om die purperval,
> 't Bankethuis, ach, verkeert genoemt,
> Om dit Banket, niet min verdoemt,
> Dan Atreus maal.

> It is called Whitehall, the place of the cross,
> [But it is] more suitable to be cursed by the name
> Redhall, because of the fall of the purple;
> The Banqueting Hall, oh, even though the meaning is different,
> Because of this banquet, it is no less cursed
> Than the meal of Atreus.

The passage is typical of Six's poetic style, with its baroque and allusive language. The cross refers to the Eleanor Cross that stood on Trafalgar Square near the old Palace of Whitehall. This refers to the cult of Charles the Martyr, according to which Banqueting House was the site of his 'crucifixion'. Six suggests that Whitehall should actually be called Redhall, thus associating the beheading of the king with sacrilege and idolatry. Atreus was the king of Mycenae, who roasted his brother's children and served them to him as an act of revenge. The message is clear. The murder on the king reveals the true nature of the English: their pathological hunger makes them no better than pagan cannibals. They 'consume' Charles I as a human sacrifice in a pagan ritual. The characterisation of the English as cannibals is a commonplace in both royalist and republican propaganda, but for Six, who was familiar with the corrupting effect of *mumia* and other human substances, the notion of cannibalism takes on a deeper meaning. In 'Afraadinge van vreede, met de teegenwoordige regeeringe van Engeland' ('Advice Against a Peace with the Present Government of England') (J98), Six portrays the English as a people 'van zoo veel seegens droncken, / Dat met het Kooninghs bloed, syn schonken / Opvulde […]' ('drunk from so many victories, a people who filled their bones with the blood of the King') (l. 142–143). Their jealousy and unfaithfulness are thus caused by their pathological bloodthirstiness. And in his ironic 'Kontrefeitsel van Olivier

of the word in Hendrick Hexham, *A large Netherdutch and English Dictionarie; Composed out of the best Netherdutch Authours*, 1658, unpaginated.

Kromwel' ('Portrait of Oliver Cromwell') (J349) Six compares 'dit hellbeest' ('beast from hell') with 'de wilden, in Guine' ('the wild people in Guinea') (l. 85–86).[65] In early modern treatises on wild people in foreign countries, cannibalism served as a means to distinguish between barbaric and civilised peoples. However, by attributing a cannibalistic hunger to the English, Six turns this hierarchical view of peoples upside down. Six bases himself on a *topos* within Calvinist literature, among others with his friend and nephew Johannes Hoornbeeck: moral standards can be found more readily among 'noble pagans' than among more and more rebellious and decadent Europeans.[66]

On this view, the brutality of the English republicans clearly goes beyond all acceptable norms. According to Six, the English republicans are guilty of a 'cannibalistic lust for power' – indeed, of fratricide when the First Anglo-Dutch War breaks out, because it is a war with a neighbouring Protestant population. That makes England a greater threat than Spain, the traditional enemy of the Republic.[67] So there is a difference in content between these texts and Six's satires on Roman Catholic Southern Europe. In these latter, Six always emphasises that he is travelling through countries where vices such as paranoia and voluptuousness are rampant. We have seen many of the examples he gives of this. But the new situation in England has changed the political and moral map of Europe. The new characteristic of the people who were neighbours of the Dutch, a rebellious English lust for power, far exceeds the sinful sensuality of the Southern Europeans.

Then we have to come back to Six's position as a trader. In this book I have looked at how Six sees foreign drugs as transformative substances. Importing them, he believes, is dangerous for the social and political well-being of the country. We remember the way Six depicts a new medicinal horn in 'Uitroep om hoornafsetters'. Its seductive appearance was a trap. In fact, this imported product represented

65 *Cf.* Six's ironic reflections on the English's hunger for bloody flesh: 'Van 't schaapevleisch te Spa, aan Raimond de Smeth' ('On the Mutton in Spa, to Raimond de Smeth') (J111), l. 29–34).

66 *Cf.* for a similar strategy, William Eamon, 'Cannibalism and Contagion: Framing Syphilis in Counter-Reformation Italy', *Early Science and Medicine*, 1998, p. 22.

67 'Dees krygh viel lastiger, dan van den Kastiljaan, / Zoo langen tyd gedraagen' ('This war was more difficult than the war with the Spanish, that lasted so long') (l. 45–46): The Eighty Years War was a war of freedom against a superior Catholic power. Before the war with England, Six said that the root of the problem lay in betrayal, first because of the division between two Protestant brothers, and second because of the internal division of the English. *Cf.* Six's epigram 'England' (J481): 'O Engeland, ghe hebt uw Engelsch hoofd onthoofdt, / Dit 's oorsaak, dat uw ryk, van Duivlen, blyft geklooft.' ('O England, you have beheaded your English head, and that is why your kingdom is divided in two by devils') – a reference to Mark 3:24. And *cf.* other texts with apocalyptic references: 'Olyfkrans, oover de verbonde handen, van Engeland, en 't vereenight Neederland' ('Olive Wreath, on the Joined Hands of England and the United Netherlands') (J379) (l. 21–36) and 'De gekneusde hoogmoed des heerschaps van de Zee' ('The Bruised Pride of the Lord of the Sea') (J618) (l. 55 and 65–73), in which the English navy is portrayed as the Beast of Revelation.

a common disease in Spain. Royal blood also has a similar corrupting effect in 'Rariteiten te koop', but with more fatal consequences. This luxury product on the Dutch market is in reality a pathogen. Its consumption in the Netherlands involves a contaminating of 'the new disease' from England: a thirst for power and status. In the early modern period, moralists claimed that the English were so addicted to novelty that it had devastating consequences for English society. Although such an addiction for new and strange things as a characteristic of the English people is not mentioned explicitly in Six's poems, it is likely that Six saw this addiction as the basis for the hunger for royal blood – an addiction that thus could also be spread to the Dutch Republic. According to these moralists, 'one of the more disturbing effects of the Englishman's flawed character was that it increased his likelihood to rebel against his monarch and the current political regim'.[68] What do we learn from this? 'Rariteiten te koop' not only highlights the political situation in England. It also emphasises the crucial role played by international merchants and importers of foreign goods. Six realises that he has a great responsibility when it comes to the welfare of his homeland. Several poems in *Poësy* reflect his need to explain his commercial trips to 'pernicious' England.[69]

The poem that perhaps most clearly thematises Six's role as an importer is 'Onweer, op weeromreis, uit Engeland, aan matroos' ('Storm, on Return from England, to the Sailor') (J457). The starting point for the text is a sea storm that Six experienced when he returned to the Republic after a commercial trip to England in the autumn of 1654. As the title shows, the text is addressed to the crew of the boat on which Six was sailing. Six's ardent identification with characters from the Bible is once again striking: he compares himself to the prophet Jonah, and the storm on the English Channel to the punishment God meted out to the sinful Jonah. Six knows what to do: 'Men werp my rustigh, oover boord, / God is alleen, op my, verstoort' ('You may safely throw me overboard, God is angry only at me') (l. 24–25). Jonah had brought God's wrath upon him because he had refused to pray for Nineveh. But according to Six, what was at stake was another transgression against God's laws: the accumulation of earthly wealth. The sailors 'wierpen de vaten, die in 't schip waren' ('threw overboard the barrels that were on the ship') to allay God's anger (Jonah 1:5).[70] Six identifies himself with these 'barrels' – throw me into the

68 See Sara Warneke, 'A Taste for Newfangledness: the Destructive Potential of Novelty in Early Modern England', *Sixteenth Century Journal*, 1995, pp. 881–896, quote on p. 887. *Cf.* also the description of the English as a 'niewsgierich' (curious) people by Dutch authors, see Meijer Drees, 1997, p. 131.

69 See 'Schrikspiegel, om niet naa Engeland te reisen' ('Reflection on my Aversion to Traveling to England' (J235), 'De Waarom, van myne vrymoedige reise, naa Engeland' ('The Reason for My Self-Assured Journey to England') (J404).

70 See the statement of Calvin on Jonah 1:5: 'Commentary on Jonah, Micah, Nahum', *Christian Classics Ethereal Library*, www.ccel.org/ (consulted 17 May 2019). See also Schama, 2004, p. 141.

sea like 'werldversmaadende offerhanden' ('sacrifices demonstrating a disregard for worldly things') (l. 46), he exhorts the sailors. By showing his contempt for earthly riches, Six hopes to achieve a blissful life (l. 31–48). I am not claiming that Six had a handkerchief with the blood of Charles as a commodity with him, but given the location of his confession of guilt – on his way to the Netherlands on a ship full of English goods – it is tempting to relate Six's conscientious objections not only to his own soul, but also to the moral health of his homeland.

The body of the Netherlands

The bodily transformation that 'Rariteiten te koop' turns on affects all social layers of Dutch society. The Republic finds itself in a collective state of ecstasy, brought about by the red wonder drug. Does Six also express elsewhere such an obsession with the health of his fellow citizens? Until now, the main concern has been the state of the individual body.

We have in fact seen a number of examples of a similar concern about the Dutch macrocosm – the idea of 'the body politic'. In 'Goudsucht' ('Desire for Gold') (J279), Six talked about the 'state body' and how it was poisoned by gold, which resulted in a morbid addiction. And the body of the city of Delft and a punishing God were central to 'Buskruids donder, en blixem, te Delft' ('The Thunder and Lightning of Gunpowder, in Delft') (J396).[71] One text that is certainly worth mentioning in this connection is 'Op langhduurigen reegen' ('On Long-Lasting Rainfall') (J149), which was probably written in response to a major flood.[72] The flooding of the polders and the devastating effect of the water have not only a natural, but a deeper religious cause, says Six: they are a heavenly punishment for the sins of the Dutch people. But this is not just a matter of meting out discipline: the punishment also serves as purification, which is expressed in medical terms. The flood is a 'plaaster' ('plaster', in the broader seventeenth-century sense of 'remedy') by which God, '[l]yk een ervaaren Sirurgyn' ('like an experienced surgeon'), is purging the Netherlands (l. 45–56):[73]

71 See also 'Klachte, oover het ooverlyden van Wilhelm Bakker [...]' ('Lament at the Death of Wilhelm Bakker [...]') (J316) (l. 59–64), where Six – with a metaphor that is part – Bibilical, part chemical – tells us how the Dutch fell out of favour with God, because their pure 'zielgoud' ('the soul's gold') has been contaminated by 'solfer, van de sond' ('the quicksilver of sin'). For the concept of 'body politic' in Dutch literature, see Helmers, 2015, pp. 97–120.

72 M.A. Schenkeveld-van der Dussen, 'Regen in het vredejaar', in: K. Porteman & K.E. Schöndorf (eds.), *Liber amicorum Kåre Langvik-Johannessen*, 1989, pp. 164–166.

73 See the lemma in the WNT.

De suivre Heemel siende ons aan,
In slyk gewentelt, en vergaan
Van sonden, wil, vol meedelyden,
Met deese plaaster van meer quaalen, ons bevryden.
Lyk een ervaaren Sirurgyn
Een arm, of been, van swart fenyn
Doorkroopen, tydigh af doet setten,
Om 't ongevoeligh vuur 't voortkruipen te beletten:
Zoo sette God de vruchten af,
Uit liefde, al was 't een swaare straf,
Op dat de kanker, van de goedren
Gesneeden, suivren mocht de leeden der gemoedren.

Pure Heaven looked at us
Wallowing in the mud, and perishing
In sins, [Heaven] will – full of compassion –
Free us from more ailments through this plaster [the flood].
Like an experienced Surgeon
Amputates on time an arm, a foot
That is infested with a black poison,
In order to prevent the insensitive flame from spreading:
In the same way, God amputates our fruits,
With love, although it is felt as a severe penalty,
So that excising the cancer from the merchandise
May purify the [remaining] parts of the mind.

God is forced to 'verlempen' ('lop off') parts of the Netherlands (l. 57), because they have been stricken with 'gangrene'. This superfluous 'dead meat' embodies a 'cancer of the merchandise' or superfluous wealth.[74] Six uses rhetoric from the Old Testament to make his point. But the importance of the large number of medical metaphors being used here should not be underestimated either. The flooding can also be said to exert a therapeutic effect, because Six associates sinful material abundance with fire, the element opposed to water. As we have seen, purging – the driving out of excess humoral fluids – by means of a water cure is a form of treatment to which Six accords special attention. I will come back to this presently. What is this sinful 'mud' (see the quotation above) in which Six's contemporaries are 'wallowing'? The somewhat cryptic last line of the poem provides the answer. Six exhorts his

74 *Cf.* the discussion of what is necessary versus what is superfluous in 'Nooddruft is genoegh' (J133), Chapter 4, pp. 129–131.

compatriots, 'Sie westwaarts slaaven op, de Son, in 't Ooste, schynen' ('Look up, slaves of the Westward [route], the Sun is shining in the East') (l. 64). By 'westward' Six means the colonial trade route to the East and West Indies via Spain and the Canary Islands. The 'slaves' from the West are his compatriots, who are addicted to exotic luxury goods, while 'in the East' in this context means Jerusalem, in keeping with the image of Christ as the rising sun.[75]

With this poem in mind, we will turn our attention to the most striking text related to Six's concern for collective well-being: 'Op den bidaavond' ('On the Prayer Evening') (J350). The text probably dates from the autumn of 1652, when the Republic was in crisis.[76] Not only was the Netherlands at war with England – it was also going through the First Stadtholderless Period and was being rocked by internal unrest. Just as in the previous text, the Calvinistic pathos is significant. By 'bidaavond' ('prayer evening'), Six means a weekly day of prayer required by the States General. On this day, work had to stop and shops had to close. In the poem, Six argues for such an evening in Amsterdam.[77] 'Op den bidaavond' is a complex poem with an allegorical-dramatic structure. It is set up as a struggle between a 'good' and an 'evil' spirit. The 'good spirit' is the first to speak. She expresses her disappointment in the Amsterdammers who surrender to their lusts and desires (l. 30), so that the 'dartle goude Noachs tyd [...] [r]aakt binnen Amsterdam in swangh / De wellust weeldert' ('the wanton Golden Age of Noah [...] is in vogue in Amsterdam, and lasciviousness grows') (l. 37–40). Earlier in the poem Six tells how this has happened: 'Het teiken, dat ghy duivels dient, / Zal weesen, dat uw beste vriend, / En locht, en aarde, en zee, en vier / Uw plaagen zal, door Gods bestier' ('The sign that you serve devils will be that your best friend, and air, and earth, and sea, and flame, will torment you, by the will of God') (l. 31–34). These last words refer to various natural disasters that had recently struck the Netherlands, each of which Six relates to one of the four elements: an epidemic, a plague of mice, a flood, and a city fire.[78] The notion of a broken friendship refers to the war with the English who were 'Protestant brothers of the Dutch' – apparently the worst misfortune of all. The 'good spirit' therefore decides to leave the city and move to 'den Heemelheer' ('the Lord of the Heavens'),

75 *Cf.* Jacobs's annotations to 'Scheepskroon [...]' (J342) and ''s Amsterdammers winter' (J96) (l. 110) and 'Spanjes en Hollands orakel' (J2, l. 10). This reading corresponds better to the contents of the text than the somewhat complicated interpretation of the lines by Schenkeveld-van der Dussen (1989, pp. 164–166), on which the date of 1648 is based.

76 Jacobs, 1991 II, p. 622.

77 These prayer evenings were held weekly throughout the year and also the following year, Jacobs, 1991 II, p. 622, referring to N.C. Kist, *Neêrland's bededagen en biddagsbrieven*. Part II, 1849, p. 194. 'I know nothing about a separate Amsterdam prayer evening, of which Six speaks. Is this evening of prayer perhaps a piece of advice from Six that was not followed?', Jacobs writes.

78 See Jacobs's notes to this poem.

leaving the population entirely to the 'evil spirit'.[79] Then the IJ Bay – the famous personification of Amsterdam – begins to speak, concerned about the opulence and decadence of its inhabitants. She urges the city dwellers to do penance and repent, among other things by organising a new weekly day of prayer. In response to this, the 'good spirit' – the 'Son ten Heemel' ('Sun in Heaven') – comes back (l. 92). She makes darkness disappear and once again fills the Dutch trading city with her life-creating light.

Naturally, we recognise the basic idea in 'Op langhduurigen reegen' and 'Op den bidaavond': the story of a chosen 'Dutch Israel' and the notion of physical plagues as punishment for disobeying God Almighty.[80] The fact that an early modern merchant links the fate of his city with that of the most important trading cities of antiquity, Nineveh and Tyrus, is hardly surprising. The recurring theme in the Old Testament stories about these cities is, after all, that idolatry and hedonistic excesses are a betrayal of God and his plans for the chosen people. In 'Rariteiten te koop', the Dutch people are tested by the worst excess there is: a hubristic hunger for the divine.

But 'Op den bidaavond' not only presents Six as a dramatic poet. He also plays the role of the diagnostician-druggist. Let us take a closer look at his description of the two opposing spirits fighting for Amsterdam (l. 1–14):

Twee geesten strydigh van natuur,
Als blusschend nat, en teerend vuur,
Als saalig goed, en doemlik quaad,
Versellen al het menschlik saad.
Elk mensch werd, van die twee, bestiert,
't Zy hy se beide, of eenen viert.
Die van den Heemel afgedaalt,
Dees van den afgrond opgehaalt,
Staan slinks, en rechts, aan ieders oor

79 The 'good spirit' has elements in common with the goddess Astraea from Greek mythology. She, too, flees to heaven because of people's cruelty.

80 The notion of a God resurrected by a larger collective, a macrocosm, is central to the work of many of the Calvinist ministers discussed in *Poësy*. In *Oeconomia Christiana* (II, p. 1108) Wittewrongel emphasises: 'De sonde van brasserye, sluyt ons uyt den hemel. Die sulcke dingen doen, en konnen het Koninckrijcke Godts, niet beërven [...] Ende sal dit ons niet genoegh zijn / om alle Christelicke Huys-vaders en Huys-moeders van alle brasserye af te schicken: Dit pock zijnde een van die grouwelen, daerom het gansche Landt dickmaels is gestraft geworden. Dese sonde heeft de eerste Wereldt, die van Sodom, ende het vleeschelicke Israël verdorven' ('The sin of gluttony excludes us from the heaven. Those who do search these things, may not inherit the Kingdom of God [...] And if this is not enough to defer all Christian House fathers and House mothers from gluttony: This pox is one of the horrors with which the whole Country often has been punished. This sin has ruined the first World, that of Gomorrah, and the fleshly Israel').

Der sinnen, in het herssenkoor.
Sy blaasen in geneegentheit,
Die recht, of op den dwaalwegh leit,
Waar deughd' de ziele kroont met vreughd,
Of ondeught loont, met ongeneught.

Two spirits, contradictory by nature,
As quenching liquid, and as devouring fire,
As blessed good, and as damnable evil,
Accompany the human race.
Each person is ruled by these two forces,
Whether they honour both or one of them.
The one that descends from Heaven,
The other that ascends from the abyss,
Are placed to the right and left of the ear of each person,
Each breathing affection into them,
Which leads them either onto the right track, or astray,
Where virtue crowns the soul with joy,
Or vice rewards the soul with sorrow.

The good spirit manifests itself as 'quenching liquid'; the evil one as 'devouring fire'. Both succeed in 'breathing' a good and a bad 'affection' into people. The latter, we then read, is 'schynsoet, maar vergalt' ('seemingly sweet, but bitter') (l. 27). It has a toxic effect on the body. Just like 'Op langhduurigen reegen', 'Op den bidaavond' is permeated with ideas borrowed from Galenic medicine. We would not be doing the text justice if we interpreted the fire metaphor merely as the 'fire of vengeance' sent down by the God of the Old Testament. The heavy therapeutic treatment Six subjects the body of the state to reminds us of the purging that Six's own body has to go through in 'Dankoffer, aan gesondheit' (J184) – a text in which there is not a single biblical reference to be found.[81] The poem tells us of the loss of the life-creating light and a subsequent fall into a fiery darkness (*cf.* 'vuurbergh', l. 22), which coincides with the battle between two humorally opposed elements, fire and water. Moreover, the excess of fire is associated in both poems with immoral behaviour: becoming healthy in both cases means finding a state of physical and mental purity.

81 For the theme of water and fire in the early modern Netherlands, with and without biblical connotations, see Schama, 2004; Marco Prandoni, 'Gijsbreght tussen water en vuur, water- en vuurmetaforiek in *Gysbrecht van Aemstel*', *Vooys*, 2004, pp. 31–47. In addition to the texts discussed in this section, see also 'Reegenrym, in de Diemermeer, op de hofstee van Katarina Jeheu' ('Rain Rhyme, in Diemermeer, on Katarina Jeheu's country house') (J311).

The course and treatment of Dutch trader's disease, the microcosm, thus lines up with that of the Dutch trading power, the macrocosm. What is striking in all these poems is the idea of physical plagues as a result of too much inner fire. We see this, too, in Six's literary self-portraits, in which he focuses on his sick body, and which I have discussed in connection with 'Dankoffer, aan gesondheit'. Six presents himself as a doomed man who is corrupted from within.[82] The same perspective, but with regard to the macrocosm, is found in another text, 'Troost aan Abraham Grenier, rechtsgeleerden, oover de dood van syn vaader' ('Consolation to Abraham Grenier, Jurist, upon the Death of His Father') (J353). Even though this is an occasional poem, it is mainly about the political and moral situation of the country. Just as he does in 'Op den bidaavond', Six refers here to the many 'physical' incidents that have struck the body of the Dutch nation so hard (the text was written in 1653, during the First Anglo-Dutch War) (l. 65–70):

Men tracht het buitendeel
Te salven, daar het lyf geheel,
Van kanker, binnen werd doorkroopen,
En uitspouwt longh, en leeverhoopen.
O! wat een duistre wolk
Hanght oover 't hoofd, van Hollands volk?

One tries to anoint
The outside, while inside the body
Is infested throughout with cancer,
Which splits up the lungs and the liver
Oh, what gloomy clouds
Hang over the heads of the Dutch?

This brings us to the third point that was central to my discussion of Six's poems about himself as a patient. As we know, his ailment was traced back to his spleen. Can we draw a parallel between the small and the large Batavian body, between Six and the Netherlands? My own view is that this is a crucial point in 'Rariteiten te koop'.

The spleen, which according to early modern medical theory was closely involved in digestion, is, together with the stomach, the gateway to the inner body. Does the market for exotic goods have the same function for the body of the country? What is striking in this regard is that 'Vraage, om aaderlaatinge, aan Simon Dilman, Geneesheer' ('Request for Bloodletting, to Simon Dilman, Physician') (J159) comes

82 'Verdorventheit der Natuure' ('Corruption of [Human] Nature') (J340) and 'Schyn bedrieght' ('Appearances are Deceptive') (J420) in Chapter 4, pp. 147–148.

just after 'Rariteiten te koop'. I have already discussed the somewhat chaotic arrangement of the texts in *Poësy*, but there are also subtle transitions between various verses in the collection.[83] The question arises, then, whether Six in 'Rariteiten te koop' is also performing a kind of 'bloodletting', but this time on the body of the state. The poem does offer clues here. We are told that the fiery miracle blood that flows through the text both figuratively and 'literally' is reprehensible, and that it was fetched from the market – the 'spleen' of the Dutch body. It is dreck. It counts as waste just as much as do the vomit and the stool in 'Vraage, om aaderlaatinge' (see 'Rariteiten te koop', l. 147–150). The self-reflection and self-criticism in Six's texts concern not only his own body, but also that of his nation. The argument has much in common with the notion of the 'glutted, unvented body' we find in Margaret Healy's work. The medical treatment of the Dutch body requires a recovery from an inner humoral imbalance as much as it does the control of external, invasive sources of infection.[84] In 'Rariteiten te koop', Six confesses that, as an importer of luxury goods, he is guilty, along with others, of morally corrupting Dutch society. But with the parallel purging of the body of the state and of his own body, Six shows that he is repentant: he is willing to sacrifice and punish himself for the sake of his country's health.

The blood of Christ

In this chapter we have looked at the most exclusive drugs from the early modern pharmacy, medicines from the human body, the creature created in the image of God. Just like the drugs in the previous chapters, Six integrates these into a process of self-examination: the druggist-poet shows that these are not only worthless forgeries, but also poisons with a corrupting effect on the bodies of individual consumers and that of the Netherlands. 'Rariteiten te koop' occupies a special position among the texts discussed in this chapter. The poem stages a moral trial with the most tempting drug an early modern druggist could ever get hold of: a divine substance, the blood of Charles I – an apparent equivalent to the miraculous blood of Christ. But in the end, this substance turns out to have the opposite effect. Does this mean that Six completely rejects a desire for the divine? No, because three texts that I will discuss in this chapter offer a different view of medical anthropophagy. Here, it is Christ's blood that is on the menu: 'Op het H. nachtmaal' ('On the Lord's Supper') (J186),

83 See, for instance, 'Bruiloftsangh, aan Joannes Abeels getrouwt met Anna de Bra' (J171) and 'Oostkappele, aan Abraham Grenier den jongen' (J172), and the placing of 'Boetsangh, op de wyse van den 130. psalm' ('Penitential Song, in the Manner of Psalm 130') (J471) as the last text of *Poësy*. *Cf.* Schenkeveld-van der Dussen, 2007, pp. 238–239.

84 Margaret Healy, *Fictions of Disease in Early Modern England: Bodies, Plagues and Politics*, 2001.

'Noodinge ten avondmaal. Op de wyse van den 24. psalm' ('Invitation to the Lord's Supper. In the manner of Psalm 24') (J409) en 'Op de woorden: My dorst. Aan Jesus Kristus aan 't kruys' ('On the Words: I Thirst. To Jesus Christ on the Cross') (J323).

Let us look at 'Op het H. nachtmaal'. The reformed character of the Lord's Supper is immediately clear. First, Six distinguishes between inner and outer wealth in approaching Christ's body: the bread and the wine of the sacrament are 'liefliker, dan hooninghraat, en melk' ('lovelier than honeycomb and milk') (l. 2), the food of the Promised Land. Second, he expresses the main Calvinist objection to Catholic communion, the doctrine of transubstantiation. At the actual Lord's Supper there is no substantive change to the body and blood of Christ, Six emphasises, in line with reformed doctrine. The body of Christ is only symbolically present – 'in teikens' ('in signs') (l. 5). This is followed by the third point: to be celebrated correctly, the Lord's Supper requires a pure mind and genuine repentance. Hypocritical repentance leads the participant in the Supper directly to hell (l. 6–10). The same three points also form the basis for 'Noodinge ten avondmaal'. The question of outer versus inner wealth is further elaborated in this poem (l. 7–10):

> Hem [de protestant] werd noch Ahasueers banket,
> Noch Heidensch Nectar voorgeset,
> Noch God in deegh der pausgenooten:
> Maar louter brood, en klaare wyn,
> Die teikens van Gods lichaam zyn,
> Aan 't kruis gekruissight, en vergooten.

> Neither the banquet of Ahasuerus,
> Nor Pagan Nectar was served to him [the Protestant],
> Nor God in the dough of the followers of the Pope:
> But pure bread and clear wine,
> Which are the signs of God's body,
> Who was crucified and who shed his blood.

'The banquet of Ahasuerus' – Six is referring to the abundant meal of King Ahasuerus (Esther 1) – and 'Pagan Nectar' could refer to the exotic luxury goods from Six's drugstore. Neither Eastern spices nor the Roman Catholic host offer humankind salvation, according to Six. But the Lord's Supper, consisting of 'only bread, and clear wine, which are signs of God's body' does – as long as Christians are prepared for catharsis: 'wie een waarde gast wilt zyn / Aan Kristus taafel, die verschyn, / Met milde, en onbesmette handen' ('he who wants to be a worthy guest at Christ's table appears with mild and uncontaminated hands' (l. 25–27). We then read that, whereas the very first people on earth, Adam and Eve, got divine food from 'vrucht, in Edens paradys' ('fruit, in the

Garden of Eden') (l. 17), the postlapsarian man can turn to the body of Christ for such food. With the death of Christ, vegetarianism, the pure diet from before the Fall of Man, has been replaced by religious cannibalism: 'Men eet den priester, in dat maal, / En drinkt hem' ('One eats the priest in that meal, And drinks him') (l. 20–21).[85] The whole physical interpretation of the processing of the flesh and blood of Christ, which is actually at odds with the Protestant doctrine of a metaphorical concept of Lord's Supper, is striking: 'Dat voedsel heilt de kranke ziel, / En maakt se, als sneeuwwit, dat varsch viel, / Des winters, langs de swarte hooven' ('That food heals the sick soul and makes it white, like snow that has just fallen in the winter over the black gardens [of sin]') (l. 22–24). The body of Christ has a healing effect on the sick body, and a purifying effect on the sinful spirit of the participant. 'Myn ziel, hoe smaakt my deesen disch! / De rotse, en 't Man der wildernis, / Kon dorst, en honger zoo niet smaaken' ('My soul, how good this meal tastes! The rock and the Manna of the wilderness, could not satisfy thirst and hunger in this way') (l. 31–33), exclaims Six at the end, and thus complements the theological argument with his personal experience of the Lord's Supper, a Christian *enthousiasmos*: 'Ik vloogh alree verheugt om hoogh, / waar Englen, in het saaligh oogh, / Der eewge Dryheit sich vermaaken' ('I flew joyfully up, where angels, in the blissful eye, of the eternal Trinity are delighted') (l. 34–36): The body and blood of Christ are the true *drug:* they make the poet healthy, ecstatic and immortal.[86]

In 'Op de woorden: My dorst', Six is even more personal. The poem is a meditation on suffering – a popular genre in the mid-seventeenth century.[87] For this poetic exercise, Six apparently chose the moment that appeals most to him from the story of Christ's passion: his last hour, when Jesus complains about his thirst and dies, after which blood and water flowed from his side, which had been pierced with a spear (John 19:28–34). The flowing of the holy blood from Jesus' side links the text to the sacramental poems discussed above. The original, and rather physical, character that Six describes also contributes to this. All the main themes from Six's poetry are covered here: self-criticism, the consumption of luxury goods, and physical and spiritual purification. And the title also prompts us to look at other typical characteristics of Six's poetry in the text: on the one hand there is the strong religious empathy – Six's dramatic identification with the suffering Christ – and on the other, there is the important place he reserves in the text for his own medical

85 For Adam and Eve's vegetarianism, see Schoenfeldt, 1999, pp. 131–167. *Cf.* also the contrasting of the blood of Christ with both the dew of the Garden of Eden, and spices of the 'warm South', in: Jeremias de Decker, *Goede vrydag ofte Het lijden onses heeren Jesy Christi*, ed. by W.J.C. Buitendijk, 1978, pp. 129 and 135.

86 In contrast to the weekly Eucharist of the Catholic Church and the frequent celebration of the current reformed Church, the Calvinist Supper only took place a few times a year in the early modern period. This may have contributed to Six's experience of it as a rare, intense event: Schenkeveld-van der Dussen & De Vries, 2007, p. 130.

87 See Porteman & Smits-Veldt, 2008, pp. 651–658.

history. These two are interwoven: according to Six, Christ, in his thirst, suffers from the same syndrome as Six does: an inner drought.

Let us turn now to the contents of the poem. Jesus' words 'my dorst' ('I Thirst) make Six think about His suffering on the cross. He realises that he is partly guilty for this, begins to feel repentance and remorse, and proposes to Christ to pay off his debt (l. 1–4):

Dorst u, helaas! o bron van 's leevens soete stroom?
  Heb ik ook schuld van zulken droogte, en geeuwen?
Wach my! drinkt dan, myn God, uit oogen, sonder schroom,
  Voor 't heilloos heir der marmere Hebreeuwen.

Do you thirst – how regrettable! O, source of the sweet stream of life?
Am I also to blame for this dryness, and your gasping?
Woe to me! Drink then, my God, of my eyes, without hesitation,
For the wicked band of the unshakable Hebrews.

What is striking is the way Six wants to pay his debt: he wants to quench Jesus' thirst with the tears flowing from his own eyes. The redemption expressed in the following lines is described in just as specific a way. Christ accepts the tears of Six and lets the repentant druggist drink the blood of his body in exchange. This is how the rest of this short poem goes (l. 5–12):

U smaakt geen spons gedoopt, in galligen asyn,
  Maar in den rouw van sonden, vet van traanen.
Die, die waardeert ghy, voor den kostelyksten wyn.
  Drinkt dan myn God, uit deese boesemkraanen.
Ai! brenght het my, op myn gesondicheit bedacht.
  Ik doe bescheid, met bloed, dat ik sie druipen,
Uit uwe sy. Dit, dit 's gesondheit toegebracht.
  Fy, dronken mensch, het ander is maar suipen.

You do not taste a sponge dipped in bilious vinegar,
But in the repentance of sins, soaked with tears,
Which you appreciate more than the most precious wine.
Drink then, my God, from these taps of my bosom.
Oh, drink to me, drink to my health,
I will toast back to you, with blood that I see dripping
Out of your side. This, this is what has brought about good health,
Shame, drunk man, the other way [of drinking] is boozing.

The content of the text makes a strange impression on the modern reader. In view of the theme of this chapter, it is striking how the repayment of guilt and the bringing of salvation are portrayed as an exchange of human 'drugs'. And what is even stranger is that this cannibalistic exchange ends with a toast to each other's health. 'Bizarre' imagery and 'curious terminology', M.A. Schenkeveld-van der Dussen rightly states in her analysis of the poem (Fig. 9.3).[88] The 'toasting' evokes associations with the festive poems Six wrote in response to various trade agreements – *cf.* 'Fooi' (J212). These verses set us on the right path to further interpretation. If we think of the mythological framework of 'Fooi', which we looked at above, we can get a better understanding of this unconventional representation of Christ's passion, combined with Six's own salvation. 'Toosten' was an important part of Bacchic orgies and sacrificial ceremonies – a fact to which our self-aware druggist, who knows only too well the religious origins of poetry and pharmacy, is apparently alluding.[89] The crucifixion of Christ and the dripping out of his blood are a break with, but also a continuation of, pre-Christian sacrificial ceremonies. We must not forget the original function of sacrifice: to assuage the anger of the gods and thus to ensure the health of the land and the people.[90]

The term 'druggist' gives us immediate insights into other aspects of the poem. The tears of the sinner as a symbol of confession, and the blood of Christ as a symbol of salvation, are commonplaces in Christian literature. But Six's emphasis on 'droogte' ('drought') (l. 2) makes a more singular impression on the reader. An etymological explanation of the words in Dutch can help us understand this: 'drogerij', 'drogist' and 'dorst' all derive from words that have to do with 'dryness'.[91] Six once again gives the name of his profession a new connotation: this time not 'sober', but 'thirsty', in the sense of longing for God. He connects the spiritual distress he expresses in the poem with his syndrome: a humoral excess of dryness. His idiosyncratic identification with Christ is best understood in light of early modern medical theories. 'Droogte' indicates a state of physical and mental imbalance. The administration of fluid can help the sick body recover both spiritually and physically. In Six's argument, the spiritual exchange of guilt and redemption thus coincides with a humoral exchange of good and bad humoral fluids. We have now come to the last element in 'Op de woorden: My dorst'. The dilemma underlying the poems discussed above on the Last Supper also marks this text. Six warns against the intake of the wrong liquid – liquid that would disrupt the spiritual

88 Schenkeveld-van der Dussen & De Vries, 2007, p. 136.

89 See Chapter 8.

90 See comment 60 to John 19:35 and comment 11 to 1. John 5:6 in the *Statenvertaling*.

91 The word 'dorst' ('thirst') is derived from 'dor', a synomym for 'droog'. Six was aware of this etymology – *cf.* 'drooghte' and 'dorst' in 'Op een boetsenmaaker' ('To a Joker') (J269). See also meaning 6 of 'droog' in the WNT.

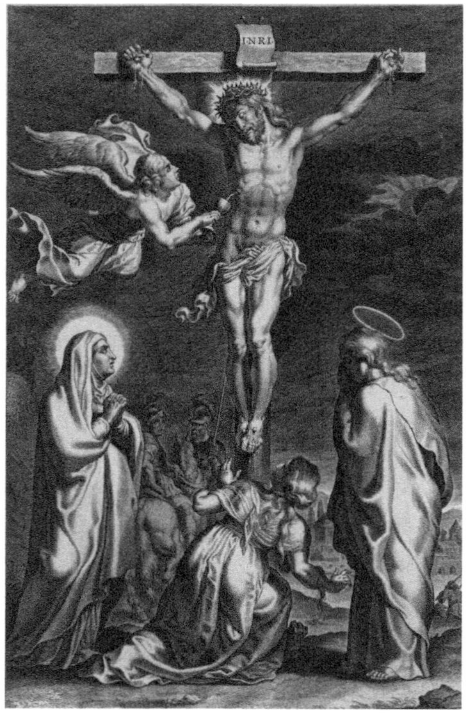

Fig. 9.3: Theodoor Galle (possibly), after Peter Paul Rubens, *Crucifixion of Jesus, with the drinking of Christ's blood*. The symbolism of Six's poem is thus also to be found in Dutch art. 1612–1616. Engraving. (© Rijksmuseum, Amsterdam).

and medical exchange mentioned above. Jesus values tears higher than 'the most expensive wine'. And Six also writes: Jesus' blood gives his body 'health', while wine is synonymous with 'boozing' – which according to early modern medical theories indeed did not quench thirst, but rather caused a physical blockage. Here, too, Six is more personal than in the other texts: in the early modern period, wine was both a medicine and a stimulant, and, as we have seen above, Six probably also sold it in his shop.[92]

Conclusion

At the beginning of this chapter, I wrote that 'Rariteiten te koop' is a culmination of themes, motifs and exotic medicines that are expressed in Six's poetry, and that it is therefore also a culmination of the presentation of topics and drugs that we have

92 See Chapter 4, p. 120.

looked at in this book. We saw this in my reading of the text, which showed the unique multifunctionality and transformative power of blood. My interpretation of blood has also shown that it is the drug in Six's *oeuvre* that has the greatest seductive power. The key to understanding the poem, then, lies in an intertextual reading of the kind I have done in this chapter. My interpretation of 'Rariteiten te koop' has demonstrated that the poem goes beyond the framework of pro-Stuart literature, and that Six's ironic eulogy to the blood of Charles I should be understood in the light of his self-portrayal as a self-critical druggist-merchant – a druggist who, in a time of crisis, diagnoses the medical and moral condition of both his own body and that of the Netherlands, and who continually examines his own actions as a druggist. This is evident from a similarity to the other human medicines discussed in this chapter. The sublime power of royal blood is related to its origins: it is not a raw material from the 'kingdom of plants, minerals and animals', nor even a substance from the human body: this substance comes from a deity, from the *sacrosanct* body of an anointed king. And unlike *mumia* and relics, it is neither about the thousand-year-old remains of an Egyptian pharaoh, nor about ancient relics of Christian saints – the authenticity of which is questionable – but about the fresh blood of a deity from the poet's own time. As we have seen, rarity and inaccessibility normally go hand in hand when it comes to drugs. The accessibility of this product is based as much on spatial proximity as on proximity in time: it comes, not from distant, exotic regions, nor from distant empires, but from the British Empire. The authenticity, freshness and vitality of this panacea make it superior to all the dry and 'dead' drugs we have looked at in this book. 'Rariteiten te koop' presents the ultimate miracle drug, a substance that is interchangeable only with the blood of Jesus Christ.

In this connection, it is worth asking whether Six really traded a handkerchief that had blood on it. In auctions in our time, handkerchiefs with the blood of Charles I on them have indeed appeared, so it is possible that Six was actually offered one.[93] But my view is that this is more of an imaginary than a real trading situation, even though the negotiation takes place in a socially and politically recognisable reality. The literary strategy underlying 'Rariteiten te koop' has many parallels with that of 'Uitroep om hoornafsetters' and other texts that Six wrote and in which Six stages the introduction to a new drug as a moral test. For Six, the execution of the king was not only an exceptional political event, but also a unique pharmaceutical phenomenon, because of the paradoxical nature of this rarity. It is an easily available *unicum*, a European *exoticum*, and nevertheless, a miracle drug that promises perfection and divinity but that in reality carries with it falsehood and immorality.

93 A handkerchief with the blood of Charles I was put under the gavel at the auction house Dominic Winter Auction, 2008. My thanks to Hans de Boeck for this reference.

Six is, however, not a stoic who rejects all forms of desire. Even the most extreme form of desire, cannibalism, belongs to human nature, Six argues, but then a cannibalism that must be understood in religious terms. It is to this context that the new interpretation that Six gives the name of his profession belongs: 'thirsty', in the sense of longing for God. The last three poems we have looked at broaden and refine our image of Six's nutritional-physiological understanding of spiritual and physical well-being. My discussion of the early modern notion of drunkenness in the previous chapter can help us understand the latter better: Six does not deny the existence of cannibalistic hunger as such, but – just as he distinguishes pagan from Christian ecstasy – he states that there is a lawful and an illicit form of anthropophagy. As we have just seen, texts that speak of salvation and healing can be as blood-red as texts dedicated to the pagan sacrificial cult and decadence.[94] The only good human remedy is the blood of Jesus Christ – as long as it is experienced as an inner force. That blood is immaterial. It has no seductive odours and colours and, moreover, it cannot be expressed in monetary terms. We could hardly be farther away from the luxurious blood in 'Rariteiten te koop'.

94 *Cf.* also 'Spasangh. Op de wyse vanden 6. psalm' ('Spa Song. In the Manner of Psalm 6') (J108), which emphasises that the consumption of water from the springs at Spa must be accompanied by the consumption of another, spiritual 'spring': 'Jesus bloedfontein' ('the spring of Jesus' blood') (l. 33).

10. Conclusion

Hoe soet zyn uw beveelen?
Vry soeter, dan het soet,
In Brasiljaansche steelen,
Van suikerriet gevoedt.

How sweet are thy words?
Much sweeter than the sweet
Of Brazilian stems,
Of which sugarcanes are fed.
– Joannes Six van Chandelier[1]

The true drug

The final poem in *Poësy* has the revealing title 'Boetsangh, op de wyse van den 130. Psalm' ('Penitential Song, in the Manner of Psalm 130') (J471). It is a chronological story about the relationship between Six and God, and deals with sin and forgiveness. Six tells how his sins have created a 'scheibergh' ('separating mountain') (l. 7) between him and God. A reconciliation between the two follows, but the situation soon deteriorates again, because Six falls back into a sinful life. This time there is no mountain, but a tower of sins that separates them from each other. But, thanks to the purifying blood of Christ, Six's sins are erased, and he finally finds grace again with God. At first glance, this allegorical confessional story seems to apply to anyone. But, upon closer examination, we recognise formulations that explicitly point to a trader in exotic drugs: Jesus' words are sweeter than Brazilian sugar cane, Six proclaims at the end of the text (see the quote above).[2]

1 'Boetsangh, op de wyse van den 130. Psalm' ('Penitential Song, in the Manner of Psalm 130') (J471, l. 121–124).
2 *Cf.* psalm 119:103, 'how sweet are thy words unto my taste! Yea, sweeter than honey to my mouth'. Like other exotica, sugar has also had beneficial powers attributed to it. But sugar was also used in Six's time as a preservative, as decoration and as a sweetener, among other things to make syrups and sweet medicines, and to make fruit into jam. *Cf.* Chapter 5, p. 174. For the import of Brazilian sugar to the

Spaans, R., *Dangerous Drugs: The Self-Presentation of the Merchant-Poet Joannes Six van Chandelier (1620–1695)*. Taylor & Francis Group, 2020
DOI 10.5117/9789462983543_CONCL

As we have seen, the order of the poems in *Poësy* makes a chaotic impression, but the place of 'Boetsangh, op de wyse van den 130. Psalm' shows once again that, behind the order in which many of the poems appear, there is a well-considered plan. As the final text in the collection, this poem emphasises, on the one hand, the confessional content of *Poësy* – a function that, as I have shown in this book, many of Six's poems have. On the other hand, this poem anticipates the book that Six would publish after twenty years of silence, a rhyming version of the psalms of David (1674).[3] 'Boetsangh' also points to a dilemma that has been central to this book: in many texts, Six describes how, as a merchant, he finds himself having to choose between morally good and bad drugs. The words with which he ends the poem are interesting in this respect. He thanks Christ: 'Myn heil, myn middelaar' ('My saviour, my mediator') (l. 136). Neither sugar nor other appealing luxury goods, but Jesus Himself is the only good spiritual mediator – He is the only good 'heilmiddel' ('remedy').

This dichotomy is also reflected in Six's rhetorical descriptions of his profession. In another confessional poem, written on commercial trips in Southern Europe, 'Op het ontbeeren van den waaren godsdienst' ('On Being Deprived of the Service of the True Church') (J76), he plays with the name of his profession and the name of his pastor in Amsterdam, Jacobus Hollebeek. Repenting for having neglected his Calvinist religion, he cries out: 'Och mocht een drupje van die koele volle beek [...] [d]e drooge tongh myn's ziels nu laaven met een preek' ('Oh, may a drop of the cool, full brook [...] now refresh my soul's dry tongue with a sermon' (l. 8–10): By 'dry' Six means 'thirsty' and 'weak', in the medical and religious senses of the word. But we have also seen that, just as in 'Het boek, aan den leeser' (J119), he defines 'dry' as 'sober' and 'rational'. It is this ambiguity that underlies Six's two self-profiling strategies as a druggist. The double identity of the druggist-poet will also be the starting point for this conclusion.

The self-aware merchant-poet

In my study of the self-presentation of Joannes Six van Chandelier, I have paid as much attention to his professional identity as to his poetry. This wholesaler of drugs and member of Amsterdam's merchant elite lived at a time when various medical

Republic, and Amsterdam as the centre for the Western European sugar industry, see A.H. Poelwijk, *'In dienste vant suyckerenbacken'. De Amsterdamse suikernijverheid en haar ondernemers, 1580–1630*, 2003.

3 'Boetsangh' is the last poem of the sixth volume of *Poësy* (the third volume of the 'Dichtbosch'), which is followed by the appendix 'Opschriften', a collection of epigrams. Six was not completely silent after the appearance of *Poësy*. As I mentioned above, he wrote a number of pamphlets, but his poetic productivity was never as high as before 1657.

professions were in a process of a demarcation. In Chapter 2, I have shown that the assessment of his poems by his contemporaries was closely related to the social prestige of his profession. From 'Op quaade tongen' (J229), it appeared that the increasingly scientifically oriented physicians and apothecaries wanted to distance themselves from the merchant-druggist. In many people's eyes, 'merchant' was synonymous with lies and cravings, especially greed, while 'druggist' was linked to the negative properties associated with the trade in foreign drugs: foreignness, wealth and disease. In addition, the ailment the poet had in this spleen also affected his social status – as we have seen in Chapter 4. For example, Six contradicts rumours in a number of poems that attribute the disease to visits to brothels during his business trips in Southern Europe, the sensual part of Europe in the view of moralists.

My analysis has shown that Six uses various strategies to cast his profession in a positive light. He defends himself against the prejudices of the new scientific *virtuosi*. His attack on the *gentlemen-virtuosi* circle does not necessarily mean that he himself has no social ambitions. He wants to be seen as a down-to-earth and humanistically educated botanist. In this context, I have pointed to the ideals that Franciscus Sylvius put forward as rules of thumb for the scientist: self-knowledge, moderation and reason. Although Sylvius is known today as a representative of new science and empirical research, he did not reject the knowledge of classical authorities. When Six presents himself as a representative of *gentlemanly codes* in the Republic, as a learned, self-aware merchant, he does so based on a solid humanist foundation – in accordance with the rules that we also found in Caspar Barlaeus's ideal of the *Mercator sapiens*, the learned merchant, and the Christian ideals of Dirk Volckertszoon Coornhert's *De Coopman*.

Self-presentation as a down-to-earth druggist

The merchandise the merchant-druggist sold also underwent a process of redefinition in the seventeenth century. As we have seen, exotic materials were a source not only of economic and scientific advancement, but also of moral unease in the Republic. This is clear from *Inleydinge tot de Hollandtsche Genees-middelen* (1642) by Johan van Beverwijck. In the early modern period, the effect of foreign drugs was debated. Moralists regarded drugs as dangerous transformative and stimulating substances. Van Beverwijck points to medical, moral and social arguments in his rejection of foreign drugs, and he defines drugs as a danger to the body, not only of the individual, but of the state. According to Van Beverwijck, exotic drugs were incompatible with the humoral 'complexion' of the Batavian body. Although the discussion of domestic versus foreign plants had no economic consequences for the Netherlands as a global trading power, it did have a social, cultural and scientific impact. These aspects are essential to my study of Six's self-presentation as a druggist-poet. The various strategies Six uses in presenting himself as a down-to-earth druggist are thus motivated not only by traditional labels linked to merchants, avarice and profit-seeking, but also by phenomena that we would associate with drug abuse: intoxication, addiction, and individual and social ailments. For Six it is important to show that in his day-to-day dealings with exotic drugs, he preserves his innate 'Dutchness', which was conceived as a physical as well as a cognitive quality. The acquisition of knowledge about these substances is presented as a physiological process. The druggist learns about their properties and their quality with the help of his senses (*cf.* Sijbrand Feitama's 'Op de vyf Zinnen'). This is why, in my research into the self-presentation of Six van Chandelier, I have adopted a method that on the one hand takes into account early modern theories about emotions, the body and the physical properties of materials and, on the other, literary concepts and ideas. I have of course also included general social and political developments of the period in my analyses.

Early modern drugs were multifunctional and were therefore used in different areas of society. This fact has shaped the structure of the second and main part of this book. We can hear quite clearly Six's unique, self-critical voice in this part. He presents himself as a learned, down-to-earth druggist who is aware of the dangers of drug use in all parts of society. In addition to the medical and culinary use of drugs and spices, social, artistic and religious applications are also subject to self-critical research – including their metaphorical use in Renaissance literature. Six shows, for example, that he distinguishes between socially useful and harmful ways in which drugs were used. He condemns the cosmetic use of drugs as 'quack colours', and he denounces miracle drugs such as amber, gold, horns and incense. This process of self-examination also includes early modern phenomena and concepts that Six associates with drugs, such as the cabinet of curiosities, *exotica* as status symbols, dyes as carriers of enchanting powers, the notion of the artist as a divine creator, and oil and incense as means to apotheosis. The latter plays an important role in the last chapters of the main part of this book, where I discuss the treatment in Six's poetry of the religious and ceremonial use of drugs. Six protests against the idealised representation of women in Petrarchan love poetry, and against royal worship – this in relation to Joyous Entries and worshipful panegyrics to people in high position. He mocks the notion of any transformative effect that drugs were supposed to have on both the one whose praises are being sung (and who is thus elevated to the status of a deity) and on the spectators (who are amazed and enraptured), by linking religious-pharmaceutical language with hubris, a lust for power, and idolatry.

The last chapter of Part two is about the transformative effect of drugs on the body of the druggist-poet. In that part I discuss texts on the theme of poetic inspiration as a source of divine insights. By linking this *furor poeticus* to the substances he sells as a druggist, Six underscores his view that poetic ecstasy is the result, not of divine revelation, but of humoral-physiological processes in his body. He links the notion of the possessed *vates* (the poet-prophet) to early modern theories about drunkenness. In this way, he is, so to speak, diagnosing the concept of *furor poeticus*. At the same time, however, he emphasises that there is also a good kind of rapture: the power of the Holy Spirit, for which no physical aids are needed.

The first 'drug poet' in Dutch literature

The fact that Six relates poetic inspiration so strongly to hallucinogenic substances is remarkable from a literary-historical perspective, and raises the question whether he can be considered the first 'drug poet' in the Netherlands. My study has had a textual starting point: we do not know whether Six was, to use a modern term, a 'drug addict', although some poems, such as 'Verrukkinge van sinnen' (J401), do seem to indicate 'consciousness-expanding' experiences, while others, such as 'Fooi' (J212), contain surprisingly precise physiological descriptions of psychoactive materials. Unfortunately, we also do not have any contemporary descriptions by other writers of drug use on Six's part. An osteological study of the poet's mortal remains – if they are still present under the floor of the Zuiderkerk in Amsterdam – could determine to what extent any chemical substances were present in his body. The discussion of drug use in Six's poetry is based mainly on *narratives* that link drugs to phenomena that we associate with drug use today: stories about sexual immorality, unreason and intoxication. And as a humanist scholar, Six found these narratives with his favourite classics, such as Horace, Persius and Pliny, alongside Christian authorities such as Augustine. Six is the first 'drug poet' in Dutch literature in the sense that he is the first to articulate the individual and social dangers of drug use. In this area, my research corresponds with Brian Cowan's study, which I discussed in the introduction, on social life around coffee in the early modern period. It is not, then, biological facts but cultural constructions linked to early modern drugs that determine their status as 'dangerous intoxicants'. One difference between Cowan's research and mine has to do with my focus on the considerable attention Six devotes to the ceremonial and religious uses of spices. That can, however, be explained in light of the presence of products such as oils and incense in 'The Gilded Unicorn'. In that respect, the special attention in Six's poetry to the Roman imperial cult, the oracle of Sibyl and the ceremonial poetry of Pindar is also worth mentioning: he apparently found explanatory models here that enabled him to give an ethical judgment on representations of the display of political power in early modern Europe – where these representations have a quasi-religious character.

What is interesting in this context is Six's emphasis on a specific Dutch humoral 'complexion'. His cold and dry disposition made him immune to the poetic fire, the *furor poeticus*. This is evident from a few texts in which he shows a physical shortcoming with regard to poetic ecstasy. For Six, then, sobriety is a moral characteristic that is not so much the result of intellectual deliberation as a physical 'instinct' of the Dutch body. The emphasis on a physical reaction is also important from an aesthetic perspective, in the view of Six's literary programme. The descriptions of ailments in Six's poetry are, in many texts, related to the pathological effects of exotic drugs. But the inadequacy of human existence does, perhaps surprisingly, have a positive value in these poems. Human weakness functions as a contrast to the high aspirations of the *vates*, and therefore as proof of the humanity of the down-to-earth druggist. This fact forms the basis for Six's rhymester poetics. It represents the natural, the indigenous and the authentic as an ideal, in contrast to the Neoplatonic, Renaissance poetics that are characterised by their desire for the divine and the perfect.

Thirst for power as a commodity

In Six's self-critical voice, we recognise the humanistic ideal of self-knowledge, but in order to really understand its meaning, we must immerse ourselves in the druggist-poet's Calvinist faith. This is evident from the fact that many of Six's self-critical poems are addressed to the erudite theologian Johannes Hoornbeeck. The aforementioned urge to scrutinise in detail all aspects of his existence as a merchant-druggist and poet makes it worth asking whether Six's authorship should be seen as a part of the Further Reformation. One characteristic of this movement was its emphasis on the impact of the messages of the Bible on all aspects of day-to-day life. The preachers of the Further Reformation called for penance and repentance. In addition to his self-profiling as a sober merchant in control of his emotions, Six often portrays himself in *Poësy* as a sinner. Another factor that plays a role here is the ailment the poet has in his spleen. Texts about his medical treatment, addressed to Simon Dilman, Six's ethically oriented doctor, show that Six attributes his illness to too much *fire* in his body, and that he sees a connection between illness and sin. This brings us to the second meaning of 'druggist', which derives in Dutch from the same word as the word for 'thirsty', and thus to the third and last part of this book, where I have discussed the kinds of drug in Six's *oeuvre* that most strongly emphasise the ethical implications of the trade in drugs, namely medicines from the human body: *mumia*, relics, and human blood.

This last substance is mentioned in the poem to which I devote the greatest attention, 'Rariteiten te koop' (J158), which was printed in red ink, and which tells of an auction of the blood of Charles I of England, who was beheaded in 1649. On the one hand, *Poësy* already contains a striking number of references to the beheading of Charles I. On the other hand, 'Rariteiten te koop' brings together all of *Poësy*'s main themes. The reason Six attributes such significant symbolic value to beheading is, in my view, that he regards this event as a culmination of several dangerous desires associated with the consumption of drugs: lust, avarice and curiosity – sentiments that, according to Six, lead to discord and revolt. 'Rariteiten te koop' describes an extreme and at the same time paradoxical situation. Since it concerns the consumption of the blood of a king – a 'deity' according to early modern state theory – the English revolt in Six's poem degenerates into thirst for power and status: the consumers of the blood are filled with the desire to be kings. But at the same time, it is about the thirst for blood, a pathological thirst that Six equates with cannibalism (*cf.* his text on *mumia*, 'Lykbalsem' (J405)). The royal ecstasy or *mania* of those who consume blood is thus presented as being diametrically opposed to reason. What makes 'Rariteiten te koop' so interesting when it comes to Six's self-portrayal is that he does not situate the auction in England, but in the Dutch Republic, a country that has been on the brink of civil war because of the conflict between the Dutch States Party and the Orangists. This brings us to the other important reason for the considerable symbolic value Six attaches to the beheading of Charles I: he trades with England and recognises that he plays a crucial role in the international dissemination of goods and ideas. In this respect, Six's search for self-knowledge has a physiological factor: the merchant-druggist is a potential source of 'infection' from dangerous desires. He realises that he is partly responsible for the health of his country. One hypothesis that can be drawn from this book, then, is related to the idea that the confessional content of *Poësy* has a corporeal foundation. For Six, preserving his 'Dutchness' is as much a physical as a spiritual process. It implies a religious-humoral purifying of both his own body (the Spa cure) and of the Netherlands itself (*cf.* 'Op langhduurigen reegen').

What is also interesting in this connection is that Six attributes to European people characteristics that many of its contemporaries might rather attribute to so-called 'primitive' peoples in the East and West Indies. Six is by no means a representative of what we would today call 'eurocentrism'. Like many moralists within the Reformed Church, he was concerned about decadent tendencies within European culture. According to 'Goudsucht' (J279), the true ideal society is not in Europe, but among the natives of Caribbean islands.[4] Six shares an ethnographic

4 This idealisation of the natives in America brings us to the concept of 'noble savages'. In the poetry of Six, and in the works of other writers of this period, we probably find a germ to the romanticisation of exotic people, but the debate on 'noble savages' belongs, as I see it, more to the sentimentalism of the 18th than the 17th century. In Six's time, the exotic was primarily associated with the fascination of the wonderful in remote lands, spices, monsters, etc.

curiosity about other cultures with theologians such as Johannes Hoornbeeck. His criticism of the English and the Spanish also reveals another important point concerning the representation of exotic commodities in *Poësy*. It is not the country from which materials originate but the history of their use that determines how Six judges them morally. In Six's renunciation of incense, for example, the Arabian origin of the product is hardly mentioned. His criticism has to do with ideas and concepts originating from Graeco-Roman religion and the Roman Catholic Church – cultural spheres with which the fragrant resin was associated over the centuries. Here, too, the humanist education of the poet comes into its own. This is why some new exotica without any European history, such as Mexican jalap, are presented in an unbiased way in the poetry of the merchant-druggist. But what about cochineal, also a novelty from Mexico? The reason for Six's criticism of the dye from these scale insects is that, through the 'annexation' of the pigment within European culture, it came to be included in a moral genealogy about imperialist red dyes. It was conceived as a continuation of Tyrian purple, so to speak.

Six's theatrical pen

There are many aspects of Six's work that will seem strange to a contemporary reader: the theory of humours, the religious pathos, and the warning against a malevolent *curiositas*. The positive revaluation of *curiositas* that took place in the middle of the seventeenth century took only partial hold in Six's *oeuvre*. Nevertheless, my own view is that he is a progressive author in many ways. His interest in native herbs and plants, his criticism of the craving for the exotic and the miraculous, and his appeal to reason and austerity can only come across as modern. But that does not mean that Six's poetry presents the true physical properties of exotic substances. Although Six's sensory approach to *materia medica* is striking, his conception of pharmaceutical substances, as I have emphasised, is not entirely separate from the methods and ideas of humanist culture. Six's opposition to the use of gold as a medicine, is mainly based, not on a real sensory perception of the metal, but on its association with greed and a lust for power.[5] Perhaps we can say that the reduction in the use of fragrances, perfumes and gemstones as medicines is related to the *intensification* of humanist and Christian arguments against exotica, such as decadence, deception, excess, and so on. This is a topic that requires more research, for in the same period, a redefinition of spices from medicines to food seasoning occurs, and spices and animal aromatics lose their significance as a social status

5 In reality, pulverised gold is not dangerous to the human body. Gold passes through the digestive system without being absorbed into the body. My thanks to Jan Karlsen for this information.

symbol. The spice trade also gradually loses ground in favour of the trade in tea and coffee. This does not mean that Christian and humanist arguments against drugs are the only explanation for the decline of the use of exotic medicine, but it is an explanatory model that deserves more attention as part of this picture.[6]

Six's *oeuvre* sees a transition from a trade in drugs based on mythical, astrological and alchemical concepts to an increasingly botanical treatment of medical plants, in which magic and fantasy are replaced by observation and systematic research. And since foreign drugs were used not only in medicine but in a wide variety of areas in early modern culture, this disenchantment also had quite some significance for other social areas that we have discussed here, such as the culture around food, theology and of course art and literature. This observation is consistent with the M.A. Schenkeveld-van der Dussen's view on Six in Dutch literary history: *Poësy* as a manifestation of a realistic-descriptive literary programme and a voice against the prevailing idealistic poetics. However, I hope this book has shown that this 'sense of reality' must be understood in the light of Six's self-fashioning as a down-to-earth druggist-rhymester. As we have seen, the drugs in which Six traded represented, in many ways, the exact opposite of realism and sobriety. While Schenkeveld-van der Dussen is right that Six often places his poems in what we could call a realistic environment, this reality is constructed in accordance with the intention of the poem. We saw this in his poems on gunpowder (J338, J383 and J396). Moreover, the study of local natural phenomena was by no means a self-evident process, but was embedded in a debate about the exotic versus the domestic. I would say that the same can be said of Six himself, with regard not only to his botanical observations, but also to his take on cultural and literary concepts. For example, the description of women as active, spirited individuals was not a commonplace in Renaissance poetry. Portraits of women were bound by the conventions of the Petrarchan-idealistic tradition. Six's description of his 'earthly' Roselle in 'Afbeeldinge en wydinge van Roselle, en haare bestraffinge' (J59–64) did not just drop out of the sky. Rather, it is closely related to his argument in the series of sonnets about the dehumanising effects of exotic aromas and dyes.

Finally, I would like to stress that the story I have outlined here of the development from druggist-poet to botanist-rhymester was by no means straightforward. The world Six lived in was characterised by conflicting interests. Among the recipients of his poems, in addition to fellow merchants from Italy who had adopted an aristocratic lifestyle, we meet rich Amsterdam traders with a predilection for

6 *Cf.* the discussion of the decline of alchemy at the end of the seventeenth century in Principe, 2012, pp. 83–92. *Cf.* also Nicholas Popper, 'The Sudden Death of the Burning Salamander: Reading Experiment and the Transformation of Natural Historical Practice in Early Modern Europe', *Erudition and the Republic of Letters*, 2016, pp. 464–490. For the decline of the spice trade, see Israel, 1989, pp. 335–336.

culinary opulence and baroque occasional poems, as well as doctors and Calvinist ministers. The author of *Poësy* is a flexible individual. His frequent use of self-irony, humour, theatricality and a rhetorical device such as *praeteritio* should be seen in this light. But this flexibility is not unlimited. Moral unease about luxury goods can be found even in many of Six's most vibrant texts. But on the other hand, Six does not deploy a litany of Protestant doctrines against wealth, make-up and mythological parades. His most beautiful poems are written with a theatrical and playful pen: Six frequently does not answer the ethical dilemmas he presents in his texts, but lets the readers come up with an answer themselves.

Appendix I: ‘Rariteiten te koop’

'Rariteiten te koop'
Alle stoffe heeft een maakler,
Andersins een vryen kaakler,
Die des Koopmans wille peilt.
Alle stoffe heeft heur venter,
Tot den almanakken prenter,
Tot die swaavelstokken veilt.
Maar nu is, op Hollands stroomen,
In myn handen, stof gekoomen,
Ongehoort, en ongesien:
Niet als quam se, uit verre landen,
Van de west, of oosterstranden,
Uit een landschap sonder liên.
Als een gomboom afgedroopen,
Als een beekjen fyn ontloopen,
Als een duuren bergh ontschaakt,
Als van boomen, of van planten,
Neevens soete waaterkanten,
Of van seldsaam kruid gemaakt.
Neen, se komt, van 't ryk der Britten,
Die niet verder van ons sitten,
Zoo de wind dient, dan een dagh,
Daar men die, om niet, kan haalen,
Of, met weinigh, hier betaalen,
Schoon de son niet duurders sach.
S'is van 't bloed van Kooningh Karel,
Schynende een robyne paarel,
Gloênden ink, en purpre verf,
Steen, en hout, en roode roosen,
Rooder dan het wroegend bloosen,
Om het kooninghlyk verderf.
Wie zal 't maakelampt bekleeden?
Die volght nu geen Judas schreeden:
Want dit bloedgeld dient de wraak,
Om wat houts, en touw te koopen,
Om syn moorders op te knoopen,

'Rarities for Sale'

All commodities[1] have a broker,
Or an independent hawker,
Who represents the interests of the Merchant.[2]
All commodities have their street-trader,
From the printer of almanacs,
To the one peddling matchsticks.
But now there has come a commodity
On Dutch waters, and in my hands,
Which no one has heard of or seen before.
It did not come from distant countries,
Of the shores of the West or the East [Indies],
From a territory without people.
As [from] a tapped rubber tree,
As [from] a nicely panned brook,
As from trees, or of plants,
By sweet water sides,
Or made of a rare herb.
No, it comes from the British kingdom.
Which is no farther away from us
Than one day's travel for the wind,
Where you can get it for nothing,
Or purchase it for a small amount of money,
Although the sun never saw a more precious thing.
It is the blood of King Charles,
Shining [as] a ruby pearl,
Glowing ink, and purple dye,
Stone, wood, and red roses,
Redder than the blushing outrage
Of the ruin of the king.
Who shall be the agent for this commodity?
He does not follow in the footsteps of Judas:
Because this blood money should be used
To buy timber and rope for revenge:
To hang the murderers of the King,

1 A more accurate translation of Dutch 'stof' would be 'stuff', 'thing' or 'matter'. The message is thus that all things get commercialized by the contact with the hands of a merchant, even the blood of a king. However, I have chosen to use the term 'commodities', which works better for present purposes.

2 The merchant, a wholesaler in international commodities, sells his goods to stores with the help of brokers. The broker serves as an intermediary, as a link between wholesaler and retailer or consumer.

Of te branden, aan een staak.
Verwers van fluweel, of laaken,
Wilt ghe schoone verwen maaken,
Fyn scharlaaken, karmosyn,
Of de kooninghlyke draghten,
Van de purpre vischgeslachten,
Kostlik, om hun weederschyn?
Gaat niet in de verwekraamen,
Van fortuin, of andre naamen,
Om den duuren koetsjenil,
Luisen van Nieuw Spanjes Inden,
Die ghe doof van kleur sult vinden,
By des Kooninghs strotaâr vil.
Salomon, in al syn praalen,
Kon gepurpert niet ophaalen
Sulken hoogen trotsen gloed.
d'Oester kon daar toe niet helpen,

Or to burn them at the stake.
Dyers of velvet or of cloth,
Do you want to produce beautiful colours,
Fine scarlet, crimson,[3]
Or as the kingly costumes,
Dyed with purple shellfish,
Precious because of its reflection?[4]
Do not go to the dyer's shops
'Good Fortune', or another name,
For the expensive cochineal,
Lice of the New Spanish Indies,[5]
Which you will find dim in colour
Compared to the cut in the King's carotid.
Solomon, in all his splendour,
Could, dressed in royal purple,[6]
not equal such a lofty, proud glow.
The purple dye from Sidon snails
Could not hold a candle to the blood either,

3 Crimson is a strong, red colour. The name refers to the colour of the kermes dye produced from the scale insect *Kermes vermilio.*

4 Six is referring to Tyrian purple, a dye extracted from the murex shellfish. The method of making Tyrian purple (also called royal or imperial purple) was known in ancient Tyre and Sidon, cities in today's Lebanon. The dye was hugely valuable for several reasons: it took thousands of shells to produce a single kilo, it was resistant to fading, and it had a changeable character: its rich deep purple seemed crimson when held to the light (Six writes about the colour's 'reflection'). Persons of high rank wore togas with a purple stripe in Ancient Rome. Compare the Roman word *purpurati*, men of military rank and power. 'It distinguishes the senate from the knighthood, it is called in to secure the favour of the gods; and it adds radiance to every garment, while in a triumphal robe it is blended with gold. Consequently, even the mad lust for the purple may be excused', writes Pliny in *Natural History*, IX, 127 (trans. by H. Rackham, 1967, pp. 248–249). The *toga picta*, which was solid purple and was embroidered with gold, was worn by generals in their triumphs in the Roman Republic, and by consuls at the time of the emperors, see Meyer Reinhold, *History of Purple as a Status Symbol in Antiquity*, 1970.

5 Cochineal refers to a red dye prepared from the dried bodies of the cochineal insects. These scale insects live, as Six writes, in the 'New Spanish Indies', in Mexico. Thanks to the Spanish trade monopoly, the insect was surrounded with mystery. During the Eighty Years War the dye was a scarce and expensive pigment; only the richest could afford to buy cochineal in a paint store like that of 'Good Fortune', For the high status of these and other red dyes, Amy Butler Greenfield, *A Perfect Red: Empire, Espionage and the Quest of the Colour of Desire*, 2005.

6 According to the *Statenvertaling*, purple clothing was worn only by kings and other great men. See comment 27 to Daniel 5:7. Six himself speaks of 'gods dressed in black and red', when talking about the nobility in Venice, 'Schetse van Venecie' (J97), l. 172. For the high status of purple and other red dyes: Reinhold, 1970; Greenfield, 2005.

Uit Sidoniaansche schelpen,
Nu vergeeten, in den vloed.
Schilders van de waapenglaasen,
Gaa niet by die winkelbaasen,
Om den Florentynschen lak:
'tWaapenglas sal hier van schynen,
Als de koolen van robynen,
Waar men solfer aan ontstak.
Wyn verkoopers, gaa niet quisten,
Om de bruindoek, by drogisten,
Weinigh ponden, voor veel geld.
Eene drup, als bloed van Santen,
Opgesopt, met neusdoek kanten,
Strekt veel schooner, als se smelt.
Bruigoms soekende juweelen,
Om aan uwe Bruids te deelen,
Gaa voor by den Juwelier:
'k Heb karbonkels, en granaaten,
Opgeraapt van Londens straaten,
En koraal, uit heur rivier.
Bisnagarsche fyne steenen,
Ook hoe gloorende, als se scheenen,
Zyn van luister, by dit bloed,
Als de kleine starren blonken,
Toen se moedigh wilden pronken,

Snails that now are forgotten in the sea.[7]
Painters of coats of arms in stained glass windows
Do not go to shops
Where they sell Florentine lacquer:[8]
The windows will shine with the King's blood,
As the ruby minerals,
Which are purified by heating them with sulphur.[9]
Wine sellers, do not waste money on
Poppy, on sale at druggists,
Where you just get a few pounds for a lot of money.[10]
A drop of the blood – like the blood of saints –
Soaked up with a handkerchief,
Is much more suitable when it dissolves [in wine].
Grooms searching for jewels
To give to their brides,
Ignore the jeweller's shop:
I have got carbuncles and garnets,
Picked up on the streets of London,
And corals[11], from London's river.
Gemstones from the Kingdom of Bisnaga.[12]
However fervently they would shine,
Compared to this blood, their lustre
Would be as blinks from small stars,
When the stars boldly would compete

7 The method of making Tyrian purple was lost in the fall of Constantinople in 1453. But that purple still stimulated the imagination in the early modern period. Apparently, there were also specimens of the purple snails in circulation among Dutch collectors of *exotica*. On his journey through the Netherlands, the German scholar Christian Knorr von Rosenroth reports that, in a cabinet of curiosities in Amsterdam, he saw 'a snail with fragrant Byzantine purple'. See R. Fuchs & J.C. Breen, 'Aus dem "Itinerarium" des Christian Knorr von Rosenroth', *Jaarboek Amstelodamum*, 1916, p. 246.

8 A lake pigment based on brazilwood that was produced in Italy.

9 Six refers to the preparation of ruby sulphur, also known under the name realgar, an arsenic sulphide mineral that played an important role in early modern alchemy. The most beautiful pieces of this material are 'golden yellow, as shiny as gold', writes Lemery (1743, p. 81).

10 A dye made from red poppy used to deepen the colour of wine – see Jacobs, 1991 II, p. 286.

11 A marine animal, but with a stony limestone skeleton that, like precious stones, was kept in curiosity cabinets. See Lemery, 1743, p. 210. Six probably means the so-called blood coral that was found in the Mediterranean. It was also used as a medicine and a religious ornament. See Marlise Rijks, '"Unusual Excrescences of Nature": Collected Coral and the Study of Petrified Luxury in Early Modern Antwerp', *Dutch Crossing*, 2017, pp. 1–29.

12 Six is probably referring to rubies and zircon stones, gems for which the Kingdom of Bisnaga in India was famous. See Wennekes, 1996, p. 198.

By de groote sonnegloed.
Meesters van de metselaaren,
Die, voor 't nieuw steehuis, gaat vaaren,
Om orduin, en marmersteen,
Genueesche berghspelonken,
Of te Bentem afgeklonken,
Duur van inkoop, maar gemeen:
Hoe dus quistigh steen genoomen,
Raad den Raad by my te koomen,
Met wat haast gereekent geld.
Ik heb Jasp, en karneoolen,
Voor doorluchter Kapitoolen,
Dan men sach op Romes veld.
Recht den bouw, op die pilaaren,
Laat den geevel zoo eens vaaren,
In den ruimen Amstellocht,
'k Wed den Hertogh van Florencen
Zoude zyn kapelle wenschen,
Zoo hoovaardigh uitgewrocht.
Waar zyn nu de nette vrouwen,
Die heur beste kaamers houwen
Netter dikwils, dan sich self?
Ik kan alle monden snoeren,
Die zoo pruts zyn, op de vloeren,
Van heur Italjaansch gewelf.
Werkers van de kabinetten
Staak de sandels, violetten,

With the glow of the great sun.
Masters of bricklayers,
Who, for the new Town Hall, travel far
To fetch blue stone and marble stone,
[the first] extracted in Bentheim,
[the second] in the mines of Genoa,[13]
which are expensive, but also ordinary:[14]
Why waste money on such stones,
Take the advice and come to me
With money you have collected in haste.
I have jasper and carnelians
For a more illustrious Capitoline
Than the one of Campus Martius [of Ancient Rome].[15]
Let the building rise on the pillars,
Let the gable be lifted high
In the spacious air of Amsterdam.[16]
I bet the Duke of Florence
Wishes that his chapel
Were just as proudly adorned.[17]
Where are the neat women,
Who often keep their rooms
Neater than themselves?
I can silence all the people
Who are so proud of the floors
In their Italian vaults.
Carpenters of cabinets,
Stop using sandalwood and rosewood

13 Marble from the Carrara mines in Italy. Although the marble is of European origin, the marble quarries of Carrara enjoyed great fame in the early modern times, as did Bentheimer sandstone. Genoa was the port from which the Carrara marble was shipped. Dutch merchants were involved in this trade; see Richard A. Goldthwaite, *The Building of Renaissance Florence. An Economic and Social History*, 1982, p. 217.

14 Materials that were used in the construction of the Town Hall. See for example *Bespiegelingen van Godt en Godtsdienst* by Joost van den Vondel, first book, l. 808, in: J.F.M. Sterck *et al.* (eds.), *De werken van Vondel. 1660–1663*, vol. 9, 1936, p. 438.

15 The temple of Jupiter Optimus Maximus, the largest and most beautiful building in Rome, was located at the Capitoline.

16 'The carnelians were in great esteem by the ancients [...] King Solomon used much of it to the beautiful Temple which he built in Jerusalem; and the Roman Emperors looked for this stone as a rare and precious substance', writes Lemery (1743, p. 176).

17 Six is referring to the Medici Chapel in Florence – see Jacobs, 1991 II, p. 287.

Of een rooder vremdgewas:
Dit wint ceders, dit wint ebben,
Indiaansche houten hebben
Geenen glans, by zoo een kas.
Wil ook imand bloeme kransen
Vlechten, van de rooseglansen,
In den winter, sonder bloem?
England dat in 't schild verkoosen
Hadde roosen, bloeit van roosen,
Nu met recht, tot Karels roem.
Waarom zouden rooselaaren
Karels bynaam niet bewaaren,
Als Narcis, en Hiacinth,
Bloemen van Apol verkooren?
Stuart is een roos herbooren,
En van Jesus hoogh bemint.
O! hoe voel ik 't hart opluiken,
By dees vroege lentparruiken,
Van dat duursaam martelbloed?
'k Wil ook selve wat behouwen,
Om daar konstigh van te vouwen,
Voor Roselle, een roosenhoed.
'k Wil ook mengen van een dropjen,
In een porceleine kopjen,
Ink, aan niemands pen, gewoon,

Or a redder plant of foreign origin:
This blood surpasses cedar and ebony.
No Indian wood has such a glow
Compared to such a cabinet.[18]
If anyone wants to make
Garlands of roses with a brilliant shine,
Now in the winter, without flowers?
England, which has chosen roses
For its coat of arms, blooms [or: bleeds],
Now rightly so, to Charles's fame.[19]
Why should rose bushes
Not be named after Charles,
As [flowers named] after Narcissus and Hyacinth,
Flowers that Apollo loved?[20]
Stuart is reborn as a rose
That is greatly loved by Jesus.[21]
Oh! How I feel my heart open
At [the sight of] the bouquet of early flowers
From that precious martyr's blood?[22]
I will also keep some of it for myself,
So that I may artfully weave
A rose garland for Roselle.
I will also mix a drop
[Of blood] in an inkwell of porcelain, –
[An ink] that outdoes everyone else's pen –

18 Red sandalwood (from the coast of Coromandel, India), rosewood (from the island of Rhodes and Cyprus), cedar (from Lebanon), ebony (from Mauritius or India) and brazilwood ('Indian wood') are all known for their reddish hue. Many of these species of wood have a pleasant smell. See Clusius's discussion of exotic woods in R. Dodonaeus, *Cruydt-boeck*, 1644, pp. 1458–1459, 1462; Lemery, 1743, pp. 398 and 629–30.

19 The coat of arms of the royal house Stuart was decorated with roses. In a macabre allegory, where Six plays with the double meaning of 'blooms' versus 'bleeds', the blood flowing from the body of the king is thus presented as an eternally blooming rose.

20 Hyacinth and Narcissus are characters from classical mythology who left their earthly existence and were 'reborn' as flowers. Just as the god Apollo is honoured with the hyacinth dedicated to him, King Charles should be immortalised by rose bushes dedicated to him. See Lemery, 1743, pp. 343 and 483; Jacobs, 1991 II, p. 288.

21 'The Rose of Stuart' is, according to the poem, similar to the bride in the Song of Songs, 'the rose of Sharon'. This bride is interpreted as Christ in biblical exegesis. See the *Statenvertaling*, comment 2 to Song of Songs 2:1. According to Holly Dugan, the rose was used as a Protestant symbol of the divine right of kingship in England, see Dugan, 2011, pp. 42–69.

22 We are in the world of ideas of the Catholic faith. Red refers to the divine suffering of saints and martyrs.

En daar meede rympjes maaken,
Om die aan de krans te haaken:
Venus krans was niet zoo schoon.
Sie hoe fraai de letters blinken,
Die alree van Karel drinken,
Op dit witte schryfpapier:
Glinstrende, als de sonnestraalen,
Uit een bron, in waaterdaalen,
d'Oogen scheemren doen, van vier.
Al myn rymen schynen dichten,
Nu heur sulke stoffen lichten,
Oovervloeit van bloenden ink.
'k Zou schier myns gelyken raaden,
Om de pen hier in te baaden,
Dat hun rymsel ook wat blink.
Wat beleeft deese eeuw Poeëten!
Die men dan alzoo zou heeten.
Werden wy zoo niet gehult,
Vrienden, wat 's er aan geleegen?
Die wat heimliks moeten veegen,
Maaken al ons rym verguldt.
Maar wat sie ik reede tongen,
Dat se slechts een prys bedongen
Voor dat wonderlyke bloed?
Voor dien ink, die verw, en roosen,
Hout, en steenen, die zoo bloosen,
Binnen Londen onder voet?
't Looven, koopers, en het geeven,
Staat er reedlik op geschreeven.
'k Wensche, dat ik maar ontfongh
Dertigh stuivers, sonder dingen,
Vry wat min, dan silverlingen,
Waar sich Judas om verhongh.

And write rhymes with the ink,
Which I will attach to the garland [of Roselle]:
The garland of Venus was not as beautiful.
See how beautifully the letters shine,
Which are drunk [from the blood] of Charles,
On this white writing paper:
Shimmering as the sun beans
[Reflected] by a water spring in valleys,
Dazzling the eyes with fire.
All my rhymes seem like poems,
Now when they are illuminated by such material,
Overflowing with bleeding ink.
I would almost recommend that my equals
Bathe their pens in the blood,
So that their rhymes would also glitter.
Oh, what Poets does this century experience![23]
Then they [the rhymesters] will be called by that name.
But if we are not praised?
Friends, what does it matter?
The ones who need to wipe their buttocks
Gild all our rhymes.[24]
But do I not already see tongues hanging out for a bargain,
So that they get a better price
For that marvellous blood?
For that ink, that colour, and roses,
Wood, stone, which 'blush' like this
Under our feet in London?
The asking price, buyers, and the purchase price
Are written on it, a moderate sum.
I wish I had just received
Thirty stivers, without bargaining,
A good deal less than the pieces of silver,[25]
For which Judas hanged himself.

23 By using miraculous kingly blood as ink, the Dutch rhymes will fulfil the classical ideal of an *aurea aetas*, a Golden Age, Six writes ironically.

24 As a consequence of using the rhymed papers as toilet paper.

25 See the *Statenvertaling*, comment 17 to Matt. 26:15, for the value that was ascribed to Judas's 30 pieces of silver in the early modern period. According to the biblical translators, 30 pieces of silver corresponds to 'ontrent een halve rijcx-daler' ('about a half *rijksdaalder*') – that is, 50 *stuivers*, so not far from the price of the handkerchief that has the blood of Charles on it.

Appendix II: Family and business network of Joannes Six van Chandelier

Joost (Justus) Six (1621–?), merchant and translator employed by the VOC, stationed in Bengal and Canton (China). Brother of the poet Joannes Six van Chandelier.

Abraham Six (c. 1632–c. 1680), merchant employed by the VOC, stationed in the East Indies. Brother of the poet.

Johannes Six van Chandelier (c. 1664–1721), merchant employed by the VOC, stationed in the East Indies. Son of Abraham Six and namesake of the poet.

Simon Dilman (1604–1666), a doctor in Amsterdam, who was Six's cousin by marriage. Dilman was married to Six's cousin, Janneke Hartgers. Her mother, Janneke Six, was the sister of Six's father, Jacob Six, and was married to Hartger Wouter. Simon Dilman included the orphans of the uncle of Joannes Six van Chandelier, Abraham Six, in his household for a period.

Jacob Dilman (1634–1663), the son of Simon Dilman, was apprenticed to the Six family business, and became a merchant-druggist.

Joost Hartgers, publisher and printer in Amsterdam, who was the son of Hartger Wouters and his third wife, Janneke van Baelbergen.

Johannes Hoornbeeck (1617–1666), a preacher and professor of theology, who was a cousin of Six and of Simon Dilman. His parents were Tobias Hoornbeeck, a merchant, and Janneke Baerts. Both were from Haarlem. Janneke Baerts was the daughter of Gillis Baert and Susanne Six, a sister to Janneke Six and Jacob Six, the father of the poet.

Hans Baert, merchant in Haarlem, was related to both Joannes Six van Chandelier and Johannes Hoornbeeck. He was the brother of Janneke Baert, thus the son of Gillis Baert and Susanne Six.

Jan Gerritsen Indies (1607–1649), a surgeon, who was married to Catharina Kemp, daughter of Catharina Juliaens, who was Six's maternal aunt, and thus a cousin by marriage to the poet.

Raimond de Smeth (1594–1661), merchant in Amsterdam. His father Joost de Smeth was married to Anna Jehu. She was the daughter of Andries Jehu, apothecary in Brussels, who was the grandfather of Catharina Jehu, the grandmother of the poet.

Joost de Smeth (1626–1704), merchant and banker in Amsterdam, married to Maria Fassin (1633–1666). Both his father and grandfather bore the same name as Joost the Younger. The first was married to Margretha Engels, while the latter was married to the beforementioned Anna Jehu.

Amsterdam City Archives:

The Ledger ('Grootboeken') of the Wisselbank, 5077:

Inv. no. 50–142 (1644-1695/96)
For the family firm of Six van Chandelier, see the years 1644-1648, fol. 368; 1648-1649, fol. 370; 1651, fol. 545; 1652, fol. 696; 1653-1664, fol. 635; 1659-1675, fol. 457; 1674-1678, fol. 995; 1679, fol. 937; 1680-1683, fol. 898; 1683-1689, fol. 1216; 1690-1695/1696, fol. 909.

Notarial deeds, Archive 5075:

Inv. no. 661, fol. 112. Notary Jan Warnaertsz. On 10 March 1627. (About trading opium in Morocco)

Inv. no. 1442, fol. 1019. Notary Cornelis Touw. On 13 November 1652. (About the delivery of Balsam of Peru from Venice. Johannes Six van Chandelier, Isaac Six van Chandelier, Jacob Dilman and Johannes van Breen testify at the request of Sara Juliens that the drugs were adulterated)

Inv. no. 2804, fol. 149-150, 153–154. Notary Hendrik Westfrisius. On 5 Febrary 1661. (About the outstanding debts for doctor's visits by Simon Dilman to Sara Juliens)

Inv. no. 2804-A, fol. 145–148. Notary Henrik Westfrisius. On 5 February 1661. (About the orphans of Abraham Six who were included in the household of Simon Dilman)

Inv. no. 2679, fol. 139. Notary Johannes van Wijningen. On 18 August 1662. (About the sale of paintings done by dr. med. Johannes Dilman, among others, a 'baars', bass, by Rembrandt)

Inv. no. 2215-A, fol. 603–604. Notary Adriaan Lock. On 19 September 1663 (About the dispute concerning the inheritance of Johanna Juliens, widow of Willem Bogaert, between Joannes Six van Chandelier, at the one side, and Pieter and Govert Bogaert, at the other side).

Inv. no. 2366, fol. 240–242. Notary Jacob de Winter. On 1 November 1669. (The last will of Maria Wijs and Gillis Hoornbeeck (1627–1688), a brother of prof. Johannes Hoornbeeck and cousin (twice removed) of the poet)

Inv. no. 3043, fol. 103. Notary H. Venkel. On 12 December 1670. (A trade clause petition sent to the King of Spain by Joannes Six van Chandelier, Sijbrand Feitama, Jan Commelin and other merchant-druggists in Amsterdam)

Inv. no. 4748, fol. 705–717. Notary David Stafmaker Varlet. On 25 August 1688. (The testament of Joannes Six van Chandelier)

Inv. no. 3961, act. nr 57. Notary Nicolaas Brouwer. On 10 September 1691 (On Six's gardener and his wife, Cornelis de Haan and Maria Heijmans)

Inv. no. 3961, fol. 222–223. Notary Nicolaas Brouwer, On 11 September 1691. (On the tax of Joannes Six van Chandelier)

Inv. no. 4759, folio 581–584. Notary David Stafmaker Varlet. On 30 September 1694. (A new version of the last will of Joannes Six van Chandelier)

Other sources:

Archive 5062, inv. no 43, fol. 139, *Ordinaris Kwijtscheldingen*. On June 1649. (About the inheritance of Jan Gerritsen Indies)

In Haarlem:

Noord-Hollands Archief, Oud-Notarieel Archief Haarlem 149, fol. 53v–54. Notary Jacob Schoudt. On 27 August 1636. (This document concerns the bankruptcy of Abraham Six (c. 1571–1636), and Maria de Haen, the uncle and the aunt of the poet)

Bibliography

Primary Sources

Amsterdamsche Vreugdtriomfe (Amsterdam: Michiel de Groot, 1660). [Bibliotheek van de Universiteit van Amsterdam, OTM Vondel 1 F 46]

Ansloo, R., *Poëzy* (Rotterdam: Joan de Haes, 1713).

Barlaeus, Caspar, *Medicea Hospes* (Amsterdam: Johan and Cornelis Blaeu, 1638).

Barlaeus, Caspar, *Blyde inkomst der allerdoorluchtighste koninginne, Maria de Medicis, t'Amsterdam*, trans. by Joost van den Vondel (Amsterdam: Johan and Cornelis Blaeu, 1639).

Beverwijck, Johan van, *Alle de wercken, zo in de medicyne als chirurgie* (Amsterdam: Ian Jacobsz Schipper, 1656).

Beverwijck, Johan van, 'Schat der gesontheyt', in: *Alle de wercken, zo in de medicyne als chirurgie.*

Beverwijck, Johan van, 'Schat der ongesontheyt', in: *Alle de wercken, zo in de medicyne als chirurgie.*

Beverwijck, Johan van, 'Inleydinge tot de Hollandtsche Genees-middelen' [1642], in: *Alle de wercken, zo in de medicyne als chirurgie.*

Beverwijck, Johan van, 'Heel-konste, ofte derde deel van de Genees-konste', in: *Alle de wercken, zo in de medicyne als chirurgie.*

Biblia, dat is: De gantsche H. Schrifture (Statenvertaling) ['States Bible translation'] (Leiden: P.A. van Ravensteyn, 1637). dbnl.org/tekst/_sta001stat01_01/index.php (consulted 17 May 2019).

Bidloo, Lambert, 'Dissertatio de re herbaria', in: Jan Commelin, *Catalogus plantarum indigenarum Hollandiae* (Amsterdam: Apud H. & viduam T. Boom, 1683).

Bidloo, Lambert, *Panpoëticon Batavûm, Kabinet, Waar in de Afbeeldingen van Voornaame Nederlandsche Dichteren* [...] (Amsterdam: Andries Van Damme, 1720).

Bos, Lambert van den, *Wegh-wyser door Italien of Beschrijvinge der Landen en Steden van Italien* (Dordrecht: Abraham Andriesz, 1661).

Brook, P., *A Brief Account, of the Nature, Vertues, Use, and Excellency of Indian Cattee* (London: Ann Arbor, 1679).

Casaubon, Méric, *A Treatise Concerning Enthusiasme* (London: Thomas Johnson, 1655).

Catalogus van een groote partij extraordinaire curieuse Rariteyten [...] *Joan Breyne*. Amsterdam; auction, 7 July 1693. [British Library 1044 a 28 (2)]

Chomel, M. Noel, *Algemeen Huishoudelijk-, Natuur-, Zedekundig- En Konstwoordenboek* [...], 7 vols. (Leiden/Leeuwarden: J.A. de Chalmot, 1778).

Clusius. Carolus, *Exoticorum libri decem* (Leiden: Raphelengii, 1605).

D.V. Coornhert, *Hert-spiegel. Godlijcker schrifturen*, in: D.V. Coornhert, *Wercken*, 3 vols. (Amsterdam: Iacob Aerfz. Kolom, 1632), vol. 1, fol. 3.

Decker, Jeremias de, *Rym-oeffeningen, verdeelt in dry Boeken, vervattende Gedichten van verscheyden styl en stoffe* (Amsterdam: Willem de Coup, Willem Lamsvelt, and Philip Verbeek, 1702).

Decker, Jeremias de, *Lof der Geldsucht*, in: Jeremias de Decker, *Rym-oeffeningen, verdeelt in dry Boeken, vervattende Gedichten van verscheyden styl en stoffe* (Amsterdam: Willem de Coup, Willem Lamsvelt and Philip Verbeek, 1702).

Dilman, Johannes, *Disputatio Medica Inauguralis de Phrenitide* (Leiden: Severinum Matthiæ, 1654). [Edinburgh University Library 1655 EUL [P.1054(12)]]

Dodonaeus, Rembertus, *Cruydt-Boeck* (Leiden: Françoys van Ravelingen, 1644 [orig. 1554]).

Drelincourt, Charles, *Cort-begryp van de dwalinghen der Roomsche Kercke*, trans. by Abraham Pietersz Wilsenius (Dordrecht: Abraham Andriessz, 1649).

Feitama, Sijbrand, *Christelijke en stigtelijke rymoeffeningen* (Amsterdam: Gedrukt voor den autheur, 1684).

Feitama, Sijbrand, *Uitbeeldingen van Staaten, Ambagten en Neeringen* (Amsterdam: Gedrukt voor den autheur, 1685).

Haes, J. de, *Het Leven Van Geeraert Brandt, Beschreven Door Joan De Haes* [...] (The Hague: Kornelis Boucquet, 1740).

Anonymous, *Hedendaagsche Historie, of Tegenwoordige Staat van Frankrijk* (Amsterdam: Isaak Tirion, 1757).

Helmont, Jan Baptista van, *Ortus medicinae* (Amsterdam: Ludovicus Elsevir, 1648).

Hexham, Hendrick, *A large Netherdutch and English Dictionarie; Composed out of the best Netherdutch Authours* (Rotterdam: Aernovt Leers, 1658).

Hoornbeeck, Johannes, *De Paradoxis et Heterodoxis Weigelianis Commentarius ubi et de Swencfeldo Aliisque Similis Indolis* (Utrecht: J. à Waesberge, 1646).

Hoornbeeck, Johannes, *Summa Controversiarum Religionis* (Utrecht: J. à Waesberge, 1658 [first edition: 1653]).

Hoornbeeck, Johannes, *De conversione Indorum et Gentilium, libri duo* (Amsterdam: Johannes Janssonius van Waesbergen, 1669).

Junius, Franciscus, *De Schilder-konst der Oude, begrepen in drie boecken* (Middelburg: Zacharias Roman, 1641).

King James Bible (London: Robert Parker, Printer of the Kings, 1611). kingjamesbibleonline.org/1611-Bible/ (consulted 17 May 2019).

Lemery, Nicolas, *Woordenboek of algemeene verhandeling der enkele droogeryen* (Rotterdam: Jan Daniel Beman, 1743).

Anonymous, *Letter sent into France to the Lord Duke of Buckingham, his Grace: of a great miracle wrought by a piece of a handkerchefe dipped in His Majesties bloud. The truth whereof, he himself saw, and is ready to despose it, and doth believe will be attested by 500 others, if occasion requires* (London, 1649). http://anglicanhistory.org/charles/letter.html (consulted 17 May 2019).

Nylandt, Petrus, *De Nederlandtse Herbarius of Kruydt-boeck* (Amsterdam: Marcus Doornick, 1670).

Oudaen, Joachim, *Poëzy, Verdeeld in Drie Deelen* (Amsterdam: Weduwe van B. Visscher en Pieter Visser, 1712).

Paré, Ambroise, *De chirurgie, ende alle de opera, ofte wercken* (Amsterdam: Cornelis van Breugel, 1636).

Pers, Dirck Pieterz., *Iconologia, of Uytbeeldinghe des Verstants van Cesare Ripa van Perugien* (Amsterdam: Dirck Pietersz. Pers, 1644).

Pharmacopaea Amstelredamensis (Amsterdam: Jan ten Hoorn, 1686).

Pieterse, Roelof, *'t Lof Des Heylighen Geestes: Dat Is: Korte Verklaringe Van Het Wesen, de Eygenschappen, ende Werckingen des H. Geestes* [...] (Amsterdam: Weduwe van Marten Jansz. Brandt en Abraham Meynartsz vanden Burgh, 1646).

Pomet, Pierre (with Nicolas Lemery and Joseph Pitton de Tournefort), *A Compleat History of Drugs, Written in French by Monsieur Pomet* [...] (London: J. and J. Bonwicke, R. Wilkin (etc), 1737).

Rodenburgh, Theodore, *Eglentiers poëtens borst-weringh* (Amsterdam: Ian Evertsz. Cloppenburgh, [1619] 1638).

Six van Chandelier, Joannes, *Vreughde-Zangen Over den eeuwigen Vreede, Tusschen Spangien En de Vereenighde Nederlanden: Daar by noch andere invallingen van den Rijmer, voor en ontrent 't sluyten der selver Vreede* [...] (Amsterdam: Joost Hartgers, 1648).

Six van Chandelier, Joannes, *Poësy. Verdeelt in ses boeken, en eenige opschriften* (Amsterdam: Joost Pluimert, 1657).

Six van Chandelier, Joannes, *Davids Psalmen* (Amsterdam: Jakob Lescalje, 1674).

Tempel, Olivier van den, *Torquato Tassoos: Vierde Gezangh. van Ierusalems Verlossinge* (Amsterdam: Joost Hartgersz, 1644).

Voetius, Gisbertus, *Oratio de pietate cum scientia conjungenda, habita anno 1634* (Gorichem: Paul Vink, 1664).

Voetius, Gisbertus, *Disputationes Theologicae Selectae*, 4 vols. (Amsterdam: Joh. à Waesberge, 1648–1669).

Vollenhove, Joannes, *Poëzy* (Amsterdam: Henrik Boom and the widow of Dirk Boom, 1686).

Vos, Jan, *Alle de gedichten van den Poëet Jan Vos*, 2 vols. (Amsterdam: Jacob Lescaille, 1662 and 1671).

Wegh-wyser, ofte reijsbeschrijvingh door de Koninckrijcken van Spanjen en Portugael [...] (Amsterdam: Nicolaes van Ravensteijn, 1650).

Wegh-Wyser, aenwijsende de besonderste vremde vermaecklijckheden die in't reysen door Vranckryck [...] (Amsterdam: Nicolaes van Ravensteijn, 1657).

Westerbaen, Jacob, *Gedichten, Verdeylt in Vijf Boecken* (The Hague: Anthoney & Iohanes Tongerloo, 1657).

Witte, Petrus de, *Delfschen donder-slagh ofte Korte aensprake aen de bedroefde gemeente van Delf* (Utrecht: Andries Hoogenhuyse, 1654).

Wittewrongel, Petrus, *Oeconomia christiana ofte Christelicke huys-houdinge*, 2 vols. (Amsterdam: Abraham van den Burgh, 1661).

Worst, Geeraard, *Disputatio medica inauguralis de Morbo regio* (Leiden: Davidis à Lodensteyn, 1655). [Edinburgh University Library 1655 EUL [P.1054(12)]]

Wright, Abraham, *Parnassus Biceps. Or Severall Choice Pieces of Poetry, Composed by the best Wits that were both the Universities before their Dissolution* (London: George Eversden, 1656).

Secondary Sources

Abrahamse, Wouter, *Het toneel van Theodore Rodenburgh (1574-1644)* (Amsterdam: AD&L, 1997).

Albala, Ken, *Eating Right in the Renaissance* (Berkeley: University of California Press, 2002).

Álvarez Francés, Lenor, 'Fascination for the "Madritsche Apoll": Lope de Vega in Golden Age Amsterdam', *Arte Nuevo: Revista de estudios áureos*, 1 (2014), pp. 1–15.

Andel, M.A. van, *Klassieke wondermiddelen* (Gorinchem: J. Noorduyn & Zoon, 1928).

Arens, J.C., 'Studies over nawerkingen van Klassieken V: Six van Chandelier tussen Horatius en David', *TNTL*, 78 (1961), pp. 114–130.

Baer, Ronnie (with contributions by Arthur K. Wheelock, Jr. and Annetje Boersma), *Gerrit Dou (1613–1675): Master Painter in the Age of Rembrandt* (Washington, D.C.: National Gallery of Art, 2000).

Bakker, Boudewijn, 'Een goddelijk schilderij: Vondel over landschap en schilderkunst in zijn *Bespiegelingen* van 1662', *Neerlandistiek*, 5 (2005), pp. 1–36.

Barlaeus, Caspar, *The Wise Merchant*, ed. and trans. by Anna-Luna Post and Corinna Vermeulen (Amsterdam: Amsterdam University Press, 2019).

Baumann, E.D., *Francois dele Boë Sylvius* (Leiden: Brill, 1949).

Beard, Mary, *The Roman Triumph* (Cambridge and London: The Belknap Press of Harvard University Press, 2007).

Beecher, Donald, 'Ficino, Theriaca and the Stars', in: Michael J.B. Allen, Valery Rees & Martin Davies (eds.), *Marsilio Ficino: His Theology, His Philosophy, His Legacy* (Leiden: Brill, 2002), pp. 243–256.

Bergvelt, Ellinoor & Reneé Kistemaker (eds.), *De wereld binnen handbereik. Nederlandse kunst- en rariteitenverzamelingen, 1585–1735*, I and II (exhibition catalogue) (Zwolle/Amsterdam: Waanders/Amsterdams Historisch Museum, 1992).

Bergvelt, Ellinoor et al. (eds.), *Verzamelen: van rariteitenkabinet tot kunstmuseum* (Heerlen: Open Universiteit, 1993).

Berkel, Klaas van, *In het voetspoor van Stevin. Geschiedenis van de natuurwetenschap in Nederland 1580–1940* (Amsterdam: Boom Meppel, 1985).

Bertelli, Sergio, *The King's Body: Sacred Rituals of Power in Medieval and Early Modern Europe*, trans. by R. Burr Litchfield (University Park: Pennsylvania State University Press, 2001).

Bie, J.P. de & J. Loosjes (eds.), *Biografisch woordenboek van protestantsche godgeleerden in Nederland*, vol. 4 (The Hague: M. Nijhoff, 1931).

Bijlsma, R., '*Oud-Rotterdamsche "Cruydenierie"*', *Rotterdamsch Jaarboekje*, 10 (1912), pp. 91–99.

Bloch, Marc, *The Royal Touch, Sacred Monarchy and Scrofula in England and France*, trans. by J.E. Anderson (London: Routledge and Kegan Paul, 1973).

Bonsdorff, Bertel von, *Abraham Six van Chandelier & consortes: en kolonisationsplan i Ingermanland 1629/30* (Helsinki: B. von Bonsdorff, 1997).

Bontemantel, Hans, *De regeeringe van Amsterdam, soo in 't civiel als crimineel en militaire (1653–1672)*, ed. by G.W. Kernkamp, 2 vols. (The Hague: Martinus Nijhoff, 1877).

Bosma-Jelgersma, H.A., *Vijf eeuwen Delftse apothekers. Een bronnenstudie over de geschiedenis van de farmacie in een Hollandse stad* (Amsterdam: Ronald Meesters, 1979).

Bosma-Jelgersma, H.A., *Poeders, Pillen en Patiënten* (Amsterdam: Sijthoff, 1983).

Bouman, Ferry, Bob Baljet & Erik Zevenhuizen (eds.), *Kruidenier aan de Amstel. De Amsterdamse Hortus volgens Johannes Snippendaal (1646)* (Amsterdam: Amsterdam University Press, 2007).

Braakman, Mario, 'Pronken met geleend licht. De Westeuropese geneesmiddelencultuur in de 16de en 17de eeuw', *Medische Antropologie*, 2 (1990), pp. 25–39.

Bredero, G.A., *Angeniet*, ed. by P.E.L. Verkuyl (The Hague: Martinus Nijhoff, 1982).

Breen, Benjamin, *The Age of Intoxication: Origins of the Global Drug Trade* (Philadelphia: University of Pennsylvania Press, 2019).

Breen, Benjamin, 'Drugs and Early Modernity', *History Compass*, 15 (2017), pp. 1–9.

Breen, Joh. C., 'Geschiedenis van het huis Keizersgracht 676', *Jaarboek van het genootschap Amstelodamum*, 13 (1915), pp. 86–94.

Breitenberg, Mark *Anxious Masculinity in Early Modern England* (Cambridge: Cambridge University Press, 1996).

Brenninkmeyer-de Rooij, Beatrijs, 'Vergoddelijkte vorsten', *Openbaar kunstbezit. Kunstschrift*, 25 (1981), pp. 46–50.

Brienen, T., *Johannes Hoornbeeck (1617–1666): eminent geleerde en pastoraal theoloog* (Goudriaan: De Groot, 2008).

Brillat-Savarin, Jean Anthelme, *Physiologie du goût* (Paris: A. Sauteret et Cie, 1826).

Brinkkemper, Simpha & Ine Soepnel, *Apollo en Christus: Klassieke en christelijke denkbeelden in de Nederlandse renaissance-literatuur* (Zutphen: Walburg Pers, 1989).

Broomhall, Susan (ed.), *Early Modern Emotions: An Introduction* (Abingdon: Routledge, 2017).

Broos, B.P.J., 'Notitie der Teekeningen van Sybrand Feitama: de boekhouding van drie generaties verzamelaars van oude Nederlandse tekenkunst', *Oud Holland*, 98 (1984), pp. 13–39.

Bruijn, Enny de, *Eerst de waarheid, dan de vrede. Jacob Revius 1586–1658* (Zoetermeer: Boekencentrum, 2012).

Bussels, Stijn, 'Theories of the sublime in the Dutch Golden Age. Franciscus Junius, Joost van den Vondel and Petrus Wittewrongel', *History of European Ideas*, 42 (2016), pp. 1–11.

Buyens, Vincent, 'Joannes Six van Chandeliers "Schetse van Venecie". Meer dan een reis-indruk', *Spiegel der Letteren*, 47 (2005), pp. 21–51.

Campen, Matthijs van, *Gans Israël: Voetiaanse en coccejaanse visies op de joden gedurende de zeventiende en achttiende eeuw* (Zoetermeer: Boekencentrum, 2006).

Cave, Terence, *Devotional Poetry in France* (Cambridge: Cambridge University Press, 1969).

Cholcman, Tamar, 'The Merchant Voice: International Interests and Strategies in Local Joyeuses Entrées. The Case of Portuguese, English, and Flemish Merchants in Antwerp (1599) and Lisbon (1619)', *Dutch Crossing: Journal of Low Countries Studies*, 35 (2011), pp. 39–62.

Cicero, *On Ends*, trans. by H. Rackham (London and Cambridge, MA: Harvard University Press, 1931).

Cook, Harold J., 'Time's Bodies: Crafting the Preparation and Preservation of Naturalia', in: Pamela Smith & Paula Findlen (eds.), *Merchants and Marvels: Commerce, Science, and Art in Early Modern Europe* (New York: Routledge, 2002), pp. 223–247.

Cook, Harold J., *Matters of Exchange. Commerce, Medicine, and Science in the Dutch Golden Age* (New Haven: Yale University Press, 2007).

Cook, Harold J. & Timothy D. Walker, 'Circulation of Medicine in the Early Modern Atlantic World', in: *Social History of Medicine*, 26 (2013), pp. 337–251.

Cooper, Alix, *Inventing the Indigenous: Local Knowledge and Natural History in Early Modern Europe* (New York: Cambridge University Press, 2007).

Coornhert, D.V., *Zedekunst, dat is wellevenskunste*, ed. by Bruno Becker (Leiden: Brill, 1942).

Coornhert, D.V., *Het roerspel en de comedies van Coornhert*, ed. by Paul van der Meulen (Leiden: Brill, 1955).

Coornhert, D.V., *De Coopman. Aanwysende d'oprechte conste om Christelyck ende met eenen gelycken moede in 't winnen ende verliesen coophandel te dryven*, ed. by S. van der Woude (Amersfoort: C.G.A. Corvey, [1580] 1969).

Corrigan, Karina H. et al. (eds.), *Asia in Amsterdam: The Culture of Luxury in the Golden Age* (Salem M.A: Peabody Essex Museum; Amsterdam: Rijksmuseum; New Haven and Londen: Yale University Press, 2015).

Corson, Richard, *Fashions in Makeup. From Ancient to Modern Times* (London: Peter Owen, 1972).

Cowan, Brian, *The Social Life of Coffee: The Emergence of the British Coffeehouse* (New Haven, London: Yale University Press, 2005).

Crenshaw, Paul, *Rembrandt's Bankruptcy: The Artist, His Patrons, and the Art World in Seventeenth-Century Netherlands* (Cambridge: Cambridge University Press, 2006).

Cruz, Joan C., *Relics* (Huntington, IN: Our Sunday Visitor, 1984).

Cummings, Brian & Freya Sierhuis, 'Introduction', in: Brian Cummings & Freya Sierhuis (eds.), *Passions and Subjectivity in Early Modern Culture* (Farnham: Asghate: 2013), pp. 1–13.

Dannenfeldt, Karl H., 'Egypt and Egyptian Antiquities in the Renaissance', *Studies in the Renaissance*, 4 (1959), pp. 7–27.

Dannenfeldt, Karl H., 'Egyptian Mumia: The Sixteenth century Experience and Debate', *Sixteenth Century Journal*, 16 (1985), pp. 163–180.

Dash, Mike, *Tulipomania: The Story of the World's Most Coveted Flower & the Extraordinary Passions It Aroused* (London: Gollancz, 1999).

Daston, Lorraine & Katharine Park, *Wonders and the Order of Nature, 1150–1750* (New York: Zone Books, 1998).

Davidson, N.S., 'Sodomy in Early Modern Venice', in: Tom Betteridge (ed.), *Sodomy in Early Modern Europe* (Manchester and New York: Manchester University Press, 2002), pp. 65–85.

Decker, Jeremias de, *Goede vrydag ofte Het lijden onses heeren Jesy Christi*, ed. by W.J.C. Buitendijk (Zwolle: Tjeenk Willink, 1978).

Dehing, Pit, *Geld in Amsterdam: Wisselbank en wisselkoersen, 1650–1725* (Hilversum: Verloren, 2012).

Deman, Albert & Christian Cannuyer (eds.), *Specerijkelijk. De specerijenroutes* (Brussels: ASLK Dienst Cultuur, 1992).

Derrida, Jacques, 'Plato's Pharmacy' in Jacques Derrida, *Dissemination*, trans. by Barbara Johnson (Chicago: University of Chicago Press 1981), pp. 61–171.

Descartes, René, *The Philosophical Writings of Descartes*, trans. by John Cottingham, Robert Stoothoff, Dugald Murdoch, and Anthony Kenny, 3 vols. (Cambridge: Cambridge University Press, 1991).

Dionysius of Halicarnassus, *The Roman Antiquities of Dionysius of Halicarnassus*, trans. by Earnest Cary, 7 vols. (Cambridge: Harvard University Press, 1950).

Dolan, Frances E., 'Taking the Pencil out of God's Hand: Art, Nature, and the Face-painting Debate in Early Modern England', *PMLA*, 108 (1993), pp. 224–239.

Drago, Elisabeth Berry, *Printed Alchemists: Early Modern Artistry and Experiment in the Work of Thomas Wijck* (Amsterdam: Amsterdam University Press, 2019).

Dudok van Heel, Sebastien A.C., '"De Gapert" van de kruidenier Hendrick Anthonisz Wissel: Damrak nr. 50', *Amstelodamum*, 63 (1976), pp. 1–11.

Dugan, Holly, *The Ephemeral History of Perfume. Scent and Sense in Early Modern England* (Baltimore: Johns Hopkins University Press, 2011).

Dupré, Sven, 'Art and Alchemy: An Introduction', in: Sven Dupré, Dedo von Kerssenbrock-Krosigk & Beat Wismer (eds.), *Art and Alchemy. The Mystery of Transformation* (Düsseldorf: Hirmer / Museum Kunstpalast, 2014), pp. 11–17.

Dupré, Sven, Dedo von Kerssenbrock-Krosigk & Beat Wismer (eds.), *Art and Alchemy. The Mystery of Transformation* (Düsseldorf: Hirmer / Museum Kunstpalast, 2014).

Eamon, William, *Science and the Secrets of Nature: Books of Secrets in Medieval and Early Modern Culture* (Princeton: Princeton University Press, 1994).

Eamon, William, 'Cannibalism and Contagion: Framing Syphilis in Counter-Reformation Italy', *Early Science and Medicine*, 3 (1998), pp. 1–31.

Earle, Rebecca, *The Body of the Conquistador: Food, Race and the Colonial Experience in Spanish America, 1492–1700* (Cambridge: Cambridge University Press, 2012).

Ebben, Maurits, *Lodewijck Huygens' Spaans Journaal. Reis naar het hof van de koning van Spanje, 1660–1661* (Zutphen: Walburg Pers, 2005).

Ebben, Maurits, 'Lodewijck Huygens' *Spanish Journal*, 1660–1661: Perceptions of Spain and Confirmation of the Identity of the Dutch Republic', in: *Dutch Crossing*, 42 (2018), pp. 118–134.

Elias, J.E., *De vroedschap van Amsterdam 1578–1795*, 2 vols. (Haarlem: Vincent Loosjes, 1903–1905).

Ellinghausen, Laurie, *Labor and Writing in Early Modern England, 1567–1667* (Aldershot, UK: Ashgate, 2008).

Es, G.A. van & Edward Rombauts, *De letterkunde van renaissance en barok*, part 2, vol. 5 of F. Baur (ed.), *Geschiedenis van de letterkunde der Nederlanden*, 7 vols. (Brussels: Standaard Boekhandel; 's-Hertogenbosch: Teulings' Uitgevers-maatschappij L.C.G. Malmberg, 1939–) (not completed).

Evans, Susanne, 'The scent of a martyr', *NUMEN*, 49 (2002), pp. 193–211.

Evenhuis, R.B., *Ook dat was Amsterdam. De kerk der hervorming in de gouden eeuw*, 5 vols. (Amsterdam: Uitgeverij W. Ten Have, 1965–1978).

Exalto, K., 'Cornelis van Niel en zijn "Welrieckende balsem" 1683', in: K. Exalto, *Beleefd geloof. Acht schetsen van gereformeerde theologen uit de 17e eeuw* (Amsterdam: Ton Bolland, 1974), pp. 102–119.

Fähler, Eberhard, *Feuerwerke des Barock. Studien zum öffentlichen Fest und seiner literarischen Deutung vom 16. bis 18. Jahrhundert* (Stuttgart: J.B. Metzler, 1974).

Faure, Paul, *Magie der Düfte. Eine Kulturgeschichte der Wohlgerüche – Von den Pharaonen zu den Römern*, trans. by Barbara Brumm (Munich/Zurich: Artemis, 1990, orig. *Parfums et aromates de l'Antiquité*, 1987).

Fleischer, Alette, 'Breyne's Botany: (Re-)locating Nature and Knowledge in Danzig (circa 1660–1730)', in: Fokko Jan Dijksterhuis, Andreas Weber & Huib J. Zuidervaart (eds.), *Locations of Knowledge in Dutch Contexts* (Leiden/Boston: Brill, 2019), pp. 107–135.

Floyd-Wilson, Mary, 'English Mettle', in: Gail Kern Paster, Katherine Rowe & Mary Floyd-Wilson (eds.), *Reading the Early Modern Passions in the Cultural History of Emotion* (Philadelphia: University of Pennsylvania Press, 2004), pp. 130–146.

Frank-van Westrienen, Anna, *De groote tour. Tekening van de educatiereis der Nederlanders in de zeventiende* eeuw (Amsterdam: Noord-Hollandse Uitgeversmaatschappij, 1983).

Frederiks, J.G. & P.J. Frederiks, *Kohier van den tweehonderdsten penning voor Amsterdam en onderhoorige plaatsen over 1631* (Amsterdam: Koninklijk Oudheidkundig Genootschap, 1890).

Freedman, Paul, *Out of the East. Spices and the Medieval Imagination* (New Haven: Yale University Press, 2008).

Frijhoff, Willem & Marijke Spies, *Dutch Culture in European Perspective: 1650, Hard-Won Unity* (Basingstoke: Palgrave Macmillan, 2004).

Fuchs, R. & J.C. Breen, 'Aus dem "Itinerarium" des Christian Knorr von Rosenroth', *Jaarboek Amstelodamum*, 14 (1916), pp. 201–256.

Geary, Patrick, 'Sacred Commodities: The Circulation of Medieval Relics', in: A. Appadurai (ed.), *The Social Life of Things: Commodities in Cultural Perspective* (Cambridge: Cambridge University Press, 1986), pp. 169–191.

Geerdink, Nina, *Dichters en verdiensten. De sociale verankering van het dichterschap van Jan Vos (1610–1667)* (Hilversum: Verloren, 2012).

Gelder, Maartje van, *Trading Places: Netherlandish Merchants in Early Modern Venice* (Leiden: Brill, 2009).

Gelder, Roelof van, 'Noordnederlandse verzamelingen in de zeventiende eeuw', in: Ellinoor Bergvelt et al. (eds.), *Verzamelen: van rariteitenkabinet tot kunstmuseum* (Heerlen: Open Universiteit, 1993), pp. 123–144.

Gemert, Lia van, 'Johan van Beverwijck als "instituut"', *De zeventiende eeuw* 8 (1992), pp. 99–206.

Gemert, Lia van, afterword in Johan van Beverwijck, *De schat der gezondheid*, ed. by Lia van Gemert (Amsterdam: Querido, 1992), pp. 164–182.

Gemert, Lia van, '"U Kunst gelt over-al": een Dordtse arts tussen West en Oost', *Literatuur: Tijdschrift over Nederlandse letterkunde*, 10 (1993), pp. 16–22.

Gemert, Lia van, 'The Power of the Weak Vessels: Simon Schama and Johan van Beverwijck on Women', Els Kloek, Nicole Teeuwen & Marijke Huisman (eds.), *Women of the Golden Age: An International Debate on Women in Seventeenth-Century Holland, England and Italy* (Hilversum: Verloren, 1994), pp. 39–53.

Georgievska-Shine, Aneta & Larry Silver, *Rubens, Velázquez, and the King of Spain* (New York: Routledge, 2017).

Gera, Judit, 'The Grocer as a Stereotype in Dutch Culture', *Praagse perspectieven*, 3 (2005), pp. 33–43.

Gier, J. de, '"Den krijg is uitgebannen". De Vrede van Münster in de poëzie', in: H.H.J. van As et al. (eds.), *Vrede, vrijheid, vaderland. Nederlandse protestanten en de Vrede van Münster* (Rotterdam: Vereniging Protestants Nederland, 1998), pp. 151–171.

Goldgar, Anne, *Tulipmania: Money, Honor, and Knowledge in the Dutch Golden Age* (Chicago and London: University of Chicago Press, 2007).

Goldthwaite, Richard A., *The Building of Renaissance Florence. An Economic and Social History* (Baltimore: Johns Hopkins University Press, 1982).

Gommans, J. & I. Loots, 'Arguing with the Heathens: The Further Reformation and the Ethnohistory of Johannes Hoornbeeck (1617–1666)', *Itinerario*, 39 (2015), pp. 45–68.

Goodman, Jordan, 'Excitantia: Or, How Enlightenment Europe Took to Soft Drugs', in: Jordan Goodman, Paul E. Lovejoy & Andrew Sherratt (eds.), *Consuming Habits: Drugs in History and Anthropology* (London: Routledge, 1995), pp. 121–141.

Gorp, H. van, D. Delabastita & R. Ghesquiere, *Lexicon van literaire termen* (Groningen/Mechelen: Wolters Plantyn, 2007).

Göttler, C. & W. Neuber (eds.), *Spirits Unseen: The Representation of Subtle Bodies in Early Modern European Culture* (Leiden: Brill, 2008).

Grafton, Anthony (with April Shelford and Nancy Siraisi), *New Worlds, Ancient Texts. The Power of Tradition and the Shock of Discovery* (Cambridge: Belknap Press of Harvard University Press, 1992).

Greenblatt, Stephen, *Renaissance Self-Fashioning: From More to Shakespeare* (Chicago: University of Chicago Press, 1980).

Greenfield, Amy Butler, *A Perfect Red: Empire, Espionage and the Quest of the Colour of Desire* (New York: Harper Collins, 2005).

Grotius, Hugo, *The Antiquity of the Batavian Republic*. With notes by Petrus Scriverius, ed. and trans. by Jan Waszink et al. (Assen: Van Gorcum, 2000).

Guépin, J.P., 'Het enthousiasme van dichters', *Bzzlletin*, 144 (1987), pp. 47–64.

Hale, David, *The Body Politic: A Political Metaphor in Renaissance English Literature* (The Hague: Mouton, 1971).

Hardin, Richard F., *Civil Idolatry: Desacralizing and Monarchy in Spencer, Shakespeare and Milton* (Newark: University of Delaware Press, 1992).

Harkness, Deborah, *The Jewel House: Elizabethan London and the Scientific Revolution* (New Haven, Connecticut: Yale University Press, 2007).

Harris, Jonathan Gil, *Sick Economies: Drama, Mercantilism and Disease in Shakespeare's England* (Philadelphia: University of Pennsylvania Press, 2004).

Harrison, Peter, *The Fall of Man and the Foundation of Science* (Cambridge: Cambridge University Press, 2007).

Harvey, Elizabeth D., 'Flesh Color and Shakespeare's Sonnets', in: Michael Schoenfeldt (ed.), *A Companion to Shakespeare's Sonnets* (Oxford: Blackwell, 2007), pp. 314–330.

Hazard, Mary E., 'An Essay to Amplify "Ornament": Some Renaissance Theory and Practice', in: *SEL*, 16 (1976), pp. 15–32.

Healy, Margaret, *Fictions of Disease in Early Modern England: Bodies, Plagues and Politics* (New York: Palgrave, 2001).

Heath, John Benjamin, *Some Account of the Worshipful Company of Grocers of the City of London* (London: Privately Printed, 1854).

Heertum, Cis van, *Alchemie aan de Amstel: Over hermetische geneeskunst. Catalogus bij een tentoonstelling in de Bibliotheca Philosophica Hermetica* (Amsterdam: In de Pelikaan, 2012).

Heijn, Nicolaas Vels, *Kleurnamen en kleurbegrippen bij de Romeinen: Colour names and colour concepts among the Romans* (Utrecht: Kemink en Zoon, 1951).

Helmers, Helmer J., *The Royalist Republic. Literature, Politics and Religion in the Anglo-Dutch Public Sphere, 1639–1660* (Cambridge: Cambridge University, 2014).

Helmers, Helmer J., 'Illness as Metaphor: The Sick Body Politic and Its Cures', in: J. Grave & B. Noak (eds.), *Illness and Literature in the Low Countries* (Göttingen: V&R Unipress, 2016), pp. 97–120.

Heyd, Michael, *'Be Sober and Reasonable': The Critique of Enthusiasm in the Seventeenth and Early Eighteenth Centuries* (Leiden: E.J. Brill, 1995).

Higby, Gregory J., 'Gold in Medicine: A review of its use in the West before 1900', *Gold Bulletin*, 15 (1982), pp. 130–140.

Hochstrasser, Julie Berger, *Still Life and Trade in the Dutch Golden Age London* (New Haven and London: Yale University Press, 2007).

Hofmeyr, J.W., *Johannes Hoornbeeck as polemikus* (Kampen: Kok, 1975).

Hofmeyr, J.W., 'Johannes Hoornbeeck, a Monumental 17th century Dutch Theologian: Continuities in His Thinking on Doctrine and Life', *Acta Theologica*, 36 (2016), pp. 19–48.

Hommes, Margriet Eikema & Elmer Kolfin, *De Oranjezaal in Huis ten Bosch. Een zaal uit louter liefde* (Zwolle: Waanders, 2013).

Hooft, Arnout Hellemans, *Een naekt beeldt op een marmore matras seer schoon. Het dagboek van een grand tour (1649–1651)*, ed. by E.M. Grabowsky and P.J. Verkruijsse (Hilversum: Verloren, 2001).

Hooft, P.C., *Reden vande Waerdicheit der Poesie*, ed. by Jeroen Jansen (Amersfoort: Florivallis, 2005).

Hoornbeeck, Johannes, *On the Conversion of Indians and Heathens*. An Annotated Translation of *De conversione Indorum et Gentilium* (1669), trans. and ed. by Ineke Loots and Joke Spaans (Leiden: Brill, 2018).

Horace, *The Odes and Epodes*, ed. and trans. by Niall Rudd. Loeb Classical Library (Cambridge, MA: Harvard University Press, 2004).

Humphreys, Humphry, 'The Horn of the Unicorn', in: *Annals of The Royal College of Surgeons of England*, 8 (1951), pp. 377–383.

Huygens, Constantijn, *Dagh-werck*, ed. by F.L. Zwaan (Assen: Van Gorcum & Comp B.V. [1658] 1973).

Israel, Jonathan, *Dutch Primacy in World Trade 1585–1740* (Oxford: Clarendon Press, 1989).

Jacob, Margaret C. & Catherine Secretan (eds.), *The Self-Perception of Early Modern Capitalists* (New York: Macmillan, 2008).

Jacobs, A.E. (ed.), *Joannes Six van Chandelier: Gedichten. Studieuitgave*, 2 vols. (Assen: Van Gorcum, 1991).

Jansen-Sieben, Ria, 'Van drogen, kruiden en specerijen', in: Albert Deman & Christian Cannuyer (eds.), *Specerijkelijk. De specerijenroutes* (Brussels: ASLK Dienst Cultuur 1992), pp. 32–41.

Jansma, Jan Reinier, *Louis de Bils en de anatomie van zijn tijd* (Hoogeveen: C. Pot, 1919).

Johnson, Christine R., *The German Discovery of the World. Renaissance Encounters with the Strange and Marvelous* (Charlottesville: University of Virginia Press, 2008).

Jonckheere, Koenraad, 'An Allegory of Artistic Choice in Times of Trouble: Pieter Bruegel's Tower of Babel', *Nederlands Kunsthistorisch Jaarboek*, 64 (2014), pp. 151–177.

Jongman, C.D., 'De historische ontwikkeling van het kruideniersbedrijf in Nederland', in: F.L. van Muiswinkel & J.C. Berk (eds.), *Het kruideniersbedrijf* (Amsterdam: Noord-Hollandsche Uitgevers Mij., 1951), pp. 3–15.

Jorink, Eric, *Reading the Book of Nature in the Dutch Golden Age, 1575–1715*, trans. by Peter Mason (Leiden: Brill, 2010).

Justi, C., *Diego Velazquez und sein Jahrhundert* (Zurich: Phaidon Verlag AG, 1933).

Juvenal, *Juvenal and Persius*, trans. by G.G. Ramsay. Loeb Classical Library (Cambridge, MA: Harvard University, 2004).

Kampinga, H., *De opvattingen over onze oudere vaderlandsche geschiedenis bij de Hollandsche historici der XVIe en XVIIe eeuw* (The Hague: Martinus Nijhoff, 1917).

Karant-Nunn, Susan, *The Reformation of Feeling: Shaping the Religious Emotions in Early Modern Germany* (New York: Oxford University Press, 2010).

Karim-Cooper, Farah, *Cosmetics in Shakespearean and Renaissance Drama* (Edinburgh: Edinburgh University Press, 2006).

Keitt, Andrew, 'Religious Enthusiasm, the Spanish Inquisition, and the Disenchantment of the World', *Journal of the History of Ideas*, 65 (2004) pp. 231–250 (consulted 17 May 2019).

Kiliaen, C., *Etymologicum teutonicae linguae*, ed. by F. Claes (Mouton: The Hague, [1599] 1972). dbnl.org/tekst/kilioo1etymo1_01/kilioo1etymo1_01_0001.php

King, Rachel, '"The beads with which we pray are made from it": Devotional ambers in early modern Italy', in: Wietse de Boer & Christine Göttler (eds.), *Religion and the Senses in Early Modern Europe* (Leiden: Brill, 2013), pp. 153–175.

Kist, N.C., *Neêrland's bededagen en biddagsbrieven*, 2 vols. (Leiden: Luchtmans, 1848–1849).

Kloek, Els, Nicole Teeuwen & Marijke Huisman (eds.), *Women of the Golden Age: An International Debate on Women in Seventeenth-Century Holland, England and Italy* (Hilversum: Verloren, 1994).

Knoppers, Laura Lunger, *Constructing Cromwell: Ceremony, Portrait, and Print 1645–1661* (Cambridge: Cambridge University Press, 2000).

Knox, D., *Ironia. Medieval and Renaissance Ideas on Irony* (Leiden: E.L. Brill, 1989).

Kopytoff, Igor & Arjun Appadurai (eds.), *The Social Life of Things. Commodities in Cultural Perspective* (Cambridge: Cambridge University Press, 1986).

Kooijmans, Luuc, 'De koopman', in: H.M. Beliën, A.Th. van Deursen, G.J. van Setten (eds.), *Gestalten van de Gouden Eeuw. Een Hollands groepsportret* (Amsterdam: Bert Bakker, 1995), pp. 65–92.

Kooijmans, Luuc, *De doodskunstenaar. De anatomische lessen van Frederik Ruysch* (Amsterdam: Bert Bakker, 2004).

Kooijmans, Luuc, *Gevaarlijke kennis. Inzicht en angst in de dagen van Jan Swammerdam* (Amsterdam: Bert Bakker, 2007).

Koopman, Frans & Frans Wetzels: 'Zijn er nog vragen? Een speurtocht in de archieven van de Oude West-Indische Compagnie', *Fumus*, 15 (2017), pp. 23–32.

Koopmans, J., 'Johan Six van Chandelier', *De nieuwe taalgids*, 9 (1915), pp. 25–49.

Koppenol, Johan, 'Een tegendraadse poëtica. De literaire ideeën van Jan van Hout', in: K.J.S. Bostoen et al. (eds.), *Jan van Hout, Voorrede tot het gezelschap. Voorrede bij zijn vertaling van Buchanans Franciscanus* (Soest: Rafaël, 1993), pp. 3–25.

Koppenol, Johan, *Leids heelal: het Loterijspel (1596) van Jan van Hout* (Hilversum: Verloren, 1998).

Kruyskamp, C., 'Poësy van J. Six van Chandelier. Bloemlezing uit zijn dichtwerk met inleiding en aantekeningen door Dr. G.A. van Es', *Tijdschrift voor Nederlandse Taal- en Letterkunde*, 72 (1954), pp. 78–80.

Kuijlen, Jos, 'De Danziger botanicus en koopman Jacob Breyne (1637–1697) en zijn betekenis voor de Hollandse plantkunde', *Tijdschrift voor de Geschiedenis der Geneeskunde, Natuurwetenschappen, Wiskunde en Techniek*, 6 (1977), pp. 116–118.

Lacey, Andrew, *The Cult of King Charles the Martyr* (Woodbridge: Boydell Press, 2003).

Lauer, Hans H., 'Zur Tradition exotischer Drogen: faufal (Areca Catechu L.) – die Betelnuß', *Sudhoffs Archiv. Zeitschrift für Wissenschaftsgeschichte*, 50 (1966), pp. 179–204.

Leonhard, Karin, *Bildfelder. Stilleben und Naturstücke des 17. Jahrhunderts* (Berlin: Akademie Verlag, 2013)

Lesger, C.M., 'Merchants in charge: The self-perception of Amsterdam merchants, ca. 1550-1700', in: Margaret C. Jacob & Catharine Secretan (eds.), *The Self-Perception of Early Modern Capitalists* (New York: Macmillan, 2008), pp. 75–97.

Lichtenstein, Jacqueline, 'Making up Representation: The Risks of Femininity', *Representations*, 20 (1987), pp. 77–87.

Lieburg, M.J. van, *De ziekte der geleerden. Een hoofdstuk uit de geschiedenis van de melancholie en hypochondrie* (Oss: Organon, 1989).

Lieburg, M.J. van, 'Voetius en de geneeskunde', in: J. van Oort et al. (eds.), *De onbekende Voetius: Voordrachten Wetenschappelijk Symposium Utrecht 3 maart 1989* (Kampen: Kok, 1989), pp. 168–180.

Lievens, Robrecht, 'Dichterlof voor de Ninoofse kloostertuin', *Land Aalst*, 51 (1999), pp. 148–159.

Linschoten, Jan Huyghen van, *Itinerario, Voyage ofte schipvaert van Jan Huygen van Linschoten naer Oost ofte Portugaels Indien 1597–1592*, ed. by H. Kern & H. Terpstra, 3 vols. (The Hague: Martinus Nijhoff, 1955–1957).

Linschoten, Jan Huyghen van, *The Voyage of Jan Huyghen van Linschoten to the East Indies.* From the English translation of 1598, ed. by A.C. Bumell and P.A. Tiele, 2 vols. (London: Hakluyt Society, 1885).

Livy, *History of Rome*, trans. by B.O. Foster. Loeb Classical Library, 14 vols. (Cambridge, MA: Harvard University Press, 1967–1984).

MacGregor, Arthur, 'Medicinal *terra sigillata*: A historical, geographical and typological review', in: C.J. Duffin, R.T.J. Moody & C. Gardner-Thorpe (eds.), *A History of Geology and Medicine* (London: Geological Society, 2012).

Marr, Alexander, 'Introduction', in: R.J.W. Evan & Alexander Marr (eds.), *Curiosity and Wonder from the Renaissance to the Enlightenment* (Burlington, VT: Ashgate, 2006), pp. 1–20.

Martial, *Epigrams*, trans. by D.R. Schackleton Baily, Loeb Classical Library, 3 vols. (Cambridge, MA: Harvard University Press, 1993).

McDermott, Jennifer Rae, '"The Melodie of Heaven": Sermonizing the Open Ear in Early Modern England', in: Wietse de Boer & Christine Göttler (eds.), *Religion and the Senses in Early Modern Europe* (Leiden: Brill, 2013), pp. 177–197.

Meganck, Tine L., *Pieter Bruegel the Elder: Fall of the Rebel Angels: Art, Knowledge and Politics on the Eve of the Dutch revolt* (Milan: Silvana, 2014).

Meijer Drees, Marijke, *Andere landen, andere mensen: De beeldvorming van Holland versus Spanje en Engeland omstreeks 1650* (The Hague: Sdu Uitgevers, 1997).

Melissen, Sipko, 'De heedendaagse Goude-eeuw', *Spektator*, 11 (1981–1982), pp. 30–60.

Meter, J.H., *De literaire theorieën van Daniel Heinsius. Een onderzoek naar de klassieke en humanistische bronnen van De Tragoediae Constitutione en andere geschriften* (Amsterdam: Adolf M. Hakkert, 1975).

Middelkoop, N. (ed.), *Kopstukken: Amsterdammers geportretteerd 1600–1800* (Amsterdam: Amsterdams Historisch Museum, 2002).

Milton, John, *Paradise Lost*, ed. by Alastair Fowler (London and New York: Routledge, 2007).

Mooij, Annet, *De polsslag van de stad. 350 jaar academische geneeskunde in Amsterdam* (Amsterdam/Antwerpen: De Arbeiderspers, 1999).

Moser, Nelleke, *De strijd voor rhetorica: poëtica en positie van rederijkers in Vlaanderen, Brabant, Zeeland en Holland tussen 1450 en 1620* (Amsterdam: Amsterdam University Press, 2001).

Nauta, Doede & Johannes van den Berg (eds.), *Biografisch lexicon voor de geschiedenis van het Nederlands protestantisme*, vol. 2 (Kampen: J.H. Kok, 1983).

Newman, William R., *Promethean Ambitions: Alchemy and the Quest to Perfect Nature* (Chicago: University of Chicago Press, 2004).

Niet, C.A. de, 'Voetius en de literatuur', *Nadere Reformatie en literatuur. Speciaalnummer van Documentatieblad Nadere Reformatie*, 1 (1995), pp. 27–36.

Noak, Bettina, 'Foreign Wisdom: Ethnological Knowledge in the Work of Franciscus Ridderus', *Journal of Dutch Literature*, 3 (2012), pp. 47–64.

Noble, Louise, *Medicinal Cannibalism in Early Modern English Literature and Culture* (New York: Palgrave Macmillan, 2011).

Norton, Marcy, *Sacred Gifts, Profane Pleasures: A History of Tobacco and Chocolate in the Atlantic World* (Ithaca: Cornell University Press, 2008).

Ommen, Kaspar van, *The Exotic World of Carolus Clusius (1526–1609)* (Leiden: Leiden University Library, 2009).

Ossa-Richardson, Anthony, *The Devil's Tabernacle: The Pagan Oracles in Early Modern Thought* (Princeton: Princeton University Press, 2013).

Oxford English Dictionary (Oxford: Oxford University Press, 2005).

Östenberg, Ida, *Staging the World: Spoils, Captives, and Representations in the Roman Triumphal Procession* (Oxford: Oxford University Press, 2009).

Parker, Grant, 'Ex Oriente Luxuria: Indian Commodities and Roman Experience', *Journal of Economic and Social History of the Orient*, 45 (2002), pp. 40–95.

Partington, James Riddick, *A History of Greek Fire and Gunpowder* (Cambridge: W. Heffer and Sons, 1960).

Partridge, Robert, *'O Horrable Murder': the Trial, Execution and Burial of King Charles I* (London: Rubicon, 1998).

Paster, Gail Kern, *The Body Embarrassed: Drama and the Disciplines of Shame in Early Modern England* (Ithaca: Cornell University Press, 1993).

Pels, Andries, *Gebruik en misbruik des toneels*, ed. by M. Schenkeveld-van der Dussen (Culemborg: Tjeenk Willink, 1987, [orig. 1681]).

Pers, Dirck Pieterz., *Suyp-stad, of Dronckaerts Leven*, ed. by J.E. Verlaan & E.K. Grootes (Culemborg: Tjeenk Willink,1978 [orig. 1628]).

Persius, see Juvenal.

Peters, Monique A.F., *Van miskend tot geprezen. Het beeld van de koopman-dichter Jan Six van Chandelier (1620–1695) in de Nederlandse literatuurgeschiedschrijving*. Bachelor Thesis (Amsterdam: Open Universiteit Nederland, 2012).

Philippa, M, F. Debrabandere, A. Quak, T. Schoonheim & N. van der Sijs (eds.), *Etymologisch Woordenboek van het Nederlands*, 4 vols (Amsterdam: Amsterdam University Press, 2003–2009).

Plato, *Plato*, trans. by H.N. Fowler, W.R.M. Lamb, P. Shorey et al., Loeb Classical Library, 12 vols. (Cambridge, MA: Harvard University Press, 1914–1935).

Pliny, *Natural History*, trans. by H. Rackham, W.H.S. Jones and D.E. Eichholz. Loeb Classical Library, 10 vols. (Cambridge, MA: Harvard University Press, 1942–1952).

Poelwijk, A.H., *'In dienste vant suyckerenbacken'. De Amsterdamse suikernijverheid en haar ondernemers, 1580-1630* (Hilversum: Verloren, 2003).

Pollard, Tanya, *Drugs and Theater in Early Modern England* (Oxford: Oxford University Press, 2005).

Popper, Nicholas, 'The Sudden Death of the Burning Salamander: Reading Experiment and the Transformation of Natural Historical Practice in Early Modern Europe', in: *Erudition and the Republic of Letters*, 1 (2016), pp. 464–490.

Porteman, Karel & Mieke B. Smits-Veldt, *Een nieuw vaderland voor de muzen. Geschiedenis van de Nederlandse literatuur 1560–1700* (Amsterdam: Bert Bakker, 2008).

Potter, Lois, *Secret Rites and Secret Writing: Royalist Literature 1641–1660* (Cambridge and New York: Cambridge University Press, 1989).

Prandoni, Marco, 'Gijsbreght tussen water en vuur, water- en vuurmetaforiek in *Gysbrecht van Aemstel*', *Vooys*, 22 (2004), pp. 31–47.

Principe, Lawrence M., *The Secrets of Alchemy* (Chicago: University of Chicago Press, 2013).

Puttenham, George, *The Arte English Poesie.* Facsimile of the 1589 edition (Menston, UK: Scolar Press Facsimiles, 1968).

Randolph, Mary Claire, 'The Medical Concept in English Renaissance Satiric Theory: Its Possible Relationships and Implications', *Studies in Philology*, 38 (1941), pp. 125–157.

Reinhold, Meyer, *History of Purple as a Status Symbol in Antiquity* (Brussels: Latomus, 1970).

Rijks, Marlise, '"Unusual Excrescences of Nature": Collected Coral and the Study of Petrified Luxury in Early Modern Antwerp', *Dutch Crossing*, 41 (2017), pp. 1–29.

Rinella, Michael A., *Pharmakon: Plato, Drug Culture, and Identity in Ancient Athens* (Plymouth: Lexington, 2011).

Rittersma, Rengenier C. (ed.), *Luxury in the Low Countries. Miscellaneous Reflections on Netherlandish Material Culture, 1500 to present* (Brussels: Pharo Publishing, 2010).

Roberts, Benjamin, *Sex and Drugs Before Rock 'n' Roll: Youth Culture and Masculinity During Holland's Golden Age* (Amsterdam: Amsterdam University Press, 2012).

Robertson, David, 'Incensed over Incense: Incense and Community in Seventeenth-Century Literature', in: Roger D. Sell & Anthony W. Johnson (eds.), *Religion and Writing in England, 1558–1689, Studies in Community-Making and Cultural Memory* (New York: Ashgate Publishing, 2009) pp. 389–409.

Robinson, Benedict S., 'Green Seraglios: Tulips, Turbans, and the Global Market', *The Journal for Early Modern Cultural Studies*, 9 (2009), pp. 93–122.

Roldanus, C.W., *Coenraad van Beuningen. Staatsman en libertijn* (The Hague: M. Nijhoff, 1931).

Ronsard, Pierre de, *La Franciade*, in: *Œuvres complètes*, ed. by Paul Laumonier, vol. 16 (Paris: Nizet, 1983).

Roodenburg, H.W. (ed.), *A Cultural History of the Senses in the Renaissance, 1450–1650* (London: Bloomsbury, 2014).

Roodenburg, H.W., 'The body in the Reformation', in: Ulinka Rublack (ed.), *The Oxford Handbook of the Protestant Reformations* (Oxford: Oxford University Press, 2017), pp. 643–666.

Rutten, A.M.G., *Blue Ships: Dutch Ocean Crossing with Multifunctional Drugs and Spices in the Eighteenth Century*, trans. by J. Wormer (Rotterdam: Erasmus Publishing, 2008).

Scaliger, Iulius Caeser, *Poetices libri septem. Sieben Bücher über die Dichtkunst*, ed. by Luc Deitz et al. (Stuttgart-Bad Cannstatt: Frommann-Holzboog, 1994).

Schama, Simon, *The Embarrassment of Riches. An Interpretation of Dutch Culture in the Golden Age* (New York: Harper Perennial, 2004 [orig.1988]).

Schenkeveld-van der Dussen, M.A., 'Theorie en poëzie: een epithalamium van Six van Chandelier', *De nieuwe taalgids*, 72 (1979), pp. 391–398.

Schenkeveld-van der Dussen, M.A., 'Joannes Six van Chandelier: Realist. Jaarrede door de voorzitter, mevrouw Dr. M.A. Schenkeveld-van der Dussen', *Jaarboek van de Maatschappij der Nederlandse Letterkunde 1981*, pp. 3–15.

Schenkeveld-van der Dussen, M.A., 'De anti-idealistische poëtica van een christen-burger, Joannes Six van Chandelier', *De nieuwe taalgids*, 76 (1983), pp. 291–316.

Schenkeveld-van der Dussen, M.A. & Hans Luijten (eds.), *Joannes Six van Chandelier: 's Amsterdammers winter* (Utrecht: HES, 1988).

Schenkeveld-van der Dussen, M.A., 'Regen in het vredejaar', in: *Liber amicorum Kåre Langvik-Johannessen*, ed. by K. Porteman & K.E. Schöndorf (Leuven: Peeters 1989), pp. 159–166.

Schenkeveld-van der Dussen, M.A., *Dutch Literature in the Age of Rembrandt: Themes and Ideas* (Amsterdam/Philadelphia: J. Benjamins, 1991).

Schenkeveld-van der Dussen, M.A., 'Najaar 1649, Jan Six van Chandelier overnacht in Toulouse – Drie anti-idealistische dichters', in: M.A. Schenkeveld-van der Dussen (ed.), *Nederlandse literatuur, een geschiedenis* (Groningen: Martinus Nijhoff, 1993), pp. 255–260.

Schenkeveld-van der Dussen, M.A., 'Ut pictura poesis: de paragone tussen dicht- en schilderkunst bij Jan Vos en Jan Six van Chandelier', *Nederlandse letterkunde*, 6 (2001), pp. 101–112.

Schenkeveld-van der Dussen, Riet & Willemien B. de Vries, *Zelfbeeld in Gedichten. Brieven over de poëzie van Jan Six van Chandelier (1620–1695)* (Amsterdam: Bert Bakker, 2007).

Scheurleer, Th.H. Lunsingh, C. Willemijn Fock & A.J. van Dissel, *Het Rapenburg. Geschiedenis van een Leidse gracht,* part IIIa (Leiden: Universiteit van Leiden, 1989).

Schivelbusch, Wolfgang, *Das Paradies, der Geschmack und die Vernunft. Eine Geschichte der Genussmittel* (Munich: Hanser, 1980).

Schrijvers, Piet, 'Een stralend nieuw lied. De Bacchus ode (3.25)', in: Piet Schrijvers, *Ik kan de Muzen niet haten* (Groningen: Historisch uitgeverij, 2004), pp. 75–98.

Schloss, Christine Skeeles, *Travel, Trade, and Temptation: The Dutch Italianate Harbor Scene (1640-1680)* (Ann Arbor: UMI Research Press, 1982).

Schmidt, Alfred, *Drogen und Drogenhandel im Alterum* (Leipzig: Ambrosius Barth, 1924).

Schmidt, Benjamin, *Innocence Abroad. The Dutch Imagination and the New World. 1570–1670* (Cambridge: Cambridge University Press, 2001).

Schoenfeldt, Michael, *Bodies and Selves in Early Modern England. Physiology and Inwardness in Spenser, Shakespeare, Herbert and Milton* (Cambridge: Cambridge University Press, 1999).

Schoenfeldt, Michael (eds.), *A Companion to Shakespeare's Sonnets* (London: Blackwell, 2007).

Schotel, G.D.J., *Het Maatschappelijk Leven onzer Vaderen in de Zeventiende Eeuw* ((Leiden: A.W. Sijthoff, reprinted 1905 [1868]).

Schwartz, Gary (ed.), *Emotions: Pain and Pleasure in the Dutch Golden Age* (Haarlem: Frans Hals Museum, 2015).

Schwyzer, Philip, *Archaeologies of English Renaissance Literature* (Oxford: Oxford University Press, 2007).

Shakespeare, William, *Complete Works*, ed. by Stanley Wells & Gary Taylor (Oxford: Oxford University Press, 1986).

Shapin, Steven, *A Social History of Truth: Civility and Science in Seventeenth-Century England* (Chicago: Chicago University Press, 1994).

Sherratt, Andrew, 'Introduction: Peculiar Substances', in: Jordan Goodman, Paul E. Lovejoy & Andrew Sherratt (eds.), *Consuming Habits: Drugs in History and Anthropology* (London, Routledge, 1995), pp. 1–10.

Sidney, Philip, *An Apology for Poetry*, ed. by Geoffrey Shepherd (London: Thomas Nelson, [1595] 1965).

Sierhuis, Freya, 'The Passions in the Literature of the Dutch Golden Age', *Tijdschrift voor Nederlandsche taal- en letterkunde*, 132 (2016), pp. 333–365.

Silva, Francisco Vaz Da, 'Sexual Horns. The Anatomy and Metaphysics of Cuckoldry in European Folklore', *Comparative Studies in Society and History*, 48 (2006), pp. 396–418.

Siraisi, Nancy G., *Medieval and Early Renaissance Medicine: An Introduction to Knowledge and Practice* (Chicago: University of Chicago Press, 1990).

Six van Chandelier, Joannes, *Poësy van J. Six van Chandelier: bloemlezing uit zijn dichtwerk*, ed. by G.A. van Es (Zwolle: Tjeenk Willink 1953).

Six van Chandelier, Joannes, see also A.E. Jacobs.

Sluijter, Eric Jan, *De 'heydensche fabulen' in de schilderkunst van de Gouden Eeuw. Verhalen uit de klassieke mythologie in de Noordelijke Nederlanden, circa 1590–1670* (Leiden: Primavera Pers, 2000).

Smith, Nigel, 'Cross-channel cavaliers', *The Seventeenth Century*, 32 (2017), pp. 433–453.

Smith, Pamela H. & Paula Findlen (eds.), *Merchants and Marvels: Commerce, Science, and Art in Early Modern Europe* (New York: Routledge, 2002).

Smith, Pamela H., *The Body of the Artisan. Art and Experience in the Scientific Revolution* (Chicago: University of Chicago Press, 2004).

Smith, Stefan Halikowski, 'Demystifying a Change in Taste: Spices, Space, and Social Hierarchy in Europe, 1380–1750', *The International History Review*, 29 (2007), pp. 237–257.

Smith, Woodruff D., 'From Coffee-House to Parlour: the Consumption of Coffee, Tea, and Sugar in North-Western Europe in the Seventeenth and Eighteenth Centuries', in: Jordan Goodman, Paul E. Lovejoy & Andrew Sherratt (eds.), *Consuming Habits: Drugs in History and Anthropology* (London: Routledge, 1995), pp. 142–157.

Smits, J., *De Verenigde Nederlanden op zoek naar het oude Egypte (1580–1780) – de traditie gevolgd en gewogen* (Groningen: Culemborg, 1988).

Snelders, H.A.M., *De geschiedenis van de scheikunde in Nederland. Van alchemie tot chemie en chemische industrie rond 1900* (Delft: Delftse Universitaire Pers, 1993).

Snoep, D.P., *Praal en Propaganda. Triumfalia in de Noorderlijke Nederlanden in de 16de en 17de eeuw* (Alphen aan de Rijn: Canaletto, 1975).

Spaans, Ronny, 'Exotica, ornaments and idolatry in the poetry of Jan Six van Chandelier (1620–1695)', *De Zeventiende Eeuw. Cultuur in de Nederlanden in interdisciplinair perspectief*, 32 (2016), pp. 115–136.

Spaans, Ronny, 'Diagnosing the Poetic Inspiration: Medical Criticism of Enthusiasm in the Poetry of Jan Six van Chandelier (1620-1695)', in: Jaap Grave, Rick Honings & Bettina Noak (eds.), *Illness and Literature in the Low Countries* (Göttingen: V&R Unipress, 2016).

Spies, Marijke, '"Op de Questye…": Over de structuur van 16e-eeuwse zinnespelen', *De nieuwe taalgids*, 83 (1990), pp. 139–150.

Spies, Marijke, 'Between Ornament and Argumentation: Developments in 16th-Century Dutch Poetics', in: Jelle Koopmans, Mark A. Meadow, Kees Meerhoff & Marijke Spies (eds.), *Rhetoric-Rhetoriqueurs-Rederijkers* (Amsterdam: Royal Netherlands Academy of Arts and Sciences, 1995).

Spies, Marijke, '"Helicon and Hills of Sand": Pagan Gods in Early Modern Dutch and European Poetry', in: H. Wilcox et al. (eds.), *Sacred and Profane: Secular and Devotional Interplay in Early Modern British Literature* (Amsterdam: VU University Press) 1996, pp. 225–236.

Stevenson, Laura Caroline, *Praise and Paradox: Merchants and Craftsmen in Elizabethan Popular Literature* (Cambridge: Cambridge University Press, 2002).

Stobart, Jon, *Sugar and Spice: Grocers and Groceries in Provincial England, 1650–1830* (Oxford: Oxford University Press, 2012).

Stoeder, Willem, *Geschiedenis der pharmacie in Nederland* (Amsterdam: Centen, 1891).

Strengholt, L., 'Tekenen van de Nadere Reformatie in de poëzie van Revius, Cats en Huygens?', *Documentatieblad Nadere Reformatie*, 11 (1987), pp. 109–125.

Strong, Roy, *Coronation: a History of Kingship and the British Monarchy* (London: Harper Collins, 2005).

Stronks, Els, *Negotiating Differences. Word, Image and Religion in the Dutch Republic* (Leiden: Brill, 2011).

Sturkenboom, Dorothee, 'Staging the Merchant: Commercial Vices and the Politics of Stereotyping in Early Modern Dutch Theatre', *Dutch Crossing*, 30 (2006), pp. 211–228.

Sturkenboom, Dorothee, 'Understanding Emotional Identities. The Dutch Phlegmatic Temperament as Historical Case Study', *BMGN*, 129 (2014), pp. 163–191.

Suetonius, Tranquillus, *The Lives of the Twelve Caesars*, trans. by J.C. Rolfe. Loeb Classical Library, 2 vols. (London and Cambridge, MA: Harvard University Press, 1913).

Sugg, Richard, *Mummies, Cannibals and Vampires. The History of Corpse Medicine from the Renaissance to the Victorians* (New York: Routledge, 2011).

Swan, Claudia, 'Collecting *Naturalia* in the Shadow of Early Modern Dutch Trade', in: Londa Schiebinger & Claudia Swan (eds.), *Colonial Botany: Science, Commerce, and Politics in the Early Modern World* (Philadelphia: University of Pennsylvania Press, 2005), pp. 223–236.

Thirsk, Joan, *Food in Early Modern England: Phases, Fads, Fashions, 1500–1760* (London: Hambledon Continuum, 2007).

Totelin, Laurence, 'Botanizing Rulers and Their Herbal Subjects: Plants and Political Power in Greek and Roman Literature', *Phoenix*, LXVI (2012), pp. 122–144.

Tummers, Anna, Elmer Kolfin & Jasper Hillegers (eds.), *The Art of Laughter: Humour in Dutch Paintings of the Golden Age* (Zwolle: Waanders B.V. Uitgeverij: 2017).

Veen, Jaap van der, '"Dit klain Vertrek bevat een Weereld vol gewoel": Negentig Amsterdammers en hun kabinetten', in: Bergvelt, Ellinoor & Reneé Kistemaker (eds.), *De wereld binnen handbereik. Nederlandse kunst- en rariteitenverzamelingen, 1585–1735* (Zwolle/Amsterdam: Waanders/Amsterdams Historisch Museum, 1992).

Veenman, René, 'De Thebaensche Swaen. De receptie van Pindarus in de Nederlanden', *Voortgang. Jaarboek voor de Neerlandistiek*, 13 (1992) pp. 65–90.

Verkuyl, P.E.L., 'Een dichterlijk pamflet naar aanleiding van de komeet van 1664', *Tijdschrift voor Nederlandsche taal- en letterkunde*, 112 (1996), pp. 30–43.

Vermeir, Koen, 'Imagination between Physick and Philosophy. On the Central Role of the Imagination in the Work of Henry More (1614–1687)', *Intellectual History Review*, 18 (2008), pp. 119–137.

Vollenhove, Joannes, *Het dagboek van Joannes Vollenhove, Engeland, 17 mei–30 oktober 1674*, ed. by G.R.W. Dibbets (Hilversum: Verloren, 2001).

Vondel, Joost van den, *Aenleidinge ter Nederduitsche dichtkunste*, ed. by Kees Blokland et al. (Utrecht: Instituut De Vooys, 1977 [orig. 1650]).

Vondel, Joost van den, *De werken van Vondel*, ed. by J.F.M. Sterck et al., 10 vols. (Amsterdam: De Maatschappij voor goede en goedkoope lectuur, 1927–1937).

Vos, Jan, *Jan Vos' toneelwerken*, ed. by W.J.C Buitendijk (Assen/Amsterdam: Van Gorcum, 1975).

Vossius, Gerardus, *Poeticarum institutionum libri tres / Institutes of Poetics in Three Books*, trans. and ed. by Jan Bloemendal (with Edwin Rabbie), 2 vols. (Leiden: Brill, 2010 [1647]).

Walker, D.P., *Spiritual and Demonic Magic: From Ficino to Campanella* (Notre Dame and London: University of Notre Dame Press, 1975).

Walthaus, Rina, 'The Sun and Aurora: Philip IV of Spain and his Queen-Consort in Royal Festival and Spectacle', in: Martin Gosman, Alasdair MacDonald & Arno Vanderjagt (eds.), *Princes and Princely Culture 1450–1650* (Leiden: Brill, 2005), vol. 2, pp. 277–308.

Warneke, Sara, 'A Taste for Newfangledness: the Destructive Potential of Novelty in Early Modern England', in: *Sixteenth Century Journal* 26 (1995), pp. 881–896.

Wätjen, Hermann, *Die Niederländer Im Mittelmeergebiet Zur Zeit Ihrer Höchsten Machtstellung* (Berlin: K. Curtius, 1909).

Weber, Gregor J.M., "t Lof van den Pekelharingh. Von alltäglichen und absonderlichen Heringsstilleben', *Oud Holland*, 101 (1987), pp. 126–140.

Wennekes, Wim, *Gouden handel. De eerste Nederlanders overzee, en wat zij daar haalden* (Amsterdam: Uitgeverij Atlas, 1996).

Westerman, Mariët, *A Worldly Art: The Dutch Republic, 1585–1718* (New York: Harry N. Abrams, 1996).

Weststeijn, Arthur, *Commercial Republicanism in the Dutch Golden Age. The Political Thought of Johan & Pieter de la Court* (Leiden: Brill, 2012).

Weststeijn, Thijs, '"Painting's Enchanting Poison": Artistic Efficacy and the Transfer of Spirits', in: C. Göttler & W. Neuber (eds.), *Spirits Unseen: The Representation of Subtle Bodies in Early Modern European Culture*, 2008, pp. 141–178.

Weststeijn, Thijs, *The Visible World: Samuel van Hoogstraten's Art Theory and the Legitimation of Painting in the Dutch Golden Age* (Amsterdam: Amsterdam University Press, 2008).

Wijnands, D.O., *The botany of the Commelins* (Rotterdam: Balkema, 1983).

Wijnroks, Eric Henk, *Handel tussen Rusland en de Nederlanden, 1560–1640* (Hilversum: Verloren, 2003).

Willebrands, Marleen. *De verstandige kok. De rijke keuken van de Gouden Eeuw* (Bussum: Pereboom, 2006).

Withington, Phil, 'Introduction: Cultures of Intoxication', *Past & Present*, 222 (2014), pp. 9–33.

Wittop Koning, D.A., *De handel in geneesmiddelen te Amsterdam tot omstreeks 1637* (Purmerend: J. Muusses, 1942).

Wittop Koning, D.A., *Compendium voor de Geschiedenis van de Pharmacie van Nederland* (Lochem: De Tijdstroom, 1986).

Woordenboek der Nederlandsche Taal (WNT). http://gtb.inl.nl/

Wuestman, Gerdien, 'Een portret van Jan Six van Chandelier?', *Maandblad Amstelodamum* 98, 2011, pp. 147–154.

Yates, Amelia, *Astrea: The Imperial Theme in the Sixteenth Century* (London: Routledge and K. Paul, 1975).

Zandvliet, Kees, *De 250 Rijksten van de Gouden Eeuw. Kapitaal, macht, familie en levensstijl* (Amsterdam: Nieuw Amsterdam, 2006).

General index

Page numbers in italics refer to figures. References to plates are indicated with the letters Pl. followed by the number of the plate. References to footnotes consist of the page number followed by 'n.' followed by the number of the note.

Index of poems by Joannes Six van Chandelier

The number preceded by a 'J' refers to the order of Six's poems in A.E. Jacobs's annotated edition of the poetry of Six van Chandelier: *Joannes Six van Chandelier, Gedichten*, 1991.

Poems by Six van Chandelier not included in Jacobs's edition of the poetry of Six van Chandelier:

For Product Safety Concerns and Information please contact our EU representative GPSR@taylorandfrancis.com Taylor & Francis Verlag GmbH, Kaufingerstraße 24, 80331 München, Germany